# HEALTH

## and Health Care Delivery in Canada

# BRIEF CONTENTS

# HEALTH
## and Health Care Delivery in Canada

**Fourth Edition**

## Valerie D. Thompson

RN, NP-PHC (Retired)
Former Professor
School of Health & Life Sciences and Community Services

Professor/Coordinator
Health Office Administration Program
School of Business and Hospitality

Conestoga College Institute of Technology and Advanced Learning
Kitchener, Ontario

ELSEVIER

Elsevier

**Health and Health Care Delivery in Canada, Fourth Edition**
**ISBN:** 978-0-323-87288-1

---

### Notice

Practitioners and researchers must always rely on their own experience and knowledge in evaluating and using any information, methods, compounds, or experiments described herein. Because of rapid advances in the medical sciences, in particular, independent verification of diagnoses and drug dosages should be made. To the fullest extent of the law, no responsibility is assumed by Elsevier, authors, editors, or contributors for any injury and/or damage to persons or property as a matter of product liability, negligence, or otherwise, or from any use or operation of any methods, products, instructions, or ideas contained in the material herein.

---

*Senior Content Strategist (Acquisitions, Canada):* Roberta A. Spinosa-Millman
*Content Development Manager:* Lenore Gray Spence
*Content Development Specialist:* Toni Chahley
*Publishing Services Manager:* Deepthi Unni
*Senior Project Manager:* Umarani Natarajan
*Design Direction:* Bridget Hoette

The cover photo was taken in Québec City, by Lise Gagne/Getty Images.

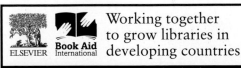

Last digit is the print number: 9 8 7 6 5 4 3 2 1

*To all the health care heroes for your dedication, sacrifices, compassion, and unwavering commitment to your professions and the work you put into helping others during these difficult times. You truly made a difference in the lives of so many people. To those entering health care professions with your eyes wide open to the challenges you face: you as well will make a difference in the lives of those you care for.*

*Also to the memory of my beloved son Spencer, who will remain forever in my heart.*

Individuals working in any facet of health care in Canada should understand the components of health and wellness and how health care is delivered. This book is unique in that the content is general in nature, providing the student with an overview of health care in Canada and a foundation from which to move forward (if desired) to related courses that are more specialized in nature. The Learning Outcomes in each chapter can be used as part of the course outline, which, upon completion, will provide the student with a suitable knowledge base for weekly class discussions. Concurrently, students can research, compare, and contrast how health care is delivered in their own region, noting currency and evolving trends.

While by no means exhaustive, *Health and Health Care Delivery in Canada*, Fourth Edition, has been extensively revised and updated to discuss the essential components of health and health care delivery from federal, provincial, and territorial perspectives, with increased use of infographics and tables. These features allow students to easily visualize and evaluate statistical topics and information among provinces and territories as they relate to a variety of subject areas.

The chapters in this book begin with the history of health care in Canada. Subsequent chapters discuss the responsibilities of the various levels of government, the cost of health and illness, the current state of health human resources, and the impact of population health initiatives from the perspective of the determinants of health. The concepts of health and illness follow, leading to an examination of the legal and ethical aspects of health care. The impacts of the COVID-19 pandemic on the health care system and on the health of Canadians are woven through the book rather than being confined to a particular chapter. In addition, this edition addresses the health and health challenges and concerns of Indigenous people in Canada in more depth than previous editions. The book's content has been carefully selected in order to highlight essential material, and each chapter expands on content in the previous chapter.

By the end of this book, students will be able to say, "I understand health care issues in Canada and how different levels of government operate in terms of health care delivery. I understand how our health care system is funded and the future issues facing health and health care in Canada." Most importantly, students will be able to say, "I understand the system that I am choosing to work in and the challenges I will be facing in a postpandemic environment."

## CONTENT

The author of this text recognizes and acknowledges the diverse histories of the First Peoples of the lands now referred to as Canada. It is recognized that individual communities identify themselves in various ways; within this text, the term *Indigenous* is used to refer to all First Nations, Inuit, and Métis people within Canada unless there are research findings that are presented uniquely to a population.

In the text, gender-neutral language is used to be respectful of and consistent with the values of equality recognized in the *Canadian Charter of Rights and Freedoms*. Using gender-neutral language is professionally responsible and mandated by the Canadian Federal Plan for Gender Equality. Knowledge and language concerning sex, gender, and identity are fluid and continually evolving. The language and terminology presented in this text endeavour to be inclusive of all peoples and reflect what is to the best of our knowledge current at the time of publication.

**Chapter 1** (The History of Health Care in Canada) provides the reader with the highlights in the history of our health care system. These include the events leading up to the implementation of the *Canada Health Act*, which is the foundation of the health care system in Canada. Students are encouraged to examine the principles of this Act in terms of their relevance in the twenty-first century—for example, how COVID-19 has affected the principle of accessibility to health care. A new section, entitled "Indigenous People: Terms and Context," clarifies how various terms pertaining to Indigenous people in Canada are used (and misused), allowing the reader to better understand various terms and use them correctly. The section discussing the history of the health and healing practices of Indigenous people in Canada from the precontact era to present day has also been expanded.

**Chapter 2** (The Role of the Federal Government in Health Care) explores the structure and function of Health Canada and the various organizations that make up Canada's health portfolio. Selected bureaus, offices, and directorates are introduced along with the major responsibilities assigned to each. The role of the federal government as a health care provider for selected groups of Indigenous people is examined, sorting through the mosaic of services also provided by provinces and territories. Services are displayed in a table format. Recent additions and changes to Jordan's Principle mandated by the Human Rights Tribunal are outlined in a boxed feature, and inequities in health care are highlighted with the introduction of Joyce's Principle (named after Joyce Echaquan, who died in an Ottawa hospital under circumstances of neglect propagated by racism). The chapter also takes a critical look at both the strengths and inefficiencies of the federal government throughout the pandemic, as well as the significant role the Public Health Agency of Canada has played.

**Chapter 3** (The Role of Provincial and Territorial Governments in Health Care) provides a current overview of the structure of the provincial and territorial health care systems, emphasizing the common elements among them and outlining significant differences. New in this edition is a more detailed look at how primary health care is delivered in each jurisdiction, contrasting the delivery of related services in the territories. The chapter follows three families, two of whom are new to Canada, addressing the challenges and barriers they face as they settle in a new country and try to understand a new health care system. Most students are likely to have had some exposure (either direct or indirect) to individuals seeking a new life in Canada and will be better able to relate to and appreciate the challenges involved with such things as finding a primary care provider, navigating the health care system, and understanding what is covered under their provincial and territorial plan.

**Chapter 4** (The Dollars and "Sense" of Health Care Funding) looks at current financial issues, where the money for health care comes from and where it goes, and what "strings" the federal government attaches to its funding for the provinces and territories. The chapter also discusses the funding provided to provinces and territories throughout the COVID-19 pandemic. Also new to this chapter is a discussion on minimum wages, how they vary among jurisdictions, and the controversial topic of "living" wages.

**Chapter 5** (Practitioners and Workplace Settings) provides the student with a balanced discussion on the controversial topic of how health care professions are categorized, with the conclusion that these categories are fluid and very much subjective. The chapter provides the student with a clear picture of the current state of our health human resources (e.g., the impact of the pandemic and related job dissatisfaction and burnout), who delivers the care, in what setting, and under what circumstances. The chapter examines how the delivery of primary health care has changed across Canada in terms of the structure and function of primary health care teams, which operate under numerous delivery models in various jurisdictions, and the expanding roles and responsibilities of numerous health care providers.

**Chapter 6** (Essentials of Population Health in Canada) explains how the government and other health care stakeholders evaluate the health of Canadians, identify risk factors, implement strategies to deal with current health problems and predict problems that are likely to arise in the future. Population health initiatives are discussed from the perspective of the determinants of health, particularly the social determinants and their sometimes devastating effects on racialized groups and other high-risk groups. New to this chapter is a discussion of the effects of racism as a determinant of health on high-risk groups.

**Chapter 7** (Health and the Individual) provides the student with an understanding of the key concepts of health, wellness, illness, disease, and disability. In this edition, spiritual and emotional wellness are emphasized along with holistic interventions and models of wellness. The concept of the Indigenous "wholistic" theory framework along with the concept of understanding the nature of balance, harmony, and living a good life are discussed. Students are encouraged to examine their own health beliefs and health behaviours and to consider how these contribute to maintaining health. The leading causes of morbidity and mortality have been revised and updated, including a section discussing the impact of COVID-19 on the health of Canadians, such as post-COVID conditions, or long-COVID.

**Chapter 8** (The Law and Health Care) analyzes legal issues, clarifying provincial, territorial, and federal boundaries in terms of health legislation and the law. Considerable discussion is devoted to medical assistance in dying (MAiD) and recent changes to the legislation, noting that there are some differences in Québec (which was the first jurisdiction in Canada to legalize MAiD). The chapter takes a critical look at the current state of private health care in Canada, with a focus on Québec legislation legalizing the right for Québec residents to purchase insurance for private health care. Current constitutional challenges regarding health care are also discussed (e.g., Dr. Brian Day and a challenge that went to the Supreme Court of Canada in 2022).

**Chapter 9** (Ethics and Health Care) highlights ethical principles and points out that health care providers are held to a higher level of ethical accountability than are those in many other professions. This chapter discusses MAiD from an ethical perspective and the rights of health professionals who are uncomfortable being involved (even indirectly) with the procedure. Racism and the rights of people to fair, unbiased health care are highlighted through discussions on the tragic experiences of Brian Sinclair and Joyce Echaquan.

**Chapter 10** (Current Issues and Emerging Trends in Canadian Health Care) discusses important challenges currently facing Canada's health care system, many of which have been compounded by the pandemic. These include an acute shortage of human health resources and dealing with the backlog of diagnostic, medical, and surgical procedures resulting from delays imposed by the pandemic. The chapter also addresses the state of mental health services, managing care for Canada's aging population, and updates on national strategies for long-term as well as home and community care. The chapter also contains a section about current challenges facing Indigenous people, such as the right to clean water.

## LEARNING FEATURES

Each chapter contains several unique features meant to stimulate student interest:
- **Learning outcomes** outline the objectives for the chapter.
- **Key terms** define challenging concepts.
- **Review questions** at the end of every chapter test student comprehension of the material.
- **Chapter summaries** cover the main topics and their key takeaways.

Each of the following boxed features encourage the student to think through facts, points of interest, and actual situations and to answer questions that promote exploration of personal views, general discussion, and, in some cases, further investigation:
- **Thinking It Through** boxes ask students to critically consider key aspects of health and health care delivery.

- **Did You Know?** boxes present real-life situations exemplifying content presented in the chapter.
- **Case Examples** provide real-life situations, exemplifying content presented in the chapters.

Additional Evolve® online resources to accompany the text can be found at http://evolve. elsevier.com/Canada/Thompson/health.

## ELSEVIER EBOOKS

This exciting program is available to faculty who adopt a number of Elsevier texts, including *Health and Health Care in Canada*, Fourth Edition. Elsevier eBooks is an integrated electronic study centre consisting of a collection of textbooks made available online. It is carefully designed to "extend" the textbook for an easier and more efficient teaching and learning experience. It includes study aids such as highlighting, e-note taking, and cut-and-paste capabilities. Even more importantly, it allows students and instructors to do a comprehensive search within the specific text or across a number of titles. Please check with your Elsevier Educational Solutions Consultant for more information.

# ACKNOWLEDGEMENTS

Writing a book of this nature cannot possibly occur in isolation. I owe a great deal to so many people, including those working with the Canadian Institute for Health Information, Statistics Canada, and Health Canada. Research teams working for these organizations have been readily available, providing me with advice, direction, and the most current information available.

I would like to express my deepest appreciation to Lana Mau, my research assistant, whose help and contributions to this edition of *Health and Health Care Delivery in Canada* cannot be overestimated. A special thanks also to Elizabeth Ralph, who, while completing a post-graduate degree, kindly volunteered some of her time to do additional research and create some tables for the book.

I am deeply grateful to Janet Daglish, National Director, Bayshore Healthcare, and Nadine Henningsen, CEO, Canadian Home Care Association for the information and sources they shared with me regarding home and long-term care in Canada. Thanks to Lyle G. Grant, RN, BComm, BSN, MSN, JD, PhD, Executive Director of Acute Care—NW Saskatchewan Health Authority, who provided me with an expert review of Chapter 8, The Law and Health Care. Thanks also to Joanna Odrowaz for her assistance with editing and research for Chapters 2, 6, and 10.

Thank you to Toni Chahley, Content Development Specialist, for her ongoing support, patience, and expert advice throughout the development of this edition of this book. Toni made working on this edition more of a pleasure than a task.

Thanks to Elsevier's reviewers, who provided helpful comments, advice, and suggestions for improvements during various stages of the manuscript. I am particularly appreciative of the expert advice from some of the reviewers regarding Indigenous content that has been added to various chapters throughout this book. Their advice and the information they provided have been invaluable, helping to ensure that Indigenous content is accurate and presented in a culturally safe manner.

ACKNOWLEDGMENTS

# REVIEWERS

**Paula Benbow, RDH, MPH, EdD**
Professor
School of Health and Community Studies
Algonquin College
Ottawa, ON

**Sandra Biesheuvel, BSc, RRT, CTE**
Instructor II
Department of Respiratory Therapy
University of Manitoba
Winnipeg, MB

**Josée Bonneau, RN, MScN**
Assistant Professor, and Associate Director
Ingram School of Nursing
McGill University
Montreal, QC

**Lorna Canada-Vanegas Mesa, PN, RPN, BSc**
Instructional Associate III
Psychiatric Nursing Department
Faculty of Health Studies
Brandon University
Brandon, MB

**Tracey Fallak, RN, BScN, MN, Certificate in Adult Education**
Curriculum Coordinator/Theory Mentor
Theory Instructor Mentor
Nursing Department
Red River College Polytechnic
Winnipeg, MB

**Caroline Foster-Boucher, RN, MN, BScN**
Assistant Professor
Faculty of Nursing
MacEwan University
Edmonton, AB

**Joy H. Fraser, BScN, MN, PhD**
Professor Emeritus
Nursing and Health Administration
Athabasca University
Athabasca, AB;
Senior Consultant
World Health Organization (WHO)

**Lyle G. Grant, RN, BComm, BSN, MSN, JD, PhD**
Executive Director of Acute Care
NW Saskatchewan Health Authority
Lloydminster, SK

**Donald W.M. Juzwishin, BA, MHSA, PhD**
Adjunct Associate Professor
Health Information Science
University of Victoria
Victoria, BC

**Jacqueline K. Rohatensky, RN, BScN, MAEd**
Lead Instructor, PN program
Saskatchewan Polytechnic
Saskatoon, SK

**Olive Yonge, RN, BScN, MEd, PhD, R. Psych**
Distinguished Professor Emeritus
Faculty of Nursing
University of Alberta
Edmonton, AB

# CONTENTS

# SPECIAL FEATURES

## CHAPTER 6

## CHAPTER 7

# The History of Health Care in Canada

*I came to believe that health services ought not to have a price tag on them, and that people should be able to get whatever health services they required irrespective of their individual capacity to pay.*

—*Tommy Douglas*

## LEARNING OUTCOMES

1.1 Discuss the early development of health care in Canada.
1.2 Understand the terms relating to Indigenous people in Canada.
1.3 Detail early Indigenous culture, traditions, and practices and the impact of colonization.
1.4 Summarize the introduction of public health, nursing, and health insurance in Canada.
1.5 Discuss significant health-related legislation leading up to the *Canada Health Act.*
1.6 Understand the terms and conditions of the *Canada Health Act.*
1.7 Explain the events, commissions, and reports occurring after the *Canada Health Act.*
1.8 Describe the agreements, accords, and other health legislation enacted between 2000 and 2022.

## KEY TERMS

| | | |
|---|---|---|
| Aboriginal | *Indian Act* | Primary health care |
| Aseptic technique | Indigenous | reform |
| Band | Innu | Quarantine |
| Block transfer | Inuit | Refugee claimants |
| *Canada Health Act* | Inuk | Reserve |
| Catastrophic drug costs | Medically necessary | Royal assent |
| Delisted | Medicare | Social movements |
| Eligible | Métis | Status Indians |
| Extra billing | Palliative care | User charges |
| First ministers | Precontact era | |
| First Nations | Prepaid health care | |
| Health accord | | |

Tommy Douglas (1904–1986) is considered by many to be the father of medicare in Canada. One can't help but wonder what advice he would have for Canadians today regarding the sustainability of medicare, how to manage it, and how to ensure that our publicly funded system can continue to equitably meet the needs of all Canadians. One might also wonder what recommendations he would have made to deliver health care equitably both during the COVID-19 pandemic and in the post-pandemic period.

This chapter looks at the evolution of health care in Canada from the precontact era to the present day. The challenges facing Canada's health care system are examined with respect to its viability within the confines of the *Canada Health Act*. Over the past century, the effects of social, economic, and technological growth have dramatically transformed health care in Canada. Every decade has brought changes to where and how people live, as well as to their views of and responses to health, wellness, and illness, in addition to the kind of treatment they both need and expect. This includes the ongoing need to address health care services and access to these services for Indigenous people in Canada, as well as adapting to meet the needs of new Canadians in a knowledgeable and culturally safe manner.

As you read this chapter, note the continuing parallels between the needs of the population and the adaptation and growth of health care services, including primary, home, and long-term care, as well as mental health services in your own jurisdiction. Be especially mindful of the effects of the COVID-19 pandemic on these services, as well as on hospitals and health human resources, in addition to the challenges resulting from the upswing in COVID-19, influenza, and RSV infections evidenced in the fall and winter of 2022–2023. Do the majority of people in your region have a primary care provider such as a family doctor, nurse practitioner, or other non-physician provider? Is your health care delivered by an interprofessional primary health care team? Are primary care services, home and community care, long-term care, and mental health services adequate? Is our health care really universal? Is health care equally accessible to all? Is it delivered to those needing it in a timely fashion? When you reach the end of the book, think about the terms and conditions of the *Canada Health Act* in particular, and ask yourself if, in your opinion, the Act still meets the needs of people eligible for health care in Canada. What about those individuals living in Canada who are not eligible for provincial/territorial health care services? At the end of Chapter 10 you will be asked to reflect back to this chapter to once again review the principles of the *Canada Health Act* with respect to the current challenges facing the Canadian health care system.

Continued debate about the quality and availability of health care has generated demands for system reform, including increased funding from the federal, provincial, and territorial governments along with improved efficiencies and cost-effective strategies to manage health care (by all levels of government). Does the *Canada Health Act* need to be restructured, or do the expectations and attitudes of Canadians need to be adjusted?

## THE EVOLUTION OF HEALTH CARE: AN OVERVIEW

The first health care systems in what is now Canada were established by Indigenous peoples hundreds of years prior to the arrival of settlers. Indigenous people lived a healthy, active lifestyle based on cooperative ideals and values, a sense of community, caring, and social responsibility. They had established systems of government, social structures, education, and health care. Health care systems included the concepts of wellness and mental health, which remain the foundation of Indigenous health today (Allen et al., 2020).

Settlers, who arrived primarily from Europe as early as the fifteenth century, initially depended on Indigenous people for advice about health issues and for traditional medicines and practices, including those related to childbirth. As time passed, and as the colonization of Indigenous lands progressed, settlers began to impose their own health care practices and policies. In doing so, the knowledge and practices related to Western medicine overtook a number of Indigenous practices (many of which, over time, were prohibited, contributing to the systematic destruction of many Indigenous cultures). Despite the repressive and inhumane restrictions that Indigenous people were subjected to, the vast knowledge base of Indigenous people was still in place during and after Confederation.

With the passage of the *British North America Act* in 1867 (renamed the *Constitution Act* in 1982), Confederation became a reality. The Dominion of Canada consisted of Ontario and

Québec (formerly Upper and Lower Canada, respectively), New Brunswick, and Nova Scotia. Sir John A. Macdonald was the Dominion's prime minister. Each province had its own representation in government, its own law-making body (which evolved into a provincial government), and its own lieutenant governor to represent the Crown. The *British North America Act* also established a federal government comprising the House of Commons and the Senate—the same structure in place today. The first census for the new Dominion, in 1871, showed a population of 3,689,257—a large enough number to warrant closer attention to people's health care needs. Legislation regarding responsibilities for health care was vague at best, but even at this early stage, responsibilities were divided between the federal and provincial governments.

## Division of Responsibilities for Health

Health matters received little attention in the *British North America Act*. The federal government was charged with responsibilities for the establishment and maintenance of marine hospitals, the care of Indigenous populations, and the management of **quarantine**. Relatively common, quarantines were imposed to prevent outbreaks of such diseases as cholera, diphtheria, typhoid fever, tuberculosis, and influenza. This remains the case today in the face of current infectious outbreaks, such as those imposed by provincial and territorial governments at the onset of the COVID-19 pandemic.

Provinces were responsible for establishing and managing hospitals, asylums, charities, and charitable institutions. Many of the provincial responsibilities regarding health care—including social welfare, which, broadly speaking, encompassed health and public health matters—were assumed by default since they were not clearly outlined in the Act as federal responsibilities.

In 1919, the federal government created the Department of Health, to assume its health care–related responsibilities, which included working collaboratively with the provinces and territories in health care matters and promoting new health care initiatives. (From 1867 to 1919, federal health concerns were managed by the Department of Agriculture.) Early projects undertaken by this new department reflected the issues faced by Canadians at that time—specifically, the increase in sexually transmitted infections (STIs) and the recognition of the importance of keeping children healthy and safe. In response, "venereal" disease clinics were established across the country, and campaigns promoting child welfare were launched.

In 1928, the Department of Health became known as the Department of Pensions and National Health. The name changed again in 1944 to the Department of National Health and Welfare, and federal responsibilities expanded to include food and drug control, the development of public health programs, health care for members of the civil service, and the operation of the Laboratory of Hygiene (a precursor to Canada's current Laboratory Centre for Disease Control). In 1993, the department was renamed Health Canada.

## The First Doctors in the Post-Contact Era

The first doctors in Canada in the post-contact era consisted of a combination of civilian and military physicians, who came with the arrival of European settlers (primarily from England and France). These doctors cared for their patients in their homes until hospitals were built early in the nineteenth century.

Only the wealthier settlers were able to afford medical attention from a doctor and to seek care in a hospital when required. Others received care through religious and other charitable organizations, or from family and friends who provided in-home care using botanical remedies and other natural medicines handed down to them by family or shared with them by Indigenous people. Some doctors cared for patients in return for payment-in-kind (e.g., farm produce, baking).

Canada's first medical school was established in Montreal in 1825. By the time of Confederation, the country had a steadily increasing number of doctors, hospitals, and medical schools, resulting in medical and hospital care that was more accessible to all sectors of the population.

## The Development of Hospitals in Canada

An order of Augustinian nuns from France who worked as "nursing sisters" established Canada's first hospital, the Hôtel-Dieu de Québec, which opened in Québec City in 1639. The nuns set up several other hospitals in the days before Confederation. In fact, with government funding often limited and unreliable, all of Canada's early hospitals were charitable institutions that relied on financial support from wealthy people and well-established organizations. It was not until the already-established Toronto General Hospital closed from 1867 to 1870 due to lack of funds that the Ontario government passed an act providing yearly grants to hospitals and other charitable institutions, laying the groundwork for the present-day provincial government funding of hospitals.

Hospitals of the early 1800s were crowded places focused on treating infectious diseases, primarily among people of the poorer classes who could not afford private care. By contrast, the wealthier segment of the population avoided hospitals by hiring doctors who would visit patients' homes to provide treatment. With the introduction of anaesthesia, **aseptic technique**, and improved surgical procedures in the 1880s, however, hospitals were finally regarded as places to go to get well, and the use of hospital facilities increased.

In the early 1900s, tuberculosis sanitariums were developed to isolate and care for patients with tuberculosis. The disease was difficult to treat, with surgical removal of diseased organs often the only viable cure, and many patients with tuberculosis died in hospital.

Special institutions to care for mentally ill people were also established. Because of the stigma associated with mental illness at the time, those who suffered from it were often forcibly admitted to these institutions by family members. Most patients never emerged back into their society.

With grants from federal and provincial governments and advances in medical care, the number of hospitals increased over the next several decades. Physician and hospital services remained out-of-pocket expenses for patients, although some had insurance protection through their employers. Charitable and religious organizations continued to assist those who could not afford health care. During this time, governments made some efforts to improve access to medical care and to provide an affordable fee structure for it (Box 1.1).

Today, most health care facilities, including long-term and community care services, in Canada are publicly operated and funded by the provincial/territorial or federal government, supported by a variety of complex funding mechanisms. This topic is discussed in Chapters 2 and 3.

### Separate Hospitals for Indigenous People

What was then termed "Indian" hospitals were initially operated by churches in the late 1800s. After World War II, the federal government's Department of Health and Welfare expanded a system of separate hospital care for Indigenous people. Some new facilities built were freestanding hospitals, others were refurbished military barracks, "out-buildings," or annexes affiliated with other hospitals. The facilities overall were underfunded and inadequately equipped, maintained, and staffed (e.g., with few kitchen and laundry facilities, few nurses proportionate to the number of patients needing care, poor heating). Initially the hospitals were established to separate Indigenous people with tuberculosis (discriminately referred to as "Indian tuberculosis"), as there was a high incidence among the Indigenous population, even

> **BOX 1.1 Innovation in Newfoundland: The Cottage Hospital System**
>
> In the 1930s, approximately 1500 communities in Newfoundland were scattered across 7000 miles of coastline. To service these communities the provincial government developed the Cottage Hospital and Medical Care Plan in 1934, which funded the building of a network of small hospitals and paid doctors and nurses to travel to port communities along the extensive coastline. One hospital was even built on a boat.
>
> Intended primarily to provide outpatient care, these small hospitals were equipped with minimal inpatient facilities (20–30 beds), an operating room, diagnostic facilities, and a well-equipped emergency department. Outpatient services offered included immunizations, prenatal and infant care, as well as patient follow-up at home. The hospitals were staffed mostly by physicians and nurses with surgical and emergency care experience. Unique to the cottage hospital system, an annual fee of $10 of $5 per person provided a family with medical care and use of the cottage hospitals, including transfer to the nearest base hospital when necessary.
>
> Not only was Newfoundland's cottage hospital system innovative and progressive for its time, but also to this day, provincial and territorial systems draw on some of its key elements, such as small clinics for rural communities.

Source: Based on Connor, J. H. T. (2007). Twillingate: Socialized medicine, rural doctors, and the CIA. *Newfoundland Quarterly, 100*(424). http://www.newfoundlandquarterly.ca/issue424/twillingate.php

in youth from residential schools (in part because of overcrowding and poor nutrition). Infected Indigenous people in the far north were transported (some by ship) to hospitals, also called *sanitoriums* in southern communities, particularly in the Prairie Provinces, Ontario, and Québec. Indigenous people were plucked from the schools, their homes, and communities if it was suspected they had tuberculosis. There was an amendment to the *Indian Act* allowing physicians to put Indigenous people in hospitals involuntarily for the treatment of infectious diseases. Horrendous records exist of mistreatment in the hospitals, including experimentation with various forms of treatment for tuberculosis, such as with vaccines and surgery (e.g., removing parts of their lungs, which necessitated removing ribs, often under local anaesthesia).

When the incidence of tuberculosis decreased, many of the Indian hospitals were transitioned into separate general hospitals operated with little regard for traditional healing practices or Indigenous culture. In Sioux Lookout Ontario, for example, there were two hospitals, the Zone (also referred to at the time as the "Indian hospital") and the Sioux Lookout General Hospital. Physicians and staff were separate (working at one or the other). Physicians working at the Zone hospital often rotated in from Winnipeg or other centres. Non-Indigenous people were rarely, if ever, admitted to the Zone hospital, and vice versa. When medicare was introduced in 1968, the federal government initiated closure of the majority of Indian hospitals, merging care of the Indigenous and non-Indigenous population into the same facilities. As an example, in Sioux Lookout, the Zone and general hospitals were moved to a new facility called the Sioux Lookout MenoYaWin Health Centre, which is a fully accredited, 60-bed acute care facility offering an additional 20 beds for extended care.

Today, many Indigenous people (justifiably) remain concerned about the different philosophies and treatment modalities among Western and traditional healing practices. All too often Indigenous people receive health care based solely on Western medical beliefs, practices, and procedures. However, a number of health centres in rural, urban, and remote settings,

---

**BOX 1.2  The Sioux Lookout Meno Ya Win Health Centre**

Andaaw'iwewin egkwa Mushkiki (Traditional Healing Practices and Medicines) is a culturally sensitive program at this hospital that incorporates traditional practices, principles, and spiritual healing ceremonies that usually take place in a specially designed ceremonial room and include vigils, smudging, and healing circles. The room has an open fire pit with circular seating. Ya Win Health Centre has a roster of traditional practitioners who are available to patients requiring their services. These practitioners must go through a process of certification administered by a traditional practitioners committee. In addition, Indigenous hospital patients can choose to be served traditional meals (game and fish), which are exempt from the inspection policies imposed on other food.

The hospital's diagnostic services include fluoroscopy, ultrasound, digital mammography, and computed tomography (CT) scans. Attached to the health centre is an extended care facility and a medical withdrawal unit to treat patients withdrawing from drug and alcohol addiction.

Source: Based on Sioux Lookout Meno Ya Win Health Centre. (n.d.). https://slmhc.on.ca/

---

although serving a general population, now focus on the needs of Indigenous people within their catchment area and incorporate traditional healing practices into their programs (Box 1.2).

In 1945, The Charles Camsell Hospital in Edmonton, Alberta (another "Indian hospital" of note), under the Authority of the Canadian Army Medical Corps and Indigenous Health Services, was converted to a tuberculosis hospital for **Inuit** and First Nations groups in Alberta, Yukon, and parts of the Northwest Territories (Leung, 2014). In addition to providing treatment for tuberculosis, it was also a site where Indigenous patients were subjected to research and where many First Nations people were sterilized (Chin, 2020). In 1964, a new hospital was constructed, and the original building was demolished in 1967.

## The Role of Volunteer Organizations in Early Health Care

In the eighteenth and early nineteenth centuries, Canadians' health care needs were attended to largely by volunteer organizations, which were also relied on heavily to raise funds for health care because there was little or no funding provided by the government or any other agency. Some of these groups are discussed below, many of which will be familiar because they still function today.

### The Order of St. John

The Order of St. John (later known as St. John's International and sometimes St. John Ambulance) provides community-based first aid, health care, and support services around the world. The organization was introduced to Canada in 1883 by individuals from England with knowledge of first aid, disaster relief, and home nursing. The organization and its volunteer responsibilities expanded over the years, providing invaluable assistance and health care to Canadians. Today, the organization provides a wide range of health care services at public events and participates in community health initiatives across Canada. They also offer a number of courses (including online) ranging from emergency and standard first aid (including pets) to family, children, and youth courses (St. John Ambulance Canada, 2022). In 2021, the organization reported having 15,000 volunteers, and 5300 medical first responders.

### The Canadian Red Cross Society

The Canadian Red Cross Society was founded in 1896. In the early 1900s, the Red Cross established a form of home care designed to keep families together during times of illness. The Red Cross gradually became involved in other public health initiatives, establishing outpost hospitals, nursing stations, nutrition services, and university courses in public health nursing. The organization also offers educational courses, including those in cardiopulmonary resuscitation (CPR), first aid, and water safety, and provides Canadians with a variety of community support services. An important role of the Red Cross is its aid and support related to disaster relief at a national and international level (e.g., 2021 disasters related to forest fires and flooding in British Columbia). The Red Cross has also been active in assisting Ukrainians with humanitarian needs and evacuation procedures during the Ukrainian-Russian war (2022).

Until 1998, the Canadian Red Cross Society also supervised the collection of blood from volunteer donors across Canada. The society was stripped of this responsibility following the contaminated blood crisis (occurring between October 1993 and November 1997). Two thousand people who had received blood and blood products contracted human immuno-deficiency virus (HIV); another 30,000 people were infected with hepatitis C.

After the 1997 report prepared by Mr. Justice Krever, *Final Report: Commission of Inquiry on the Blood System in Canada*, two independent not-for-profit organizations were formed, Héma-Québec for the province of Québec, and Canadian Blood Services for all other jurisdictions. Both organizations deliver similar services.

### Canadian Blood Services and Héma-Québec

Canadian Blood Services (CBS) became operational in 1998, through a "memorandum of understanding" between the Government of Canada and its provincial/territorial partners (Canadian Blood Services, 2022). CBS assumed full responsibility for the Canadian blood system outside of Québec (Héma-Québec for the province of Québec). CBS is separate from the government, although the organization is almost entirely funded by the Ministers of Health of the provinces and territories. CBS is overseen by a board of directors appointed by the Ministers of Health. CBS is regulated by Health Canada, as a biologics manufacturer within the sphere of blood and blood products such as plasma and stem cells. CBS is also a registry for stem cells in all provinces/territories except Québec. The organization is responsible for a national registry for organ retrieval and sharing (including Québec). Héma-Québec, although fully integrated with the Québec health network, is a separate agency from the government. It is overseen by a board of directors chosen from individuals working across the Héma-Québec system (including blood donors and recipients). Héma-Québec adheres to the safety standards outlined by Health Canada and collaborates with CBS (Héma-Québec, n.d.).

### Victorian Order of Nurses

The Victorian Order of Nurses (VON) was founded in 1897 and was one of the first groups to identify the health care needs of the population, particularly of women and children in remote areas of the country, and to provide services to these groups. For many years, VON was the largest national provider of home care, in addition to providing a wide range of health and wellness services. In November 2015, ongoing financial difficulties forced the organization to terminate services in Alberta, Saskatchewan, Manitoba, New Brunswick, Newfoundland and Labrador, and Prince Edward Island. With restructuring, the VON continues to operate branches in Nova Scotia.

## THINKING IT THROUGH

### The Role of Volunteers in Canadian Health Care

Volunteers have played a major role in the development of health care in Canada over the years. Today, in the face of widespread shortages of human health resources in health care services, both in hospitals and in the community, the health care system increasingly depends on volunteers.

1. What roles do volunteers continue to play in health care? Identify four areas that would benefit from the contributions of volunteers.
2. How do you think current social and demographic trends will affect the roles of volunteers and volunteer organizations?
3. If you were interested in volunteer work, what organization would you choose, and why?

### Children's Aid Society

The Children's Aid Society (CAS) of Toronto was created in 1891 by John Joseph Kelso. He initiated the *Act for the Prevention of Cruelty to and Better Protection of Children,* in 1893, which provided the first social safety net for the many abandoned and homeless children in the city. The CAS was established with the mandate to legally provide protection for these impoverished children. The CAS was granted the legal right to care for abandoned and neglected children, to supervise their care, and to transfer guardianship from the parents' care to the CAS when necessary (Until the Last Child, 2014). However, the initial focus was providing food and shelter to disadvantaged children. Children at risk for harm or abuse and needing protection were removed from the family environment and placed in foster homes or orphanages, with little thought given to maintaining the family unit.

Originally, the CAS acted as board members and assumed duties that paid professionals now perform. Today, the provision of a secure and caring environment for the child is still paramount, but keeping families together is also a priority. The CAS oversees many of the adoptions in Canada.

Governed by the *Child and Family Services Act,* children's aid societies in most jurisdictions continue to provide child protection services under provincial legislation. The government provides funding and monitors children's aid societies. It also develops policies to support child welfare programs and licenses children's group homes and foster homes.

## INDIGENOUS PEOPLE: TERMS AND CONTEXT

To appreciate the history of health care in Canada as it relates to the Indigenous people of Canada, it is important to understand the various terms used to reference them and the context in which such terms are used (Box 1.3). Some terms are confusing as they overlap; others have fallen out of favour and are no longer used unless there is a legal connotation. **Aboriginal** and **Indigenous**, for example, both pertain to the original inhabitants of a land. **First Nations** and *Indian* apply to the same groups of people in Canada, but the terms *Indian* and *Aboriginal* are no longer acceptable to use in Canada, outside of references to federal or provincial/territorial legislation.

## BOX 1.3    Indigenous Peoples in Canada: Explaining the Terms and Concepts

*Aboriginal* (similar to *Indigenous*) refers to people who were the earliest inhabitants of this land. Widely adopted in Canada to refer to First Nations, Inuit, and Métis Peoples, the term became popular in the 1980s, replacing *Indian* and *native*. This term was eventually replaced by the term *Indigenous*. "Aboriginal" is still used in the Canadian Constitution and "Indian" is still present in the *Indian Act* of 1872. The *Indian Act* has been amended several times over the years, but the language used in the Act remains much the same as in its original form.

*Indian* is a term that was applied to Indigenous people in the Americas, thought to be coined by Christopher Columbus in the last part of the 1400s, believing he had landed in Asia. For many years, the term was applied liberally to all Indigenous people in North, Central, and South America (it did not apply to the Inuit in northern regions such as the Arctic).

*Indigenous* is a term used by the United Nations to reference groups of people who, with their descendants, are the original inhabitants of a geographic area (Crown-Indigenous Relations and Northern Affairs Canada, 2022). These groups are distinct from other societies and maintain their own culture, political structure, health practices, and policies. In 2016, the Canadian government accepted the United Nations Declaration on the Rights of Indigenous Peoples without qualifications. Since then the term *Indigenous* has been widely used in Canada to collectively refer to First Nations, Métis, and Inuit peoples. In Canada, *Indigenous* is used as an umbrella term for these unique population groups. Although there are some commonalities, there are also differences. For example, it is inaccurate to say that Indigenous people in Canada live on **reserves**, or in **bands**. This is specific to some (but not all) First Nations communities.

*First Nations* encompasses all those who lived in the land now known as Canada, except for those in the Arctic communities, who are referred to as *Inuit*, whose peoples were the original inhabitants of the land, and their descendants (Office of Indigenous Initiatives, 2019). The term *Indian* (as described above) applied to this population group for many years. *First Nations* began replacing the term *Indian* in the 1970s and is now the preferred usage. Most First Nations people find the term *Indian* both outdated and offensive, especially as the term relates to their traumatic history of colonization and residential schools. It is worth noting that not all First Nations people are legally considered Indians and unless they have Indian status as outlined in the *Indian Act*.

*Indian* (as defined in 1876 by criteria set out in the *Indian Act*), refers to the legal identity for those who meet this criteria (McCue, 2020).

*Status Indians:* Indian status is the legal standing of a First Nations person who is registered under the *Indian Act*. Registered First Nations are eligible for selected benefits and rights and are eligible for numerous programs and services offered by the federal and provincial/territorial governments, including health care, under Canadian law (Indigenous Services Canada, 2022b). First Nations who are registered under the *Indian Act* are referred to as **Status Indian**, despite the fact that the term *Indian* is no longer considered acceptable.

A *non-Status Indian* is a person who identifies as Indian (and may be part of a band) but is not registered with the federal government and therefore not legally recognized as Indian under the *Indian Act*.

*Treaty Indians* are Status Indians who belong to a First Nations community or band who have signed treaties with the Crown (in England). There are approximately 640 recognized First Nations in Canada representing more than 50 nations and 50 languages. Although there are many common threads, First Nations communities across Canada differ in terms of size, structure, and how they govern, as well as in the health practices and ceremonies they use.

The **Métis** people in Canada have a distinct history and culture that originated as long ago as the early 1600s, according to the Métis Nation of Canada (n.d.). However, Library and Archives Canada (2020) states that the Métis people originated in the 1700s when European fur traders (e.g., from France and Scotland) married Indigenous women and had families. Their descendants form the Métis communities in Canada. This population group has been recognized as Indian under Canadian law only since 1982. At that time, the 1982 Canadian Constitution, Section 35 (2) stated that "aboriginal peoples of Canada" includes Indian, Inuit, and Métis peoples of Canada. The Supreme Court in Powley held that the Métis have "full status as a distinctive rights-bearing peoples," a characteristic they share with the Indian (First Nation) and Inuit peoples of Canada (Library and Archives Canada, 2020).

It is important to note that this decision did *not g*rant Indian status to the Métis and/or non-Status Indians. In 2016, the Supreme Court of Canada passed a ruling stating that the federal government (not provincial governments) held the responsibility to pass legislation on matters related to the Métis people and non-Status Indians. This has been considered an important ruling, possibly opening the door to future legislation related to Métis rights.

*Inuit* is a term that refers to the Indigenous people living in the Arctic regions of Greenland, Alaska, and Canada (**Inuk** is singular for Inuit). In Canada, Inuit people live in the Inuit Nunangat—which broadly stated, means "Inuit homeland"—which is geographically divided into four regions (First Nations Studies Program, University of British Columbia, 2009). The previously used term *Eskimo* was replaced by the term *Inuit* in the 1980s when it was sanctioned by the Inuit Circumpolar Council to represent Inuit population groups across the circumpolar geographic regions. *Eskimo* is thought to be a racial slur and derogatory for a variety of reasons (Parrott, 2008).

*Band* is a term that was imposed on Indigenous people in Canada under the *Indian Act* (1876). It defines a "governing unit" of Indians under the Act. Groups of First Nations peoples living on designated lands were given limited governing responsibilities. The overriding purpose was to gain control over Indigenous communities and assimilate "Indians" into colonial society (Crey, 2009). Today, bands are also referred to as First Nations (communities). In 2020, the government of Canada formally recognized 619 First Nations. Although the Department of Indigenous-Crown Relations and Northern Affairs oversees some matters relating to First Nations, they function as local governments managing most of their own affairs, including education and (increasingly) health care and social matters (e.g., child welfare).

*Reserve* describes a section of Crown land put aside by the federal government (under the *Indian Act*) exclusively for use by a group of registered First Nations people (Status Indians) (Indigenous Awareness Canada, n.d.). Some reserves were assigned to First Nations with a treaty, others were not. Much of the land was taken by the government without negotiation or the consent of First Nations peoples, which is ironic since, in the precontact era, Indigenous peoples had traditional rights and use of all the land and water in what became Canada (Wilson & Hodgson, 2018). Eighty percent of the reserves assigned to First Nations were in remote areas where the land is undesirable and far from basic services. Restrictions imposed by governments across Canada and a lack of autonomy over their land and resources deepened socioeconomic disparities and inequities suffered by First Nations peoples. In 1985, an amendment to the *Indian Act* loosened restrictions, allowing non-Status Indians to live on reserves at the discretion of band leaders.

**DID YOU KNOW?**

*Early Reserves in Canada*

While there is controversy as to when the earliest reserves were established, there are records indicating that some of the earliest ones appeared as early as 1637 in New France. They were established by Catholic missionaries in an attempt to impact the nomadic lifestyle of some Indigenous peoples, such as the **Innu** and Algonquin, and convert them to the Catholic faith. These reserves lacked the political components of the reserves later created under the *Indian Act*.

## Treaty 6 and The Medicine Chest Clause

Treaty 6 was the only treaty that included a clause related to the provision of any type of health care for those bands who signed the treaty (the Medicine Chest). The clause remains controversial today, as it comes nowhere near meeting the current health care needs of the population groups for whom the treaty was signed.

Treaty 6 was an agreement between the Crown and numerous bands of Cree and Stoney First Nations, signed in 1876 at Fort Carlton, Fort Pitt, and Duck Lake (Saskatchewan). Numerous amendments were made to the original treaty over subsequent years. Some bands held out, negotiating for better terms. The Treaty covered geographic areas in parts of what are now Alberta and Saskatchewan (Beal, 2005). Treaty 6 contained many of the standard clauses found in other treaties, such as surrender of Indigenous land rights, moving bands onto reserves, and numerous other promises made by the government (many of which were not kept). The treaty was unique in that the negotiators provided for inclusion of a clause specifying that a "medicine chest" be available for each band who signed the treaty (Beal, 2005). The medicine chest was to be kept at the house of an Indian Agent, who was a government official placed in charge of people on reserves. The Indian Agent had extensive powers, including managing use of the medicine chest. Thus, Indigenous people had little control over use of the medicine chest and little or no power when dealing with the Indian Agent on other matters (Maskwacis Cree Foundation, 2018).

As time went on, the Indigenous peoples involved in the treaty recognized the medicine chest as an agreement to provide necessary health care and benefits to eligible recipients. The bands would keep their traditional health care practices but recognized that, at times, they would require assistance.

## INDIGENOUS TRADITIONS AND PRACTICES

### The Precontact Era

Indigenous peoples in Canada had a complex and effective health care system for thousands of years before coming into contact with outsiders (the **precontact era**). For years, knowledge about healing ceremonies and health practices was passed down from one generation to another by healers, both orally and through "hands-on" experiences. Very little information was actually documented, resulting in few written resources.

Most cultural practices were rooted in holistic and spiritual beliefs, along with an integral relationship with nature (Alberta Regional Professional Development Consortium, n.d.). Indigenous people depended on their environment for their very existence, developing an intimate knowledge of, relationship with, and respect for their environment (sometimes referred to as *Mother Earth*, which is not a term generated by Indigenous people). The lives of Indigenous people thus were intertwined with nature and all it had to offer. As such, Indigenous people connected spiritually with the world around them enabling them to survive.

At the time, Indigenous healers went by many names, including *Medicine Man* and *Shaman*. There were also midwives, typically women known as life-givers, and spiritual and herbal healers (Chapter 5). The role of healer was not exclusive to men; in fact, in many Indigenous cultures, women and other gender roles had long been recognized as powerful healers and community leaders. Groups called their healers different names (many terms have been anglicized and, in some cases, assumed colonized views of the roles healers played). Contrary to some common beliefs, Indigenous people often had different types of healers—not just a person who oversaw the health care within their community. Medical care and ceremonies, along with advice about relationships and living in general, were intertwined, resulting in a truly holistic model of health care. An individual would seek a number of different healers, depending on their specific needs and what aspect of their being was out of balance (which is not very different from the concept of interprofessional health care teams practised widely in Canada today).

## DID YOU KNOW?

### Gender Variance in Indigenous Communities

Historically, many Indigenous groups have had multiple genders, acknowledging anywhere between three and five gender roles. These include female, male, Two Spirit female, Two Spirit male, and transgender. Gender variance was welcomed among First Nations, and individuals were treated with reverence and respect. Traditionally, a person was not judged on gender identity but on their character and contributions to their community. Some tribes believed that the ability to view the world through the eyes of both a man and a woman was a gift from the Creator. Some tribes dressed their children in gender-neutral clothing until the child decided their gender identity. Not surprisingly, there was little to no tolerance for gender variance by Europeans and settlers, who demanded conformity with their religious and moral beliefs. Although tribes had their unique names to identify various gender roles, collectively, many tribes formally adopted the term "Two Spirited" from the Ojibwe language, in Winnipeg, Manitoba in 1989 as a standardized term.

Source: Based on Brayboy, D. (2018, September 13). Two spirits, one heart, five genders. *Indian Country Today*. https://indiancountrytoday.com/archive/two-spirits-one-heart-five-genders

Contributing to the excellent health of Indigenous people were active lifestyles and nutritious diets. Their sources of food were from the land, through hunting, fishing, and harvesting local vegetation. Depending on their geographic area, some bands moved seasonally to maximize their sources of food. The few illnesses that Indigenous people had were sometimes attributed to evil spirits, or to an imbalance or disharmony between such entities as the body, mind, community, and nature. History indicates that Indigenous people had arthritis and jaw abscesses. Indigenous healers had their own traditions, an understanding of healing, and the use of herbal medicines. A variety of rituals, ceremonies, and spiritual practices were used to treat some of these disorders, whereas other disorders were treated with an assortment of plants, herbs, roots, and fungi. For example, Indigenous healers used the bark of the willow tree—which contains the ingredient in aspirin—to treat headaches. Parts of the dandelion were used for skin ailments such as boils, abscesses, rashes, and inflamed joints. Rock moss was used for open sores that would not heal. Gooseberries helped with constipation. Today, many traditional medicines have been incorporated into contemporary Western medicinal practices. Treatments used by Indigenous people were also geographically motivated. The Inuit, for example, had treatments for frostbite.

Traditional rituals and spiritual ceremonies include the sweat lodge, healing circle, smudging ceremonies, and the medicine wheel, and many of these are still used today. Each of the rituals is described below, explaining the holistic and spiritual nature of traditional healing practices. Elements of these ceremonies differ from one group to another in terms of what and how ceremonies and healing practices are performed. For example, not all communities utilize sweat lodge ceremonies. European religion in some communities affected traditional practices, some encouraging a more Indigenous focus than others, resulting in a mix in beliefs.

### Sweat Lodge

In some communities, the *sweat lodge* was one of the most valued methods of traditional healing, and it is still used by many communities today. It is a cleansing and healing ceremony. Preparations for the ceremony vary. The person being treated may, for example, be required to fast for a period of time prior to the ceremony. This is thought to weaken the (powerful) physical self, rendering the person vulnerable and thus more receptive to advice and teachings from the spirit world. Today, in other regions, Indigenous persons seeking healing from a sweat lodge ceremony might still be required to fast prior to the ceremony, others may not. Some lodge keepers may ask that a participant refrain from using drugs or alcohol for a period of time before the ceremony. The desired outcome is to have those who are participating in the ceremony complete it with a renewed sense of self and life's direction. Although these ceremonies were most often associated with cleansing and healing, ceremonial leaders could assign a different purpose to each ceremony—for example, to work out any family issues and, in more recent years, deal with addictions (substance use disorders).

### Healing Circle

The configuration of the *healing circle* (or sharing circle) is an important part of Indigenous culture. It was structured to promote open communication. Participants include individuals who are dealing with difficulties and problems in their everyday lives. This ceremony sometimes begins with *smudging*—the burning of medicine such as sage or sweetgrass. Smudging requires that participants sweep the smoke toward their faces (eyes, ears, mouth) and all over their bodies. The smoke is believed to help participants to see, hear, and understand things in a positive manner; speak wisely, carefully, and truthfully; and create a loving environment (Mehl-Madrona & Mainguy, 2014). Emotional and spiritual healing occur through the talking circle as well as healing and strengthening of relationships.

Traditionally, any time prayers are said, and smudging occurs in the context of a talking circle, it is believed that spiritual energy from unseen forces are at work (along with human energy). Often individual prayers are followed by a group prayer that is said to be carried to the Creator by the smoke. Then a facilitator makes group introductions and explains the rules and how the session will be conducted. For some ceremonies, the facilitator passes out an eagle feather wand or a talking stick. The person who has possession of the feather or stick is allowed to speak (everyone in the group is given the opportunity to speak if they wish).

Sources: Rice, W. (January 18, 2016). *Eagle feathers now on hand for oaths at Ottawa courthouse.* http://www.cbc.ca/news/canada/ottawa/eagle-feathers-now-on-hand-for-oaths-at-ottawa-courthouse-1.3409212; Royal Canadian Mounted Police. (October 27, 2017). *Media advisory: Nova Scotia RCMP to unveil eagle feather initiative.* https://www.grc.gc.ca/en/news/2017/media-advisory-nova-scotia-unveil-eagle-feather-initiative; Thatcher, A. (October 3, 2017). Eagle feather flies into Nova Scotia detachments. *Gazette, 79*(4). https://www.rcmp-grc.gc.ca/en/gazette/eagle-feather-flies-nova-scotia-detachments

### Medicine Wheel

With similar concepts to the holistic model of wellness discussed in Chapter 7, Indigenous people have historically adopted a holistic approach to health and wellness that considers the mental, physical, cultural, and spiritual well-being of not only the individual person but also the entire community. The holistic framework incorporates the *medicine wheel* (Fig. 1.1). The

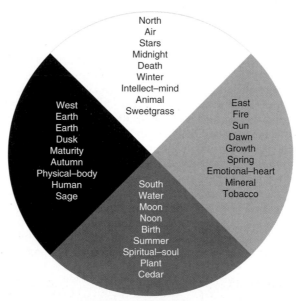

**Fig. 1.1** Indigenous medicine wheel. Source: Joseph, B. [2013]. *What is an Aboriginal medicine wheel?* [Web log post]. *Working effectively with Indigenous Peoples.* https://www.ictinc.ca/blog/what-is-an-aboriginal-medicine-wheel. The link provided here gives you information about the structure, function, and use of the medicine wheel. A short video about the medicine wheel is at: https://youtu.be/S7nb4rJ_N14

medicine wheel has been used by Indigenous people for centuries for teaching, learning, health, and healing.

The medicine wheel is typically a circle divided into four quadrants, representing four directions, beginning in the east and moving methodically through the south, west, and then to the north. The east addresses the realms of spirit and vision; the south addresses the value and importance of relationships, community, and heart; the west concentrates on Indigenous knowledge and the importance of continuing knowledge production; and lastly, the north encompasses concepts and ideas about healing, movements, and actions that guide practice (Bell, 2014). The directions can also represent various entities such as the stages of life, seasons of the year, or the four parts of a person—spiritual, physical, cognitive, and emotional. In this case the person must acknowledge responsibility for themselves in all categories to regain health. Sometimes there is a small circle in the center of the larger circle (not shown in Fig. 1.1) representing holism, balance, and harmony.

The circle itself represents wholeness and the interconnectivity of the self, the individual, the family, the community, society as a whole, and creation. Another part of the holistic concept is understanding the nature of balance, harmony, and living a good life. An individual who experiences altered health, evidenced by symptoms or presenting problems, is considered to be out of balance or experiencing disharmony.

Each quadrant is a different colour: black (or blue) represents the north, red represents the south, yellow represents the east, and white represents the west.

### Contact With Outsiders

Some of the initial documented contacts with Indigenous people were as early as the 1500s with Russian, French, Spanish, and British traders and explorers, as well as settlers. Contact in the interior was primarily with traders who worked for the Hudson's Bay Company. They brought with them numerous diseases previously unknown to this part of the world. Indigenous people had no natural immunity to these diseases, and traditional rituals and practices were largely ineffective as treatment options. Such illnesses included smallpox, tuberculosis, influenza, whooping cough, and measles. The effect on the Indigenous population was disastrous, resulting in the deaths of thousands, including Indigenous healers and elders with knowledge about cultural and healing practices. As a result, much valuable information about health care practices that depended on oral history was lost with them. The large numbers of deaths over decades ultimately resulted in the collapse of many population groups. In addition, the smallpox vaccine discovered at the turn of the century was (initially) rarely available to the Indigenous population, in part because there was little vaccine available, geography, and the logistics of distributing the vaccine. This situation improved in the mid-1700s as availability of vaccines increased. By 1800, advances in the vaccination along with public health interventions helped to control the spread of the disease.

The *British North American Act* (1867) and the *Indian Act* (1876) set the stage for the assimilation of Indigenous people, applying numerous restrictions to their practices and ways of life. The inability of Indigenous healers to successfully treat the newly introduced diseases allowed non-Indigenous people to discredit traditional healing ceremonies and the legitimacy of traditional healers. These two Acts were clearly discriminatory, which is in contrast to an earlier proclamation issued by King George III.

---

**DID YOU KNOW?**

### *The Royal Proclamation—1763*

The Royal Proclamation issued by King George III established guidelines for European settlements in Western regions of what became Canada. This land was surrendered to England by France after the Seven Years War (1763). Among other agreements, the Proclamation established the structure for treaty negotiation with Indigenous people inhabiting large sections of Canada with the exception of the Maritimes, Québec, and Southern Ontario. The Proclamation stated that settlers could not claim First Nations land unless it was first purchased by the Crown (and only the Crown could purchase land from First Nations). It prohibited settlement on Indian territory, ordered those settlers already there to withdraw, and restricted future settlements (Editors of Encyclopaedia Britannica, 2022).

The Proclamation is part of the *Constitution Act* (section 25), which, as part of the Charter of Rights and Freedoms, guarantees that nothing can terminate or diminish the Indigenous rights outlined in the document (such as the right to self-determination, self-government, and the right to practise one's own culture and customs, including language and religion). Because of this, the Proclamation is sometimes referred to as the "Indian Magna Carta."

The Indigenous population also suffered from the devastating effects of being in residential schools. The intergenerational trauma and suffering from these experiences continue today, impacting almost every aspect of their lives, from their physical and mental health to socioeconomic disparities. The discovery of unmarked graves on the grounds of former residential schools in 2021 (an ongoing process) has added further emotional pain and trauma to Indigenous people (Chapter 10). For more information about residential schools see Box 1.4.

---

### BOX 1.4  Residential Schools

Residential schools were church-run boarding schools, funded by the federal government, which essentially assumed custodial rights of Indigenous children (primarily between the ages of 7 and 16 years), although children as young as 4 years old were also taken from their homes. An estimated 150,000 children attended residential schools. Attendees of these schools were primarily First Nations children but also included some Inuit and Métis children (Union of Ontario Indians, 2013). The attendance of Métis children at the schools was inconsistent, sometimes depending on how absorbed they were into Indigenous lifestyles, the community in which they lived, and the policies and religious denomination of the church running the school (Logan, 2020). Larger numbers of Inuit children went to residential schools in the 1950s after they were officially incorporated into the residential school system (Truth and Reconciliation Commission, 2015a).

The government had two goals in mind when it established residential schools: to educate Indigenous youth, and (perhaps the overriding goal) to absorb Indigenous children into Euro-Canadian/Western culture and society, with the end goal being to assimilate them into the "white man's" world (Hanson et al., 2020).

One of the first schools opened in 1831 in Brampton, Manitoba, and the last one closed in Punnichy, Saskatchewan in 1996, long after the horrors and injustices these children suffered had become well known. Children were torn from their families and communities and stripped of their identities, language, and culture. They were subjected to varying levels and types of abuse. Mistreatment, inadequate nutrition, and denial of proper care also resulted in the deaths of large numbers of the children. As mentioned earlier, "Indian hospitals" were often aligned with residential schools that provided the hospitals with many of their patients, who experienced mistreatment and were subjected to experimental treatments, often resulting in death.

The Indian/Indigenous Residential Schools Settlement in 2007 resulted from lobbying and pressure from Indigenous people who had attended residential schools. This was followed by a formal apology by then Prime Minister Harper in 2008. The settlement acknowledged the suffering and resulting damage done to former students and established a multimillion-dollar fund for individual compensation packages to help former students seek treatment and work toward recovery through, among other resources, the Aboriginal/Indigenous Healing Foundation. The settlement also included the establishment of the Indian/Indigenous Residential Schools Resolution Health Support Program to provide support for those suffering mental health and emotional trauma. Providers include an interprofessional team of health care workers, including Indigenous elders, social workers, and psychiatrists. The settlement was not without problems and criticisms regarding unethical use of the money and unethical fees charged by lawyers. The Truth and Reconciliation Commission of Canada was established at this time to investigate what happened in residential schools, create a historical account, and promote healing and reconciliation between Indigenous and non-Indigenous people in Canada. It was headed by Justice Murray Sinclair. The report was released in 2015 with 94 calls to action. Of the report, TRC Chief Commissioner Murray Sinclair said, "We have described for you a mountain, we have shown you the path to the top. We call upon you to do the climbing" (Canadian Friends Service Committee, n.d.).

Many First Nations children never returned home, with vague or no explanations given as to what happened to them. First Nations people have claimed for years that these children died from neglect, abuse, and starvation. In 2021, a First Nations community in British Columbia produced evidence of what potentially happened to some of the missing children: unmarked graves containing the remains of a large number of bodies, most presumed to be missing children, were found on the grounds of a residential school. Ground-seeking radar was used to reveal the graves' locations. Since then, numerous other unmarked grave sites have been found on the grounds of residential schools in other locations, again revealing the remains of what appears to be predominately children. These, for the moment, are being considered "undocumented deaths." As other grave sites are found, the federal government along with some provinces have pledged millions of dollars to Indigenous communities to further search efforts to find and identify these children. There is much that is unknown, which may take years to uncover. The response to these discoveries was summed up by Rose Anne Archibald, the National Chief of the Assembly of First Nations (elected in 2021): "For many Canadians and for people around the world, these recent recoveries of our children—buried nameless, unmarked, lost and without ceremony are shocking, and unbelievable" (Austen, 2021).

In September 2021, an apology by the Canadian Conference of Catholic Bishops was issued for their role in the atrocities that occurred in Catholic-run residential schools. This was the first time an apology was issued by the Catholic Church, despite previous pressures. In the spring of 2022, a group of First Nations, Inuit, and Métis delegates (including residential school survivors) travelled to Rome for a private meeting with Pope Frances. The goal of the delegation was to promote reconciliation between Indigenous people and the Catholic Church and to obtain an apology from the Pope for the role the Catholic Church played in residential schools. The apology was issued, accepted by some, and not so much by others in the Indigenous community. The issue of compensation remains outstanding. The Pope agreed to come to Canada (in response to an invitation by the Canadian Conference of Catholic Bishops) to, at least in part, promote healing and reconciliation with the Indigenous people of Canada. The Indigenous community wanted the Pope to apologize for the role the Catholic Church played in residential schools while he was on Canadian soil.

The long-awaited apology came on Monday, June 18, in Maskwacis, Alberta. Translated into English, the Pope said, "I am sorry. I ask forgiveness, in particular, for the ways in which many members of the Church and of religious communities co-operated, not least through their indifference, in projects of cultural destruction and forced assimilation promoted by the governments of that time, which culminated in the system of residential schools." This apology was welcomed by some and received mixed reviews from others, feeling that the Pope did not go far enough with this apology. For example, he excluded the specifics of types abuses that occurred in the institutions and did not acknowledge the deaths of so many children.

Source: Based on First Nations Health Authority. (n.d.). *Our history, our health.* https://www.fnha.ca/wellness/our-history-our-health; Anderson, C. (2022, July 27). 'The real work begins now': Three Indigenous leaders on the Pope's apology. *TVO Today.* https://www.tvo.org/article/the-real-work-begins-now-three-indigenous-leaders-on-the-popes-apology?gclid=Cj0KCQjw39uYBhCLARIsAD_SzMSVhGWWUcvbitcbfYQ0wODt-R7rr1hcmOSv0f-0UWfR1OSTRdAf5igaApEIEALw_wcB

Over the years, Western medical practices have largely replaced traditional healing. In addition, providing access to health services in more remote communities is an ongoing challenge. Services are also often limited in terms of health human resources and access to diagnostic and other services as well as supplies (Chapter 5), and at times they do not meet the criteria outlined in the *Canada Health Act.* Few of the goals and standards outlined in Health Canada's determinants of health have been met, which remains a growing concern, with inequities particularly related to the social determinants of health (Chapter 6).

However, there are recent movements to return the responsibility of health care to Indigenous communities and to honor the value of traditional health practices. Many hospitals, clinics, and community health centres now integrate traditional health practices with Western medical practices.

Currently, the conditions most affecting Indigenous populations include diabetes, heart disease, tuberculosis, cancer, mental illness, and drug and alcohol use. Indigenous people were hit hard by the SARS-CoV-2 (COVID-19) virus for several reasons, not the least of which were crowded living conditions on reserves and in more remote communities, comorbidities, and, to some extent, vaccine hesitancy related to a (well-founded) mistrust of Western medicine and interventions.

## DID YOU KNOW?

### *Residential Schools in Newfoundland and Labrador*

Thousands of Indigenous children from Newfoundland and Labrador were removed from their families and communities between 1949 and 1979 to go to residential schools. Many suffered physical and emotional abuses similar to those suffered by children in other residential schools. They also lost their language and culture. When Prime Minister Stephen Harper issued his apology regarding residential schools, he did not include the survivors of residential schools in Newfoundland and Labrador because they were not run by the federal government itself. The apology to these survivors came from Prime Minister Justin Trudeau in November 2017.

**THINKING IT THROUGH**

*Health-Related Traditions and Cultural Practices*

Health professionals should be knowledgeable about health-related traditions and cultural practices that are important to the people and families in their communities. Honouring such practices whenever possible will contribute to a positive patient experience, improve health outcomes such as understanding treatment plans, and contribute to the patient's well-being.

1. Identify individuals or groups of people within your community who would benefit from culturally specific approaches to health care.
2. Considering cultural traditions or practices, explain three ways in which you could improve the health care experience of at least one of the groups you identified.

## THE ROAD FORWARD: PUBLIC HEALTH, NURSING, AND PUBLIC HEALTH INSURANCE

At the beginning of the nineteenth century, the prevalence of infectious diseases peaked. In 1834, William Kelly, a British Royal Navy physician, suspected a relationship between sanitation and disease and deduced that water was possibly a major contaminant. Although how disease spread was not clearly understood, many recognized the effectiveness of quarantine practices in limiting the spread of some diseases.

Upper and Lower Canada each established a board of health in 1832 and 1833, respectively. These boards of health enforced quarantine and sanitation laws, imposed restrictions on immigration (to prevent the spread of disease), and stopped the sale of spoiled food. Some health care measures met tremendous public opposition. For example, in the mid-1800s, a doctor in Nova Scotia attempted to introduce a smallpox vaccine, which had been discovered and proven successful in England around the turn of the century. Public resistance was strong despite proof that the vaccine protected individuals from the disease. Consequently, the value of smallpox vaccinations was not fully appreciated until the 1900s.

In the early 1900s, the provinces began establishing formal organizations to manage public health matters. A Bureau of Public Health was established in Saskatchewan in 1909 and became a government department in 1923. The provinces of Alberta, Manitoba, and Nova Scotia likewise established Departments of Health in 1918, 1928, and 1931, respectively. These public health organizations assumed responsibility for public health matters, including activities such as pasteurizing milk, testing cows for tuberculosis, managing tuberculosis sanatoriums, and controlling the spread of STIs. Maternal and child health care became a focus of public health initiatives at the beginning of the twentieth century. Both doctors and nurses actively promoted such things as immunization clinics and parenting education.

### The Role of Nursing in Early Health Care

Nursing care has been an essential part of health care in Canada since before Confederation, when the Hôtel-Dieu Hospital in Québec launched the first structured training for North American nurses in the form of a nursing apprenticeship (Canadian Museum of History, 2004).

In 1873, the first school of nursing was established at Mack's General and Marine Hospital in St. Catharines, Ontario (Mount Saint Vincent University, 2005). Another nursing school opened at Toronto General Hospital in 1881. Over the next 50 years, many hospital-based schools of nursing were established, and in 1919, the University of British Columbia offered the first university degree program for nurses.

The Canadian National Association of Trained Nurses (CNATN) became Canada's first formal nursing organization in 1908, with a mandate to provide support for nurses graduating from formal programs. In most jurisdictions, graduates of hospital-based programs held a diploma in nursing and were eligible to write provincial/territorial examinations to become registered nurses (RNs). Over time, hospital-based schools of nursing closed, transferring nursing education to other post-secondary facilities (colleges and universities). For example, in 1973, the Ontario government closed all hospital-based nursing programs. Schools of nursing at Woman's College Hospital, Wellesley Hospital, and the Hospital for Sick Children merged, forming a nursing program at what was at that the time Ryerson Polytechnical Institute (now Toronto Metropolitan University). Graduates still wrote provincial/territorial examinations and held either a diploma or a degree in nursing (program specific).

In the 1990s, diploma programs for RNs were phased out with entry to practise now at the baccalaureate level, except in Québec, where students can still graduate with a college diploma (DEC [Diploma of Colleges]) (Ordre des infirmieres et infirmiers du Québec, n.d.). Now there are transfer degree programs in which students may begin in a community college and enter into a university-degree program to complete their degrees. Today, some community colleges affiliate with universities for completion of a degree in nursing; other community colleges are now offering degree programs independent of affiliation with a university.

Nurse practitioners (NPs) were first introduced in Canada in the 1960s. Today NPs practise in all jurisdictions in a variety of settings (see Chapter 5).

## The Introduction of Health Insurance

Concerned about the continued shortage of physicians within their community, in 1914 the residents of the small municipality of Sarnia, Saskatchewan devised a plan, without government approval, to offer a local doctor $1500 (from municipal tax dollars) as an incentive to practise medicine in the community rather than join the army. The scheme proved successful, and over the next several years attracted a number of doctors to the area. In 1916, the provincial government passed the *Rural Municipality Act*, formally allowing municipalities to collect taxes to raise funds for retaining physicians and administering and maintaining hospitals. By 1931, 52 municipalities in Saskatchewan had enacted similar plans. Not long afterward, the provinces of Manitoba and Alberta followed suit.

In 1919, the first federal attempt to introduce a publicly funded health care system formed part of a Liberal election campaign. However, once in power, the Liberals were unsuccessful in their negotiations for joint funding with the provinces and territories and the plan was not carried out.

In the aftermath of the Great Depression in the 1930s, public pressure for a national health program mounted. Canadians realized that a more secure, affordable, and accessible health care system was necessary.

### First Attempts to Introduce National Health Insurance

In 1935, the Conservative government of R. B. Bennett pledged to address social issues such as minimum wage, unemployment, and public health insurance. Bennett's government proposed the *Employment and Social Insurance Act* on the advice of the Royal Commission on Industrial Relations. Under the Act, the federal government would gain the right to collect taxes to provide social benefits. However, the Act was declared unconstitutional by the Supreme Court of Canada and the Privy Council of Great Britain on the grounds that it violated provincial and territorial authority.

Although employment and social insurance were deemed the responsibility of provincial and territorial governments in 1937, shortly thereafter the federal government began to secure some gains in overseeing social programs. In 1940, under Prime Minister Mackenzie King, the provincial and federal governments agreed to amend the *British North America Act* to allow the introduction of a national unemployment insurance program. By 1942, this program was fully operational. Two years later, in 1944, the federal government passed another piece of legislation introducing family allowances for each child aged 16 and under (often referred to as "the baby bonus"), paving the way for more social programs, the modification of existing ones, and formalized health insurance.

## Post—World War II: The Political Landscape

Major changes in Canada's political landscape followed World War II. Provinces and territories began to exercise more authority over the social and economic lives of their populations. A shift in thinking, largely due to the devastating effects of the Depression, resulted in the idea that governments were responsible for providing citizens with a reasonable standard of living and acceptable access to basic services, such as health care. Canadians wanted the security and equity that a publicly funded health care system would bring.

Canadians, particularly the middle class, had felt the impact of not having access to appropriate health care. The rich could afford proper care; the poor could turn to charities. The expanding middle class was caught in between.

At the same time, medical discoveries were advancing treatment, care, and diagnostic capabilities. A shift from home- to hospital-based care, particularly when complex medical procedures were involved, created a perceived need for a more organized approach to health care. Various **social movements** advanced this agenda, because people believed the involvement of the federal government would result in more stable and equitable funding, which would then support and promote medical discoveries and treatment options.

In 1948, the federal government set up a number of grants to fund the development of health care services in partnership with the provinces. In 1952, these grants were supplemented by a national old-age security program for individuals 70 years of age or older. That same year, the provinces and territories introduced financial aid for people between the ages of 60 and 69, provided on a cost-sharing basis with the federal government. In 1954, legislation permitted the federal government to finance allowances for adults who were disabled and unable to work. All of these measures contributed to Canadians' health and well-being.

Despite increasing public requests for a nationally funded health care system, the provinces, the territories, and the federal government continued to struggle over how the system would be implemented. Who would be in charge of what, and how much power would the federal government hold over matters under provincial and territorial control?

The federal government, looking for a workable solution, ultimately decided to offer funds to the provinces and territories to help pay for health care costs; however, it also set restrictions on how the funds could be spent.

## Progress Toward Prepaid Hospital Care

The National Health Grants Program of 1948 marked the first step that the federal government took into the provincial and territorial jurisdictions of health care. Through this program the federal government offered the provinces and territories a total of $30 million to improve and modernize hospitals, to provide training for health care providers, and to fund research in the fields of public health, tuberculosis, and cancer treatments. Welcomed in all jurisdictions, these grants resulted in a hospital building boom that lasted nearly 30 years.

The next decade saw little progress in the introduction of comprehensive insurance plans in the provinces and territories. Then, in 1957, the federal government, under John Diefenbaker, introduced the *Hospital Insurance and Diagnostic Services Act*. The Act proposed that any province or territory willing to implement a comprehensive hospital insurance plan would receive federal assistance in the form of 50 cents on every dollar spent on the plan, literally cutting in half the province's or territory's expenses for insured services—an appealing offer indeed! Five provinces, along with the Northwest Territories and Yukon, bought into the plan immediately. All remaining jurisdictions were on board by 1961.

Even with the financial aid of the federal government, some provinces and territories were not able to implement comprehensive services, primarily because of population distribution. To rectify this problem, the federal government introduced an equalization payment system through which richer provinces would share revenue with poorer provinces to ensure all could offer equal services. This program remains in place today, but not without controversy (Chapter 2).

The *Hospital Insurance and Diagnostic Services Act* stated that all residents of a province or territory were entitled to receive insured health care services upon uniform terms and conditions. The Act provided residents with full care in an acute care hospital for as long as the physician felt necessary. It also included care provided in outpatient clinics, but not in tuberculosis sanitariums, mental institutions, or long-term care facilities.

Services for some allied health workers (e.g., physiotherapists) and other nonmedical professionals, as well as diagnostic procedures, were covered by provincial and territorial health insurance plans only if the care was provided in a hospital setting and under the direction of a physician. This coverage paved the way for a huge increase in hospital admissions, some more necessary than others. If **prepaid health care** was available with no out-of-pocket fee in the hospital, why would a patient go elsewhere where they would have to pay? As a result, spending for hospital services increased dramatically. A good example is the fact that some physicians admitted patients simply for weight loss. An individual could spend weeks in the hospital on a calorie-reduced diet until a designated number of pounds were lost. In addition, patients were admitted prior to surgery, sometimes for several days for diagnostic tests related to the surgery, costing the health care system millions.

## PROGRESS AND LEGISLATION PRECEDING THE *CANADA HEALTH ACT* AND PREPAID MEDICAL CARE

Tommy Douglas, known as the father of **medicare** (although this remains controversial— Justice Emmett Hall is also sometimes referred to as Canada's father of medicare), was the premier of Saskatchewan from 1944 to 1961 (Tommy Douglas Research Institute, n.d.). Douglas long campaigned for a combined comprehensive hospital and medical insurance plan that everyone could afford. He firmly believed that the implementation of a social health insurance plan was a government responsibility and that private insurance plans, although useful, discriminated against those with lower incomes, disabilities, and serious health issues.

In 1939, the Saskatchewan government enacted the *Municipal and Medical Hospital Services Act*, permitting municipalities to charge either a land tax or a personal tax to finance hospital and medical services—a precursor to comprehensive hospital insurance in the province. Eight years later, in 1947, Tommy Douglas's government passed the *Hospital Insurance Act*, guaranteeing Saskatchewan residents hospital care in exchange for a modest insurance premium payment.

In 1960, Douglas was ready to take the next step of providing Saskatchewan citizens with comprehensive, publicly funded medical care, in addition to hospital insurance. His initial attempts to introduce medical care insurance inspired fierce opposition from Saskatchewan doctors, who worried they would be controlled by the province. Douglas fought an election campaign with a platform promising to introduce the health insurance program and was re-elected in 1960. The following year, Douglas left Saskatchewan to lead the New Democratic Party in Ottawa. Under his successor, Premier Woodrow Lloyd, the *Saskatchewan Medical Care Insurance Act* was passed in 1961 and took effect in July 1962.

The day the medicare law came into effect, the doctors in Saskatchewan launched a province-wide doctors' strike, which lasted 23 days. In early August of 1962, the Saskatchewan government revised the *Medical Care Insurance Act* in an attempt to repair the relationship with the province's doctors. One amendment allowed doctors the option of practising outside the medical plan, but within 3 years most doctors were working within the plan, finding it the easier route to follow. Billing patients separately and collecting money owed proved expensive and time-consuming and resulted in only a marginal difference in remuneration. Most other provinces and territories adopted similar plans over the next few years. Today, physicians are remunerated in several ways, particularly those working within primary care teams (e.g., capitation-based funding and salaried positions [see Chapter 8]).

---

### THINKING IT THROUGH

#### *Socialized Medicine and Imposed Fee Schedules*

The *Saskatchewan Medical Care (Insurance) Act*, enforced socialized medicine and imposed fee schedules. It is a funding formula that persists across the country today. This means physicians are paid a calculated amount for each patient assessment, dependent on the complexity of the assessment, where the assessment takes place (e.g., office or patient's home), and when (e.g., evenings or weekends). This is called *fee for service*. Other funding mechanisms used today include salaries and paying doctors a set amount per year for each patient (used often in conjunction with primary care teams). The number of times a doctor sees a patient is irrelevant (see Capitation- or Population-Based Funding, Chapter 4).

1. Do you know how your physician is paid?
2. Do you think paying physicians for every service is more cost-effective than paying them a lump sum per patient, per year ?

---

The federal government remained committed to a comprehensive health insurance program. Box 1.5 summarizes the Hall Report, the *Medical Care Act*, and the *Established Programs and Financing (EPF) Act*, all of which played a significant role leading up to the *Canada Health Act*.

### Events Following the Introduction of the *EPF Act*

In the few years following the introduction of the *EPF Act*, health care spending continued to increase dramatically, resulting in provincial and territorial overspending and necessitating cuts to health care. Hospitals had to make cuts—some staff were let go, some medical services were either **delisted** or cut altogether, and doctors' fees were capped. In response, in 1978, outraged doctors began billing patients over and above what the provincial or territorial plan paid (in accordance with the negotiated fee schedule). For example, if the public insurance plan paid $25 for a doctor's visit, the doctor added an extra amount—say $10—and asked the patient to pay out-of-pocket for that service. This practice was called **extra billing** and contravened the principles of the *Medical Care Act*.

Opposition to extra billing was swift, with the public claiming that the fees unfairly limited access to health care. Tensions rose between physicians and the public sector. Once again,

## BOX 1.5   Legislation Leading up to the *Canada Health Act*

**The Hall Report (1960)—Royal Commission on Health Services**
- Investigated the state of health care in Canada and was instrumental in passing the *Medical Care Act* (1966)
- Passed in the House of Commons December 8, 1966
- Supported the introduction of a national medicare
- Required the federal government to share the cost of health care plans implemented by jurisdictions meeting the Act's criteria (a funding formula created by Tommy Douglas)
- Suggested the construction of new medical schools and hospitals
- Recommended that the number of physicians in Canada be doubled by 1990
- Recommended that private health insurance companies in the country be replaced by 10 provincial public health insurance plans
- Recommended that the federal government retain strong control over health care financing but allow provinces and territories some authority over the implementation of their health care services

**Implementation of the *Medical Care Act* (1968)**
- Implemented on July 1, 1968, and accepted by all provinces and territories by 1972
- Allowed all jurisdictions to administer the plan as they saw fit as long as they adhered to the criteria of universality, portability, comprehensive coverage, and public administration (mirroring the *Canada Health Act*)
- Covered only in-hospital care and physicians' services
- Caused the federal government, provinces, and territories to recognize the need for community-based care and restructuring of the funding formula because of soaring costs of physician and hospital care

**The *Established Programs Financing Act* (1977)**
- Introduced a new funding formula to allocate money to health care and to postsecondary education
- Replaced the previous 50/50 cost-sharing formula with a **block transfer** of both cash and tax points
- Reduced restrictions on how jurisdictions could spend money, allowing them to fund community-based services
- Provided more transfer money for an extended health care services program, which covered intermediate care in nursing homes, ambulatory health care, residential care, and some components of home care

Justice Emmett Hall was asked to lead a health care services review, with the assistance of Dr. Alice Girard from Québec. The mandate was to scrutinize issues that had risen since the previous Hall Report, including the legality of extra billing.

Hall's conclusions were released in 1980 in a report called *Canada's National—Provincial Health Program for the 1980s*. The report stated that extra billing violated the principles of the *Medical Care Act* and created a barrier for those who could not afford to pay. Hall recommended an end to extra billing and suggested that, instead, doctors be allowed to operate entirely outside of the *Medical Care Act*. This allowed patients the choice of avoiding a doctor who was not working within the boundaries of the provincial or territorial insurance plan.

Physicians opting out of the public insurance plan would bill patients directly for their services; patients would then have to collect money from their provincial or territorial insurance plan. Alternatively, the doctor could bill the plan for services, the plan would pay the patient, and the patient would pay the doctor with the money received, plus any amount the doctor charged above the plan's allowances. It was a lengthy and cumbersome process.

Hall also advised that national standards be created to uphold the principles and conditions of the *Medical Care Act*, that the criterion of accessibility be added to the Act, and that an independent National Health Council be established to assess health care in Canada and to suggest policy and legislative changes when needed.

The recommendations from the second Hall Report were taken seriously but put on hold until the Parliamentary Task Force on Federal–Provincial Arrangements completed its review the following year. This task force was to review the funding arrangements under the *EPF Act* and the other subsidies the federal government provided to the provinces and territories. The task force's recommendations included adjusting equalization payments, introducing federal responsibility for income distribution, and separating health care funding from higher education funding.

Together, the Hall Report and the report of the Parliamentary Task Force on Federal–Provincial Arrangements prompted the *Canada Health Act*, new and comprehensive legislation that replaced both the *Hospital Insurance and Diagnostic Services Act* and the *Medical Care Act*.

## THE *CANADA HEALTH ACT* (1984)

The *Canada Health Act* became law in 1984 under Prime Minister Pierre Trudeau's Liberal government. It received **royal assent** in June 1985 and is still in place today, governing and guiding—and perhaps limiting—our health care delivery system. The Act's primary goal is to provide equal, prepaid, and accessible health care to **eligible** Canadians (Box 1.6) and thereby meet the objectives of Canadian health care policy (Box 1.7).

### Criteria and Conditions of the *Canada Health Act*

The *Canada Health Act* established criteria and conditions for the delivery of health care. To qualify for federal payments, the provinces and territories must adhere to the five criteria discussed below, and also to two additional conditions (Box 1.8).

### Public Administration

The *Canada Health Act* stipulates that each provincial and territorial health insurance plan be managed by a public authority on a nonprofit basis. That is, the health insurance plan must not be governed by a private enterprise and must not be in the business of making a profit. The public authority answers to the provincial or territorial government regarding its decisions about benefit levels and services and must have all records and accounts publicly audited.

---

**BOX 1.6   Eligibility for Health Care Under the *Canada Health Act***

To be eligible for health care in Canada, a person must be a lawful resident of a province or territory. The *Canada Health Act* defines a resident as "a person lawfully entitled to be or to remain in Canada who makes his home and is ordinarily present in the province, but does not include a tourist, a transient, or a visitor to the province" (Government of Canada, 1985). Each province or territory determines its own minimum residence requirements.

Source: Government of Canada (1985). *Canada Health Act*, R.S.C., 1985 c. C-6. https://laws-lois.justice.gc.ca/eng/acts/c-6/page-1.html

---

**BOX 1.7    The Primary Objectives of Canadian Health Care Policy**

"To protect, promote and restore the physical and mental well-being of residents of Canada and to facilitate reasonable access to health services without financial or other barriers."

Source: Government of Canada. (2020). *Canada Health Act.* https://www.canada.ca/en/health-canada/services/health-care-system/canada-health-care-system-medicare/canada-health-act.html

---

**BOX 1.8    The *Canada Health Act*: Criteria and Conditions**

| Criteria | Conditions |
|---|---|
| 1. Public administration | 1. Information |
| 2. Comprehensive coverage | 2. Recognition |
| 3. Universality | |
| 4. Portability | |
| 5. Accessibility | |

Source: Tiedemann, M. (2019). *The Canada Health Act: An overview and options.* Library of Parliament. https://lop.parl.ca/sites/PublicWebsite/default/en_CA/ResearchPublications/201954E

---

To meet the criteria of the Act, health plans must be overseen by the Ministry of Health, the Department of Health, or the equivalent provincial or territorial government department. Services provided under the umbrella of the relevant department are distributed via different vehicles, primarily via regional health authorities or the equivalent.

### Comprehensive coverage

Provincial and territorial health insurance plans allow eligible persons with a medical need to access prepaid, medically necessary services provided by physicians and hospitals. Select services offered by dental surgeons, when delivered in the hospital setting, are also covered. Services included under the provincial or territorial plan must be equally available to all insured residents of the province or territory; there must be no barriers to access.

Each province or territory has the latitude to select which services will be covered under its specific plan. Coverage may include components of home care or nursing home care, chiropractic care, eye care under specific conditions, and pharmacare for designated population groups. Comprehensive coverage of these provincially or territorially tailored services must be offered to every eligible resident in the jurisdiction. Procedures that are considered cosmetic are generally not covered; if the procedure was required for a medical reason, however, it would be covered (Case Example 1.1).

---

**CASE EXAMPLE 1.1    Coverage for Certain Services for Baby B.K.**

Baby B.K. is 3 days old. His mother would like him to be circumcised. This procedure is not considered elective or medically necessary so would not be covered under a public plan in most jurisdictions. If, down the road, Baby B.K. developed a medical condition (phimosis) requiring that he be circumcised for medical reasons, the procedure would be covered under a provincial/territorial plan. The procedure in this case would be deemed medically necessary.

## Universality

All eligible residents of a province or territory are entitled, on uniform terms and conditions, to *all* of the insured health services that are provided under the provincial or territorial health insurance plan.

The federal government allowed the provinces and territories to decide whether they would charge their residents insurance premiums. Where premiums were charged, however, a citizen's inability to pay could not prevent their access to appropriate medical care. The province or territory would then be able to subsidize premiums for those with low incomes but could not discriminate on any basis—for example, on the individual's previous health record, current health status, race, or age. *Universality* means that no matter how young or old, or rich or poor a person is, or what their health condition is, that person is eligible for the same insured health services as anyone else (Case Example 1.2).

---

### CASE EXAMPLE 1.2 Premiums and Access to Care for J.N.

J.N. lives in British Columbia, a province where residents are not required to pay health care premiums. J.N. needs knee replacement surgery, which is covered by the provincial health care plan. Ontario charges health care premiums. If J.N. lived in Ontario, was unemployed, and was on social assistance, would the same surgery be covered?

---

## Portability

Canadians moving from one province or territory to another are covered for insured health services by their province of origin during any waiting period in the province or territory to which they have moved, under the Reciprocal Agreement (see Chapter 3). Most jurisdictions enforce a 3-month wait before public health insurance becomes active. Under the Act, the waiting period cannot exceed 3 months. Individuals moving to Canada may also have to endure a waiting period of up to 3 months and therefore are encouraged to have private insurance in place in the interim (see Chapter 7).

Canadians who leave the country will continue to be insured for health services for a prescribed period of time. Every province or territory sets its own time frame (usually 6 months less a day, or 183 days). Ontario states that a person may be out of the country for a maximum of 212 days in any given year, while Alberta, British Columbia, Manitoba, and New Brunswick state that a person must remain in the province for at least 6 months to retain coverage. In Nova Scotia, with permission and under certain conditions, a temporary absence of up to 1 year is allowed. Newfoundland and Labrador offer out-of-province coverage for individuals who remain in the province for only 4 months of the calendar year—the lowest residency requirement of all jurisdictions, in part due to the number of migrant workers in the province. In addition, every jurisdiction offers coverage for special situations, such as absences for educational or work purposes. Although Canadian residents are covered for necessary care (i.e., urgent or emergency care) while absent from their home province (e.g., for business or a vacation), they are not permitted to seek elective surgeries or other planned care in another province or territory. In some cases, prior approval for coverage may be granted for elective surgery (Case Example 1.3). Usually approval is not given unless the procedure cannot be performed within benchmark timelines determined by the person's province jurisdiction of origin. The websites of the provincial and territorial ministries of health offer information about the particulars of each jurisdiction's health care coverage.

---

### CASE EXAMPLE 1.3   Coverage for Surgery in Another Jurisdiction for N.R.

At 69 years old, N.R. is booked for elective hip replacement surgery in 6 months in their home province of Nova Scotia. However, they decide to visit their sister in British Columbia and have their hip replaced there because surgical wait times are shorter. To ensure that the Nova Scotia government will cover the cost of N.R's surgery in British Columbia, they have to contact the Nova Scotia Department of Health for *prior approval*. If N.R has the surgery without requesting approval from the Nova Scotia Ministry of Health, or if they are denied approval, they will have to pay for the surgery out-of-pocket. However, if N.R falls down the stairs and breaks their hip while they are visiting their sister, the surgery would be done in British Columbia, and the total cost would be covered by their province of origin without question.

Conversely, if N.R, while visiting a sister, had a skin rash or a sore throat, they could seek medical attention in British Columbia and the cost of the visit (and any treatment) would be covered by the Nova Scotia health plan through the reciprocal agreement. The British Columbia medical care plan would bill the Nova Scotia health plan directly.

---

Insured services received outside the person's province of origin will be paid at the host province's rate, except by Québec (Chapter 8).

### Accessibility

The criterion of accessibility was added to the *Canada Health Act* in an attempt to ensure that eligible individuals in a province or territory have reasonable access to all insured health services on uniform terms and conditions. *Reasonable access* means access to services when and where they are available. A service may not be available to a person because of where they live—for example, in a more remote or rural community (Case Example 1.4). Or a service may be unavailable because of a shortage of beds or lack of health care providers to supply the service. Individuals needing a service that is not available must be granted access to that service in the closest location it is offered—whether in another town or city, in another province, or in the United States (Chapter 3).

Accessibility applies to wait times as well. Some jurisdictions have established maximum wait times for certain procedures. If a person has to wait for a procedure (e.g., a hip

---

### CASE EXAMPLE 1.4   Access to Services for M.T.

M.T. is a 40-year-old Indigenous woman living in Pickle Lake, Ontario. She has just been diagnosed with breast cancer, and after her surgery she requires a series of 21 radiation treatments. She had her surgery in Thunder Bay, Ontario and was able to return home to recuperate. Her community does not have access to radiation therapy, so M.T. will have to return to Thunder Bay for these treatments, staying for nearly a month away from her community, as the treatments are daily. In accordance with the accessibility criterion, M.T. would be sent to Thunder Bay for her treatments. If radiation therapy was not available in Thunder Bay—or if the wait time was excessive—M.T. would be sent to Winnipeg, Manitoba.

replacement or cardiac bypass surgery) beyond that set time limit, the province or territory will send the person somewhere else for the procedure (see Case Example 1.3). Note, as previously mentioned, that a province or territory would pay for a patient to receive an available service only at the closest alternative location, not a location farther afield or one that the patient prefers.

There are situations wherein a person scheduled for surgery that is considered time sensitive has their surgery postponed if the services they require are not readily available. This has been a frequent occurrence throughout the COVID-19 pandemic. Even during the fourth wave of the pandemic the hospitalization rates for individuals with COVID-19 were high in many jurisdictions, including Alberta and Saskatchewan. In order to increase Critical Care Unit (CCU) or Intensive Care Unit (ICU) capacity, in September 2021, Alberta Health Services cancelled all elective surgeries and outpatient procedures, acknowledging that the move could have a serious impact on patients, some of whom might suffer serious consequences (e.g., postponed surgery for cancer) (Alberta Health Services, 2021). The hospitals were functioning beyond capacity, especially in terms of providing acute care and CCU beds. There was also a shortage of health professionals with the skills to care for these patients. Situations such as this, although both necessary and unfortunate, impact the concept of accessibility (Case Example 1.5). Note that during the COVID-19 pandemic, almost all jurisdictions faced similar circumstances at one point or another.

The interpretation of *reasonable access* is controversial. A person living in Churchill, Manitoba, will not have the same access to health care as a person living in Halifax, Toronto, or Vancouver. Today, service availability varies even between rural and urban settings. For the purposes of the *Canada Health Act*, accessibility has been interpreted as access to services where and when available. It does not, in the true sense of the word, guarantee "equality" of services across Canada.

The following two conditions were imposed on provinces in the *Canada Health Act*:
- *Information.* Each province or territory must provide the federal government with information about the insured health care services and extended health care services for the purposes identified in the *Canada Health Act*.
- *Recognition.* The provincial and territorial governments must publicly recognize the federal financial contributions to both insured and extended health care services.

### Interpreting the *Canada Health Act*

**Medically necessary** is a subjective term that has been hotly debated within the context of the *Canada Health Act* (also see Chapters 2 and 8). Typically, a physician or other health care provider eligible to bill the provincial or territorial plan makes a clinical judgement to provide the patient with specific medically necessary services, which usually include assessment, diagnostic tests, and treatment. Note, however, that some jurisdictions may not cover all

---

**CASE EXAMPLE 1.5    Prioritizing Care for A.P.**

A.P. was scheduled for cardiac bypass surgery. Their surgery was cancelled because the hospital was over capacity treating patients with COVID-19. All CCU beds were full in surrounding hospitals. Although A.P.'s surgery was time sensitive, it was not considered an emergency, so they would have to wait until the services they needed were available. Patients with COVID-19 who required CCU beds would be sent to other facilities in other provinces, if necessary, where there was a bed available. Because COVID-19 patients' condition was acute, their cases would have priority over A.P.'s.

diagnostic tests and treatments. The *Canada Health Act* does not outline what services should be insured, allowing for some variability among jurisdictions. That said, what is considered medically necessary is reasonably consistent across the country. Supplementary services are determined by each jurisdiction and may vary more.

Medical services (e.g., Caesarean delivery) must not be provided simply for the convenience of the patient or physician. And when more than one treatment is available, a physician must consider cost-effectiveness. For example, when faced with two treatment options that have similar outcomes, a physician must recommend the less expensive option. In some jurisdictions, diagnostic tests done for preventive purposes have guidelines as to when they should be done and for whom. These guidelines may include the patient's age and risk factors.

What one doctor considers medically necessary another doctor may not. Consider breast reduction: a surgeon in Manitoba might determine that this surgery is medically necessary for a particular patient with large breasts because of the backaches and muscle strains the person suffers. Another surgeon may not think breast reduction is medically necessary for this patient, meaning that the patient would have to pay for the surgery, since it would then be considered a cosmetic procedure.

### THINKING IT THROUGH

#### *Medically Necessary Procedures and Services*

The term *medically necessary* appears in the *Canada Health Act* to identify procedures and services that are covered by provincial and territorial health insurance.

1. Look up the term *medically necessary* in two sources.
2. Do you think that the term is too subjective? Think of two examples.
3. Are there health services in your province or territory that you feel should be covered but are not?

Physicians, through their governing body, and government officials—usually from the Ministry or Department of Health—select which services are medically necessary and are, therefore, insured. At designated intervals, the provinces and territories review their lists of insured services, sometimes adding services, sometimes removing them.

For example, a few years ago many jurisdictions removed elective newborn circumcision from the list of insured services because evidence showed no medical reason for this procedure and found other reasons (e.g., a belief that a person who is circumcised is cleaner, or that the baby should resemble his father), to be invalid. However, circumcision is still insured when a valid medical reason exists for doing it (see Case Example 1.1).

Also addressed in the *Canada Health Act* are extra billing and **user charges** (or user fees; also addressed under the *Medical Care Act*)—a fee imposed for an insured health service that the provincial or territorial health care insurance plan does not cover (Tiedemann, 2019). Currently, under the Act, extra billing and user charges are not allowed because they create a barrier to seeking medical care. If a province or territory nevertheless permits extra billing or user charges, the federal government will total the amount of money the province or territory has collected and will deduct that amount from the next transfer of funds. Proponents of user charges believe they play a useful role in today's health care climate. For example, charging people who use the emergency department for nonurgent complaints (Case Example 1.6) is an example of how user charges could be implemented.

---

**CASE EXAMPLE 1.6   User Fees for K.J.**

K.J., who lives in Alberta, went to the emergency department because they had a bad cold. The provincial plan would cover the cost of the visit, but the hospital charged K.J. an additional fee because they came to the emergency department instead of going to their doctor. The extra fee is a user charge.

---

### Services Not Covered Under the Act

Long-term care, homecare services, and extended services are *not* included under the *Canada Health Act* and therefore are not available to Canadians on a universal basis. These services are subject to each province's or territory's health insurance plan (see Chapters 3 and 5). Some jurisdictions, for example, will provide a certain number of home care hours per week. Once the limit is reached, the patient must pay a home care agency for additional care. The legislation prohibiting user charges and extra billing does not apply to extended health care services. Each province and territory chooses which optional services (i.e., services that are not medically necessary) will be covered under its health plan.

The amount of coverage for optional services will vary. For example, a province's plan may cover up to $200/month in physiotherapy services. Services in excess of this amount are subject to user charges and extra billing, which, as mentioned, are permitted for services deemed not medically necessary under the Act.

## AFTER THE *CANADA HEALTH ACT:* COMMISSIONED REPORTS AND ACCORDS

Most of the resistance to the Act came from physicians and those affected directly by the restrictions set out in the Act. In 1986, Ontario physicians participated in a 25-day strike in opposition to the Act, arguing that the key issue was not money but professional freedom, a claim not well received by the public. That same year, the Canadian Medical Association opposed the implementation of the *Canada Health Act* on the grounds that it violated the *Constitution Act* of 1982. The case went to the Supreme Court of Canada but did not proceed.

Just prior to the introduction of the Act, most of the provinces and territories had established some form of extra billing, user charges, or both as a result of events leading up to the implementation of the *Canada Health Act*. These extra fees could not be removed overnight. Over the next 2 years, the federal government imposed monetary penalties to noncompliant jurisdictions, again fueling resentment and opposition. The federal government decided to reimburse provinces that took corrective action against extra billing and user charges within 3 years. Most jurisdictions complied, but these practices were not entirely eliminated. Even today, some provinces and territories defy this part of the Act, each year resulting in withheld funding primarily related to user charges at private clinics deemed by the federal government to be operating outside of the law (see Chapter 8).

In the decade following the implementation of the *Canada Health Act*, the health care system in Canada experienced increasing difficulties that persist today. At first, hospitals had trouble functioning within their allotted budgets. Provinces and territories pushed for more money to sustain reasonable levels of care, yet federal funding continued to dwindle. In the early 1990s, hospitals restructured, downsized, redistributed beds, laid off staff, cut services, and closed. Doctors and nurses left the country, and fewer graduates pursued careers in these roles (especially in nursing), leading to widespread shortage of health human resources.

Some provinces and territories responded proactively by establishing innovative and alternative health care strategies (Box 1.9). Home care and eventually community care became

## BOX 1.9   Alternative Health Care Strategies

New Brunswick was one of the first jurisdictions to predict the problems related to funding shortfalls, cutbacks, population changes, and an increased need for hospital beds. The province led the move toward community-based care, called "a hospital without walls," and established the Extra-Mural Program, which focused on shortening hospital stays and providing the appropriate care and support to meet health care needs in home and community settings. This concept was actually introduced in 1979, 5 years before the *Canada Health Act* was passed.

Throughout the 1980s and 1990s, various provinces and territories completed investigations into the state of health. These include the Royal Commission on Health Care in Nova Scotia (1989), the Commission on Directions in Health Care in Saskatchewan (1990), the Premier's Council on Health Strategy in Ontario (1991), and the Health Services Review in British Columbia (1999).

National reports were also commissioned; for example, the first, second, and third reports on the health of Canadians, released in 1996, 1999, and 2003, respectively, examined and summarized the health status of Canadians. A 2016 report on the health of Canadians focused on the growing number of Canadians with heart disease.

By 2002, public confidence in health care was at an all-time low, with health care topping the list of Canadians' concerns. Following this concern were those regarding services (or lack thereof) for mental health, community care, and the omission of a national pharmacare strategy. Provinces and territories introduced a variety of commissions to study varying concerns regarding health care within their own jurisdictions, some coming to fruition, others not.

On a national level, over a number of years, responding to gaps in mental health and home care services became a priority. In 2006, the Senate Standing Committee on Social Affairs, Science, and Technology completed a Canada-wide study on mental health and illness, recommending, among other things, establishing a Canadian Mental Health Commission to address shortcomings in mental health services. The Mental Health Commission of Canada (chaired by the Honourable Michael Kirby) was created the following year to provide and oversee mental health services at a national level. Creation of the Mental Health Commission of Canada was supported by all jurisdictions, except Québec.

In 2017, the federal government provided targeted funding for both mental health and community care initiatives. In response to national pressure to provide dignity for persons with terminal illness, medical assistance in dying (MAiD) was legalized. The associated procedures were deemed to be the responsibility of primary care practitioners and overseen by family physicians and nurse practitioners. MAiD has undergone several changes over the past few years. In March 2021, changes made to MAiD became law, particularly in relation to eligibility criteria (discussed in Chapters 8, 9, and 10).

How primary care is delivered continues to evolve, affected greatly by the COVID-19 pandemic. Jurisdictions have implemented fee-for-service codes allowing providers to submit claims for a wider variety of virtual appointments (see Chapters 3, 5, and 10). Today the need to increase the capacity for mental health services has never been more acute, given the upswing in mental health issues and substance use across all age groups as a result of the pandemic, including among children and youth (see Chapters 2, 3, 5, and 10).

Source: Based on South East Regional Health Authority. (n.d.). *Extra-mural program.* https://www2.gnb.ca/content/gnb/en/services/services_renderer.8975.Extra-Mural_Program.html

| TABLE 1.1 The Goals of Primary Care | |
| --- | --- |
| **Medical Model of Health Care** | **Goals of Reformed Primary Care Models** |
| Physician-based care | Team-oriented care |
| Illness-focused | Emphasis on disease prevention and health promotion |
| Hospital-based care | Community-based care |
| Curative (in relation to disease) | Treating maladies, which sometimes results in living healthy lives with chronic conditions |
| Problems are isolated | Care is comprehensive and integrated (i.e., holistic) |
| Health care provider—dominated | Collaborative care involving interprofessional teams, the patient, family, and loved ones |

a priority across Canada; the concept of "health care teams" reflecting how primary care is delivered today was introduced; access to primary care services was expanded (e.g., through after-hours clinics, telephone helplines, and extended office hours); and **primary health care reform** began to take place. In addition, nurse practitioners and other care providers assumed more responsibilities in providing primary care within their areas of expertise (Chapter 3) (Table 1.1).

### DID YOU KNOW?

#### Québec and Medical Aid in Dying

Québec was the first jurisdiction in Canada to legalize Medical Aid in Dying. Bill 52 passed in June 2014, which was an Act respecting end-of-life care. Québec was the fourth jurisdiction in North America to pass such legislation; the others were in the United States: the states of Washington, Vermont, and Oregon.

## Social Union

In 1997, the provincial and territorial **first ministers** met with their federal counterparts to form a social renewal program that required that all governments work collaboratively on what the first ministers called a *social union* (Canadian Intergovernmental Conference Secretariat, 1999). The agreement acknowledged the need to establish national standards for social rights and associated related policies.

The principals of the covenant included being recognized equally for all Canadians. All Canadians should be treated with fairness and dignity and equality of rights; they should be afforded equal opportunities and provided appropriate assistance for those needing it; and they should be afforded mobility within Canada. *Mobility* means Canadians can move freely within the country to seek opportunities, and governments will remove any residency-based barriers. Canadians have the opportunity to use monetary transfers from social support programs such as health care.

Difficult negotiations followed, primarily around the federal funding formula and the amount of autonomy provinces and territories would have with respect to where and how to spend the money (e.g., cancer treatments, improvements to emergency departments, long-term care). The final agreement was signed by all jurisdictions, with the exception of Québec, on February 4, 1999 (Asselin, 2001). Québec was unwilling to sign any agreement that did not clearly support the province's right to unconditionally opt out of programs supported by or initiated by the federal government, which the social union did not provide.

In the final agreement, the union agreed to maintain the five criteria of the *Canada Health Act* and to work continuously to improve health care. Also included was a commitment to work collaboratively with Indigenous people, their governments, and their organizations to improve health care and social programs. The federal government then promised to boost health care spending by $11.5 billion over the next 5 years, which began in the 1999–2000 fiscal year.

The success of the social union today is questionable at best. Federal funding formulas changed (see Chapter 8), and the agreement drove a wedge between Québec and the federal government; certainly inequities related to social programs are evident. Consider the rise in the rate of tuberculosis among Inuit living in Inuit Nunangat: it is 300 times the rate for non-Indigenous Canadians (Indigenous Services Canada, 2022a).

## Commissioned Reports

By the end of 2002, three major reports on the status of health care in Canada had been commissioned and released: the Mazankowski Report, the Kirby Report, and the Romanow Report. See Box 1.10 for the key points of each of these reports.

The *Truth and Reconciliation Commission of Canada: Calls to Action* (Truth and Reconciliation Commission of Canada, 2015b) also addresses health matters relating to Indigenous people in Canada, specifically Calls to Action numbers 18–24. The Calls to Action address current inequities in health care for Indigenous people. Call to Action #18 states that "the health of Aboriginal peoples is a direct result of previous Canadian governments policies, including residential schools, and to recognize and implement the healthcare rights of Aboriginal people as identified in international law, common law and under the Treaties" (TRCtalk (a), n.d.). The other Calls to Action under "Health" range from asking that the government close the gaps and inequities between non-Indigenous and Indigenous people to addressing the health care needs of the Métis, Inuit, and off-reserve Indigenous peoples by honouring their requests for funding for Indigenous health centres and respecting "healing practices and [using] them in the treatment of Aboriginal patients" (TRCtalk (b), n.d.). This is to be done in collaboration with Elders upon request. Call to Action #23 asks the government to increase the number of Indigenous health care providers, and #24 states that health-related education facilities need to ensure that students in nursing and medical schools take a course on Indigenous health issues and the legacy of residential schools. The Calls to Action are detailed on this website: https://www2.gov.bc.ca/assets/gov/british-columbians-our-governments/indigenous-people/aboriginal-peoples-documents/calls_to_action_english2.pdf. Please take the time to read and discuss them.

### Impact of the Romanow Report

Following the release of the Romanow Report, the federal government under Prime Minister Jean Chrétien stated that the report would provide the foundation for the direction of health care over the next several years. In 2004, the federal government earmarked $10 billion for health care to be distributed over a 10-year time frame to address the problems identified in the report.

Several of Romanow's recommendations have been implemented. On April 1, 2004, the Canada Health Transfer (CHT) and the Canada Social Transfer (CST) replaced the Canada Health and Social Transfer (CHST), a set amount of money (a block transfer payment) from

---

**BOX 1.10** **Three Major Reports on the Status of Health Care in Canada**

**The Mazankowski Report:** *A Framework for Reform* **(2001)**
*Commissioned by former Alberta premier Ralph Klein in August 2000 and chaired by Donald Mazankowski, former Cabinet member in the Mulroney government.*
   **Purpose**: to provide strategic advice to the premier on the preservation and future enhancement of quality health services for Albertans

*Key Points*
- Supported private health care in that it recommended that doctors be allowed to work in private health care venues after devoting a specific amount of time to the public sector
- Recommended, after review, delisting selected services currently covered under the provincial plan
- Recommended implementation of province-wide electronic health records and electronic health cards
- Suggested that taxes be used as a source of increased revenue and that Albertans pay higher health premiums (not well received)

   **Significant Outcomes**: By 2003, Alberta had implemented a province-wide electronic health record initiative, becoming the first Canadian province to do so.

**The Kirby Report:** *The Health of Canadians—The Federal Role* **(2002)**
*Led by Senator Michael J. Kirby*
   **Purpose**: to examine the state of the Canadian health care system and the role of the federal government in it

*Key Points*
- Bore important similarities to the Mazankowski Report
- Claimed the health care system was unsustainable with existing levels of funding
- Recommended the implementation of new taxes or insurance premiums that were paired to income
- Recommended setting limits to wait times; once the limit was reached, stated that the government should pay for the patient to receive treatment elsewhere, even in the United States if necessary
- Recommended a government-funded assistance plan for medications under certain circumstances related to the cost of medications proportionate to a person's (or a family's) income
- Recommended an immediate outlay of $2 billion for information technology, including the development of a national system for electronic health records, and another $2.5 billion over 5 years for advanced medical equipment
- Suggested government incentives encouraging health care providers to return to Canada, and outlay of funds to recruit and train doctors and nurses

   **Significant Outcomes**: This report was not as widely accepted as the Romanow Report. However, Ontario did adopt payment premiums for health care.

**The Romanow Report:** *Building on Values: The Future of Health Care in Canada* **(2002)**
*Led by Roy Romanow, former premier of Saskatchewan and chair of the Commission on the Future of Health Care in Canada*
   **Purpose**: to present recommendations to ensure the survival of Canada's health care system and to consider health promotion and disease prevention initiatives

*Key Points*
- Bore important similarities to the Mazankowski Report
- Gathered information and advice from Canadians through public forums and meetings held across the country
- Believed that health care was sustainable but that immediate action was necessary by all levels of government (funding and revision)
- Opposed privatization of health care, stating that any new plans creating private health care initiatives should be discouraged
- Recommended the creation of the Health Council of Canada to oversee improvements to health care, to conduct regular reviews of the health care system (e.g., home- and community-based care, primary care reform initiatives, human health resources, implementation of drug plans, wait times), and to report findings to the public
- Recommended that reform initiatives be paid for by the federal government's surplus or by raising taxes (e.g., the federal government could establish a dedicated cash-only Canada Health Transfer)
- Recommended adding the criterion of accountability to the *Canada Health Act*
- Recommended extending coverage for home care, diagnostic testing, **palliative care**, and mental health care
- Suggested that employment insurance benefits and job security be extended to family members and friends who choose to care for sick or dying loved ones at home
- Recommended that **catastrophic drug costs**, subject to certain terms and conditions (e.g., ability to pay), be covered
- Recommended that a national body control the price of medications, provide a centralized list of medications covered by public health plans, monitor the safety and cost of new medications seeking federal approval for use, and review the efficacy and outcomes of medications in use
- Recommended the establishment of another independent agency to review and approve prescription medications and to ensure that Canadians have clear and concise information about the medications they are taking
- Advocated the organization of a central body to monitor and streamline wait lists, but did not recommend a limit on wait times

**Significant Outcomes**: See Impact of the Romanow Report, later in the chapter.

Sources: Kirby, M. J. L. (2002). *The health of Canadians—The federal role. Final report.* https://publications.gc.ca/site/eng/398166/publication.html; Mazankowski, D. (2001). *A framework for reform: Report of the Premier's Advisory Council on Health.* https://open.alberta.ca/dataset/a2a779b1-9539-4d31-b6cf-399901520575/resource/098ed295-c86b-464b-9900-51c4c73feaa7/download/mazankowski-report-2001.pdf; Romanow, R. (2002). *Building on values: The future of health care in Canada.* https://publications.gc.ca/collections/Collection/CP32-85-2002E.pdf; Until The Last Child. (2014). *The history of child welfare in Canada.* https://www.untilthelastchild.com/the-history-of-child-welfare-in-canada/

the federal government to the provinces intended to pay for health care, postsecondary education, and welfare. See Chapter 4 for further discussion.

Health promotion campaigns have been maintained and further promoted by all levels of government. Limits on wait times were implemented across the country, and current wait times were required to be posted on the Internet. The Health Council of Canada was created as a result of the 2003 First Ministers' Accord but was subsequently disbanded by the federal government in 2014. At the 2004 first ministers' meeting, Canada's first ministers agreed on more funding and initiatives for health care renewal, including funding for family members to remain at home to care for ill relatives. Primary health care reform initiatives have been tested, implemented, and revised across Canada. That process is ongoing as various primary health care delivery models are continually improved to be cost-effective and meet the needs of the communities they serve. Funding was made available for information technology and electronic health records in all regions. In some jurisdictions the money was used effectively, but in others it was not. The implementation of electronic medical records and their effectiveness remain fractured from a national perspective, although improvements have been made. A national catastrophic drug plan (see Chapter 4) has not been implemented, although most jurisdictions now have one of their own. Drug coverage is inconsistent across the country. Canada is still the only industrialized nation with universal health care that does not have a national pharmacare.

See the interview with Roy Romanow on Evolve in which he talks about shortcomings in medicare today and gives his thoughts about the recommendations in his report that were not carried out.

---

**THINKING IT THROUGH**

### A National Drug Plan for Canada

Despite past recommendations to establish a national drug plan (e.g., The Romanow Report) to date, this has not been done. Some claim that a national drug plan would be cost prohibitive; others claim that a national plan would be cost-effective and save billions of dollars. The federal government, as part of the 2018 budget, announced the creation of an Advisory Council on the Implementation of National Pharmacare to assess the impact that such a plan would have for Canadians and the health care system.

1. In your opinion, is health care as we know it sustainable?
2. Do you think a national paid-for drug plan and increased coverage for home care would be cost effective?

---

## Accords

The following summaries of first ministers' meetings highlight the most recent **health accords** between the federal government and the provincial and territorial governments.

### First Ministers' Meeting, 2000

In September 2000, the first ministers met and agreed to work together to identify the significant issues facing health care in each province and territory, to prioritize these concerns, and to pledge to work collaboratively to address these concerns on both a provincial or territorial and national level. The major issues identified at this meeting included health promotion, timely access to services, the state of primary care services, the shortage of health professionals, lack of funding and services for home and community care, inefficient management of health records, aging diagnostic equipment, lack of equipment, and the high cost of medications for the many Canadians without a drug plan.

A number of meetings followed. Agreements were achieved, commitments were made, and funding was pledged to address concerns. The renewed commitment at subsequent meetings built on the promises made at the September 2000 first ministers' gathering.

### First Ministers' Accord on Health Care Renewal, 2003

In February 2003, the prime minister and the premiers of seven provinces met in Ottawa to outline the immediate direction for health care in Canada. The overriding commitment made was to preserve universal health care under the current *Canada Health Act*. Most of the concerns are the same as those discussed in the First Ministers' Meeting in 2000 (Health Canada, 2003).

A key component of this accord was establishing standards of care for Canadians, including access to health care providers 24 hours a day, 7 days a week; prompt access to diagnostic services and treatments; the implementation of a nationwide electronic health record system; and financial assistance for those who need medications but cannot afford them.

Over a 5-year time frame the Health Reform Fund, created at this meeting, channeled money into primary care, a catastrophic drug plan, and home care services. Through this fund the federal government transferred money to the provinces and territories so that they could address the specific needs of their residents.

The ministers also addressed the unique needs of Indigenous people. The federal government pledged to work more closely with provincial and territorial governments and Indigenous leaders to bring health care services for Indigenous people on par with those provided to other Canadians.

The equalization payment program was re-examined to ensure that all provinces had adequate funding to provide comparable health care services to their citizens. As previously mentioned, it was through this accord that the *Canada Health Transfer* was created, separating the funding formula that had combined federal funding for both health care and post-secondary education.

In this accord, the federal government also pledged to introduce a *compassionate care benefit package* through the Employment Insurance program, along with job protection through the Canada Labour Code (as recommended in the Romanow Report), to provide financial security and job protection for individuals who temporarily leave their place of employment to care for a seriously ill or dying parent, spouse, or child. This recommendation was implemented in 2012.

In 2016, the federal government extended paid benefits to 26 weeks from 6 weeks. Nova Scotia, the first province to align its labour code with federal legislation, extended the leave to 28 weeks in 2016, followed by Saskatchewan, and Newfoundland and Labrador.

In addition, the Health Council of Canada was created and given the responsibility to report to Canadians on health outcomes (it was disbanded in 2014, according to the federal government, having served its mandate).

### First Ministers' Meeting on the Future of Health Care, 2004

The First Ministers' Meeting on the Future of Health Care was convened to follow up on agreements made in 2003, discuss progress, and move forward with other proposals (Health Canada, 2004). At this meeting, the prime minister and premiers signed a second agreement, with the federal government pledging $41 billion for health care services over a 10-year time frame. Once again, the first ministers renewed their commitment to building on the criteria of the current *Canada Health Act* and to working together in a constructive and open manner. They promised to share information and to be more accountable to the public about progress being made. The Health Council of Canada was given increased responsibilities to report to Canadians on health outcomes.

The prime minister, first ministers, and Indigenous leaders established the Aboriginal Health Transition Fund, which provided $200 million for improving Indigenous health care services to meet the needs of Indigenous people across Canada.

### Annual Conference of Ministers of Health, 2005

At the Annual Conference of Ministers of Health in 2005, particular consideration was given to the catastrophic drug coverage mentioned at previous meetings. The ministers of health discussed measures to move forward with previous recommendations to standardize the price of medications across Canada and pledged to have better control over the pharmaceutical industry's relationship with provincial and territorial health insurance plans (Government of Canada, 2005).

### The Kelowna Accord, 2006

The first ministers met again in Kelowna, British Columbia, where the federal government promised to spend $5 billion over 5 years to improve health, housing, and education for Indigenous people (Patterson, 2006). The ministers also established the *Blueprint on Aboriginal Health*, a plan aimed to bring the health outcomes of Indigenous people in line with those of the general Canadian population—although provinces and territories have yet to commit to the plan.

A few days after the meeting, the Paul Martin minority Liberal government fell, and the promises outlined in the Kelowna Accord were never met.

### The Mental Health Commission of Canada (MHCC), 2007

The Standing Senate Committee (the Kirby Report) recommended the creation of a mental health commission to focus attention on mental health in Canada. The MHCC identifies issues related to mental health and makes recommendations for improvement. Such issues include addictions (e.g., drugs and alcohol) and homelessness (often homelessness goes hand in hand with addictions and other mental health issues). Support includes that for inmates with mental health issues, housing, health care, and supporting individuals with mental illness as well as their families. More recently, the focus has been on coping with the opioid crises exploding across the country, supporting addicts with harm reduction centres and rehabilitation programs.

The MHCC provides annual reports on its progress and accomplishments and identifies new strategies. The latest report is *Advancing the Mental Health Strategy for Canada: A Framework for Action (2017—2022)* (MHCC, 2016).

The consultations that took place in 2015 included individuals from across Canada with a variety of roles and backgrounds. The common denominator was an interest and investment in mental health by many stakeholders (e.g., politicians and policymakers, health care providers, caregivers, concerned individuals, the Indigenous community, and people who have interfaced with the mental health system).

Continuing priorities include developing strategies to address current mental health concerns, from dealing with the opioid crisis to providing mental health and support to the surge of refugees and **refugee claimants** who have come to Canada over the past few years (MHCC, 2016).

---

**DID YOU KNOW?**

### *Mental Health Support for New Canadians*

The mental health and well-being of refugees is a priority for the Canadian Mental Health Association (CMHA). Supporting new Canadians in need is a complex affair that must consider culture, adjusting to a new way of life, and, for many, coming to terms with previous trauma experienced (e.g., post-traumatic stress disorder [PTSD]). Communities across the country are including treatment for mental health at clinics as well as specialized centres. For example, in 2016, Woman's College Hospital in Toronto (Crossroads) collaborated with the CMHA and created a mental health and wellness program called New Beginnings. Saskatoon includes mental health assessment and treatment at its Refugee Engagement and Community Health Clinic. One resource claims that up to 80% of the women and children accepted into Canada require mental health support. Refugees are provided with basic medical health services under the Federal Interim Health Program. Provision of other types of medical services such as mental health care is left to individual provinces and territories to decide how refugees should access these services.

### The 2014 Health Accord

In 2011, the federal finance minister announced a new formula for the CHT. Under the terms of the new accord (from April 1, 2014 to March 31, 2024), the federal government would continue paying the transfer payments at 6% annually until the 2016–2017 fiscal year. After that time (and at least until 2024) the transfer dollars would be tied to the rate of the gross domestic product (GDP) and be guaranteed not to fall below 3%. In addition, under this accord, provincial and territorial CHT transfers were adjusted so that payments were to be allocated on an equal per capita *cash* basis only (excluding tax points). There were no strings attached as to how the money was spent. This accord was crafted unilaterally by the federal government—the provinces and territories had no say in the legislation, which resulted in unrest and discord and divided the provinces and territories. The hope was that if a new government was elected in 2016 that a new agreement would be negotiated. The new government was formed under Prime Minister Justin Trudeau in 2016.

### The 2017 Health Accord

The federal minister of health met with first ministers late in 2016 to initiate talks on a new Canadian Health Accord. The federal finance minister and minister of health presented a unilaterally drafted offer of a 3.5% annual increase in Canada health transfers and $11.5 billion over a 10-year time frame to be spent on mental health and home care initiatives. All jurisdictions initially rejected the offer, wanting further negotiations. Presenting a unified front, the first ministers countered, asking for an annual increase in CHT transfers of 5.2%. They also wanted the federal government to retract any conditions on how the money was spent. The federal government refused to negotiate, stating that it was a take-it-or-leave-it offer but indicated that the provinces and territories could approach the federal government and negotiate privately. Nova Scotia (receiving $287.8 million), New Brunswick (receiving $230 million), and Newfoundland and Labrador (receiving $160 million) were the first provinces to break the unified front, negotiating their own terms of agreement for a new accord (New Brunswick, Office of the Premier, 2016). Next came deals with Nunavut, Yukon, and the Northwest Territories, following with Saskatchewan, which, in addition to receiving extra funding, addressed an ongoing dispute with the ministry over Saskatchewan's policy of allowing private (for purchase) magnetic resonance imaging (MRI) examinations, which contravened the terms and conditions of the CHA. The province had to prove that this policy is not a disadvantage to the public system and had to guarantee a publicly funded MRI for each private one purchased.

British Columbia's agreement (February 2017) included receiving $1 billion for home care and mental health services, plus $10 million to put toward addressing the opioid crisis the province was facing (see Chapter 10), which at the time had not spread significantly to other jurisdictions.

In March 2017, Ontario signed a 10-year agreement worth $4.2 billion, plus additional funding for home care for $2.3 billion, and mental health initiatives of $1.9 billion (Health Canada, 2017). Alberta agreed to an agreement giving the province $10.3 billion over 10 years, with $703.2 million for home care and $586 million for mental health. Québec's agreement was completed after Ottawa agreed to recognize Québec as a distinct region, removing guidelines on how the money was to be spent (recognizing Québec as a province of "asymmetry"). Manitoba was the last province to sign the accord. The terms included a one-time payment in 2017 of $5 million to be used to help manage the province's opioid crisis as well as kidney disease, and additional support for home care programs (Dacey & Glowacki, 2017).

In all cases, additional funding received (in addition to the 3% CHT) had to be spent as per the terms of each agreement (e.g., split between home care and mental health services). In addition, all jurisdictions were free to apply for extra funding as circumstances dictate. For example, the Northwest Territories received additional funding for medical transportation and innovation.

In November 2022, the first fact-to face-to-face meeting of Federal, Provincial and Territorial Ministers of Health since in Vancouver B.C. to discuss the challenges facing the healthcare system faced by Canadians, many of which were mitigated by the COVID-19 pandemic.

Provincial and territorial health ministers continue to engage in discussions and negotiations aimed at improving and transforming Canada's problematic healthcare system. Key to their demands is a commitment from the federal government to provide all jurisdictions with increased and sustained funding (Chapter 10).

## SUMMARY

1.1   Indigenous people inhabited what became Canada for thousands of years before contact with outsiders (called the *precontact era*). They had effective health care practices and treatments. European settlers brought doctors and nurses (many of them with the military) to the country in the 1500s and 1600s and integrated some of their practices with those of Indigenous people. In the 1700s and early 1800s, volunteer organizations played a key role in the delivery of health care in Canada. The concept of public health emerged in the early 1800s, and with the passage of the *British North America Act* in 1867, federal and provincial governments shared responsibilities for health care, which, over time, became more structured and formalized. As a result, some government funding of hospitals began around this time, and the first school of nursing was established in 1873 in St. Catharines, Ontario.

1.2   In order to truly understand the history of health care in Canada as it relates to Indigenous people, it is important to understand the various terms used to reference them, the context in which these terms are used, and the concepts of "bands" and "reservations." Some terms are confusing, as they overlap; others have fallen out of favour and are no longer used unless there is a legal connotation. *Indigenous* refers to First Nations, Métis, and Inuit people. *Inuit* replaced the term *Eskimo* in the 1980s. First Nations regarded as Status Indians were assigned blocks of land called *Reserves* to live on, which came with certain rights. In terms of health care for Indigenous people, Treaty 6 was the only treaty that included a clause related to the provision of any type of health care for those bands who signed the treaty. The clause remains controversial today, as it comes nowhere near meeting the current health care needs of the population groups for whom the treaty was signed.

1.3   Indigenous peoples in Canada had a complex and effective health care system for thousands of years before the precontact era. For years, knowledge about healing ceremonies and health practices was passed down from one generation to another by healers, both orally and through hands-on experiences. Very little information was actually documented. As a result, there are few written records of these practices. Most cultural practices were rooted in holistic and spiritual ideals and beliefs, as well as an integral relationship with nature and "Mother Earth" (which is actually not a term that originated with Indigenous people). With colonization, Western medicine and knowledge soon overtook the traditional ceremonies and practices of Indigenous populations, invalidating much of their knowledge and traditional ceremonies (many of which have re-emerged and remain effective today). As colonization progressed, Indigenous people in Canada suffered greatly, particularly from the unspeakable and tragic abuses and atrocities they experienced at residential schools. Their grief has been compounded by the recent discovery of unmarked graves on the grounds of residential schools revealing the remains of many individuals, the majority appearing to be children.

1.4    In the early part of the nineteenth century, a Royal Navy physician began to suspect a connection between sanitation and infection, paving the way toward public health measures and the establishment of formal public health organizations in the provinces. Concurrently, formal educational facilities for nurses were founded. In 1873, the first school of nursing was established at Mack's General and Marine Hospital in St. Catharines, Ontario. In 1916 the Saskatchewan government passed the *Rural Municipality Act*, formally allowing municipalities to collect taxes to raise funds for retaining physicians and administering and maintaining hospitals. The road toward health insurance began with the first federal attempt to introduce a publicly funded health care system in 1919. Following World War II, governments began thinking that they had an obligation to provide Canadians with a better standard of living, including access to quality health care. Prepaid hospital care was introduced in 1948 and was well received by all jurisdictions. Shortly afterward, Saskatchewan spearheaded an organized push to integrate both medical and hospital care into the public health care system.

1.5    With the federal government committed to a comprehensive national health care system, a number of reports and pieces of legislation followed. The Hall Report, the *Medical Care Act*, and the *Established Programs and Financing Act* all played significant roles leading up to the passage of the *Canada Health Act*. In 1957, the federal government introduced the *Hospital Insurance and Diagnostic Services Act*, which was the precursor to prepaid health care for all Canadians. Prepaid health care as we know it today came into effect in 1984 with the passage of the *Canada Health Act*.

1.6    The five criteria established by the *Canada Health Act* of 1984 for the delivery of health care are public administration, comprehensive coverage, universality, portability, and accessibility. The two conditions included in the Act are information and recognition. The *Canada Health Act* specifically outlines extended health care services that are considered medically necessary and are thus insured. *Medically necessary* is a subjective term that has been debated within the context of the *Canada Health Act*; *extra billing* and *user charges* are permitted only for services deemed not medically necessary under the Act. The provinces and territories are responsible for establishing guidelines for what other services are covered (those not considered medically necessary under the *Canada Health Act*).

1.7    Opposition to the *Canada Health Act* was expressed by physicians and the Canadian Medical Association on the grounds that it restricted extra billing and user charges and violated professional freedom. In the decade that followed implementation of the Act, increasing difficulties in the health care system led some provinces and territories to establish innovative health care strategies, and primary health care reform began to take place. In 1997, the first ministers met with the federal government to work toward a social union and clarify the role of the federal government with respect to funding. By the end of 2002, three major reports on the status of health care in Canada had been commissioned and released: the Mazankowski Report, the Kirby Report, and the Romanow Report. Several first ministers' meetings over the past 15 years have resulted in the creation of new health accords.

1.8    The health accord negotiated under Prime Minister Paul Martin provided provinces and territories with a funding model lasting until 2014. Federal transfers guaranteed jurisdictions an increase of 6% per year until that time. The Harper government, in 2014, unilaterally imposed an accord that reduced the Canada Health Transfer (CHT) amount to 3% per year, or to the percentage of the GDP.

The 2017 accord negotiated (again unilaterally) by the Trudeau government kept the same formula for the CHT but offered additional funding aimed at specific services (home care and mental health). Provinces and territories initially presented a unified front, refusing the terms of this take-it-or-leave-it deal. The federal government offered to negotiate privately with each jurisdiction, and slowly, provinces and territories signed individual agreements. The provinces and territories worked together to support health care services during the COVID-19 pandemic. Initiatives are in place to address the inadequacies related to long-term care that became apparent during the pandemic. Other issues that the federal government has pledged to work with the provinces and territories on include concerns about mental health services and climate change.

## REVIEW QUESTIONS

1. What were the health care responsibilities of the federal and provincial governments outlined in the *British North America Act*?
2. What organizations attended to the health care needs of Canadians in the eighteenth and nineteenth centuries?
3. What are three traditional healing practices of Canada's Indigenous population? Briefly describe them.
4. Explain Treaty 6 and the Medicine Chest.
5. How and when was health insurance first introduced in Canada?
6. How and when was the concept of prepaid hospital care introduced in Canada?
7. List and describe three pieces of legislation that played significant roles leading up to the creation of the *Canada Health Act*.
8. What are the criteria and conditions of the *Canada Health Act* and what do they mean?
9. What is meant by the terms *medically necessary*, *extra billing*, and *user charges*, and how do they relate to each other in the context of the *Canada Health Act*?
10. What were the goals of primary care reform?
11. Why was the Indigenous population in Canada so affected by disease when non-Indigenous people came to Canada?
12. Describe two healing ceremonies important to First Nations people in Canada. Which ones are practised today?
13. How did residential schools affect the Indigenous population in Canada?
14. List and describe three major reports on the status of health care in Canada.

## REFERENCES

Alberta Health Services. (2021, September 3). *AHS postpones scheduled surgeries due to COVID-19.* https://www.albertahealthservices.ca/news/Page16174.aspx.

Alberta Regional Professional Development Consortium. (n.d.). *Conversation guide: History of First Nation Peoples in Alberta.* https://www.albertaschoolcouncils.ca/public/download/documents/57305.

Allen, L., Hatala, A., Ijaz, S., et al. (2020). Indigenous-led health care partnerships in Canada. *CMAJ : Canadian Medical Association Journal = journal de l'Association medicale canadienne, 192*(9), E208—E216. https://doi.org/10.1503/cmaj.190728.

Asselin, R. B. (2001). *The Canadian social union: Questions about the division of powers and fiscal federalism.* Library of Parliament. https://publications.gc.ca/Collection-R/LoPBdP/BP/prb0031-e.htm.

Austen, I. (2021, June 7). *How thousands of Indigenous children vanished in Canada.* New York Times. Updated March 28, 2022 https://www.nytimes.com/2021/06/07/world/canada/mass-graves-residential-schools.html.

Beal, B. (2005). Treaty 6. *Indigenous Saskatchewan Encyclopedia.* University of Regina Press. https://teaching.usask.ca/indigenoussk/import/treaty_6.php.

Bell, N. (2014). *Teaching by the medicine wheel.* https://www.edcan.ca/articles/teaching-by-the-medicine-wheel/.

Canadian Blood Services. (2022). *About Canadian Blood Services.* https://www.blood.ca/en/about-us.

Canadian Friends Service Committee. (n.d.) Truth and Reconciliation. https://quakerservice.ca/our-work/truth-and-reconciliation/.

Canadian Intergovernmental Conference Secretariat. (1999). *A framework to improve the social union for Canadians: An agreement between the Government of Canada and the governments of the provinces and territories.* https://scics.ca/en/product-produit/agreement-a-framework-to-improve-the-social-union-for-canadians/.

Canadian Museum of History. (2004). *A brief history of nursing in Canada from the establishment of New France to the present.* https://www.historymuseum.ca/cmc/exhibitions/tresors/nursing/nchis01e.shtml.

Chin, J. (2020, July 4). The chilling history of the hospital that's been abandoned for 24 years in Edmonton. *Malone Post.* https://malonepost.com/posts/abandoned-hospital-edmonton.

Crey, K. (2009). *Bands. First Nations and Indigenous Studies.* The University of British Columbia. https://indigenousfoundations.arts.ubc.ca/bands/.

Crown-Indigenous Relations and Northern Affairs Canada. (2022). *Indigenous peoples and communities.* https://rcaanc-cirnac.gc.ca/eng/1100100013785/1529102490303.

Dacey, E., & Glowacki, L. (2017). *Manitoba final province to sign health-care pact with feds.* CBC News. https://www.cbc.ca/news/canada/manitoba/funding-health-manitoba-1.4255391.

Editors of Encyclopaedia Britannica. (2022, September 16). Proclamation of 1763. *Encyclopaedia Britannica.* https://www.britannica.com/event/Proclamation-of-1763.

First Nations Studies Program, University of British Columbia. (2009). Royal Proclamation, 1763. https://indigenousfoundations.arts.ubc.ca/royal_proclamation_1763/#:~:text=The%20Royal%20Proclamation%20is%20a,won%20the%20Seven%20Years%20War

Government of Canada. (1985). *Canada Health Act.* R.S.C., 1985, c. C-6. https://laws-lois.justice.gc.ca/eng/acts/c-6/page-1.html

Government of Canada. (2005). *Annual conference of Federal—Provincial—Territorial Ministers of Health.* https://www.canada.ca/en/news/archive/2005/10/annual-federal-provincial-territorial-ministers-health-conference.html.

Hanson, E., Gamez, D., & Manuel, A. (2020). *The residential school system.* Indigenous Foundations. https://indigenousfoundations.arts.ubc.ca/residential-school-system-2020/.

Health Canada. (2003). *First ministers' accord on health care renewal.* https://www.hc-sc.gc.ca/hcs-sss/delivery-prestation/fptcollab/2003accord/nr-cp_e.html.

Health Canada. (2004). *First ministers' meeting on the future of health care 2004: A 10-year plan to strengthen health care.* https://www.canada.ca/en/health-canada/services/health-care-system/health-care-system-delivery/federal-provincial-territorial-collaboration/first-ministers-meeting-year-plan-2004/10-year-plan-strengthen-health-care.html.

Health Canada. (2017). *Canada reaches health funding agreement with Ontario* [Press release]. https://www.canada.ca/en/health-canada/news/2017/03/canada_reaches_healthfundingagreementwithontario.html

Héma-Québec. (n.d.) *Blood management in Québec.* https://www.hema-Québec.qc.ca/hema-Québec/profil/gestion-du-sang-au-Québec/index.en.html.

Indigenous Awareness Canada. (n.d.). What is a reserve? https://indigenousawarenesscanada.com/indigenous-awareness/what-is-a-reserve/.

Indigenous Services Canada. (2022a, March 24). Inuit Tapiriit Kanatami and the Government of Canada share commitment to end tuberculosis in Inuit Nunangat. https://www.canada.ca/en/indigenous-services-canada/news/2022/03/inuit-tapariit-kanatami-and-the-government-of-canada-share-commitment-to-end-tuberculosis-in-inuit-nunangat.html.

Indigenous Services Canada. (2022b). *About Indian Status.* https://www.sac-isc.gc.ca/eng/1100100032463/1572459644986.

Leung, C. (2014). *Charles Camsell Indian Hospital.* Eugenics Archive. https://eugenicsarchive.ca/discover/institutions/map/543a2cb5d2e5248e4000001a.

Library and Archives Canada. (2020, September 29). *Métis Nation.* https://www.bac-lac.gc.ca/eng/discover/aboriginal-heritage/metis/Pages/introduction.aspx.

Logan, T. E. (2020). Métis experiences at residential school. *The Canadian Encyclopedia.* https://www.thecanadianencyclopedia.ca/en/article/metis-experiences-at-residential-school.

Maskwacis Cree Foundation. (2018). *Submission of the Maskwacis Cree to the Expert Mechanism on the Rights of Indigenous Peoples Study on the right to health and Indigenous Peoples with a focus on children and youth* (pp. 6, 13, 17, 18, 20, 23). https://www.ohchr.org/sites/default/files/Documents/Issues/IPeoples/EMRIP/Health/MaskwacisCree.pdf

McCue, H. A. (2020, May 11). *Indian. The Canadian Encyclopedia.* https://www.thecanadianencyclopedia.ca/en/article/indian-term.

Mehl-Madrona, L., & Mainguy, B. (2014). Introducing healing circles and talking circles into primary care. *The Permanente Journal, 18*(2), 4–9. https://doi.org/10.7812/TPP/13-1.

Mental Health Commission of Canada (MHCC). (2016). *Advancing the mental health strategy for Canada: A framework for action (2017–2022).* https://www.mentalhealthcommission.ca/wp-content/uploads/drupal/2016-08/advancing_the_mental_health_strategy_for_canada_a_framework_for_action.pdf.

Mount Saint Vincent University. (2005). *Formal training for nurses, the beginning.* https://www.msvu.ca/library/archives/nhdp/history.htm.

New Brunswick, Office of the Premier. (2016, December 22). *Revised: Canada—New Brunswick health accord signed.* [Press release]. https://www2.gnb.ca/content/gnb/en/news/news_release.2016.12.1242.html.

Office of Indigenous Initiatives. (2019). *Terminology guide.* Queen's University. https://www.queensu.ca/indigenous/ways-knowing/terminology-guide#:~:text=Inuit%20are%20another%20Aboriginal%20group,legally%2Ddefined%20Indians%20and%20M%C3%A9tis.

Ordre des infirmieres et infirmiers du Québec. (n.d.). How to obtain a nursing permit from the Ordre des infirmieres et infirmiers du Québec. https://www.oiiq.org/sites/default/files/uploads/pdf/admission_a_la_profession/infirmiere_formee_hors_Québec/obtain_nursing_permit.pdf.

Parrott, Z. (2008). Eskimo. *The Canadian Encyclopedia.* https://www.thecanadianencyclopedia.ca/en/article/eskimo.

Patterson, L. L. (2006). *Aboriginal roundtable to Kelowna Accord: Aboriginal policy negotiations (2004–2005).* https://caid.ca/AboPolNeg2006.pdf.

St. John Ambulance Canada. (2022). *About St. John Ambulance.* https://sja.ca/en/about-us/st-john-ambulance.

Tiedemann, M. (2019). *The Canada Health Act: An overview.* Library of Parliament Research Publications. https://lop.parl.ca/sites/PublicWebsite/default/en_CA/ResearchPublications/201954E?#a2-2.

Tommy Douglas Research Institute. (n.d.). About the Tommy Douglas Institute. https://www.georgebrown.ca/about-the-tommy-douglas-institute.

TRCtalk (a). (n.d.). Call to Action #18. http://courseware.acadiau.ca/trctalk/call-to-action-18/.

TRCtalk (b). (n.d.). Call to Action #22. http://courseware.acadiau.ca/trctalk/call-to-action-22/.

Truth and Reconciliation Commission of Canada. (2015a). *Canada's Residential Schools: The Inuit and Northern Experience. The Final Report of the Truth and Reconciliation Commission of Canada, Volume 2.* McGill-Queen's University Press.

Truth and Reconciliation Commission of Canada. (2015b). *Truth and Reconciliation Commission of Canada: Calls to action.* https://www2.gov.bc.ca/assets/gov/british-columbians-our-governments/indigenous-people/aboriginal-peoples-documents/calls_to_action_english2.pdf.

Union of Ontario Indians. (2013). *An overview of the Indian residential school system.* https://www.anishinabek.ca/wp-content/uploads/2016/07/An-Overview-of-the-IRS-System-Booklet.pdf.

Until the Last Child. (2014). *The history of child welfare in Canada.* https://www.untilthelastchild.com/the-history-of-child-welfare-in-canada/.

Wilson, K., & Hodgson, C. (2018). *Pulling together: Foundations guide.* BCcampus. https://opentextbc.ca/indigenizationfoundations/.

# 2

# The Role of the Federal Government in Health Care

## LEARNING OUTCOMES

2.1 Explain the objectives and responsibilities of Health Canada.
2.2 Discuss the health care that the federal government provides for Indigenous people.
2.3 Explain the organizational structure of Health Canada.
2.4 Describe the agencies within Canada's health portfolio.
2.5 Discuss the internal organization that Health Canada collaborates with.
2.6 Summarize Canada's response protocol to infectious diseases.

## KEY TERMS

| | | |
|---|---|---|
| Branch | Indigenous people | Patented medicines |
| Bureau | Inuit | Severe acute respiratory |
| Hypoglycemic reaction | Pandemic | syndrome (SARS) |

Canada's health portfolio consists of a number of agencies and organizations that are headed by the Minister of Health and the Minister of Mental Health and Addictions (who also serves as the Associate Minister of Health). The health portfolio itself is comprised of Health Canada, the Public Health Agency of Canada (PHAC), The Canadian Institute of Health Research (CIHR), the Patented Medicine Prices Review Board, and the Canadian Food Inspection Agency (Health Canada, 2017). Collectively, the health portfolio operates on an annual budget in excess of $3.8 billion and employs about 12,000 people.

The federal government, working collaboratively with federal and nongovernment agencies, Indigenous partners, and other stakeholders, has designated responsibilities in areas that both directly and indirectly impact the health and health care of Canadians.

That said, the federal government has little or no power over decisions made regarding the day-to-day management of health care services affecting most Canadians, and no legal power over the health care delivered in provincial and territorial jurisdictions. The provinces and territories fiercely guard their authority over health care in their individual relationships with the federal government. On the other hand, the provinces and territories want and need federal financial support, which comes with stipulations, most of which are grounded in the *Canada Health Act* as discussed in Chapter 1.

This chapter examines the structure and function of the various organizations that make up Canada's health portfolio, as well as some of the responsibilities Health Canada has as a care provider to **Indigenous people** in Canada. Included here is discussion of Health Canada's mission statement, philosophy, and commitment to health care in Canada. These pledges provide the foundation on which the ministry was built and the values with which it strives to function. Despite the best of intentions, many issues are not addressed effectively and consistently, and problems with the Canadian health care system persist. Some of these vulnerabilities have become more apparent since the onset of the COVID-19 **pandemic**, not the least of which is an acute shortage of human health resources, including doctors and nurses, impacting patient care units in hospitals and emergency departments (EDs; resulting in long wait-times and even the temporary closure of EDs in some regions).

## HEALTH CANADA: OBJECTIVES, RESPONSIBILITIES, AND LEADERSHIP

Health Canada's detailed mission statement includes information about its purpose, values, and activities. Health Canada's website describes this federal institution as "responsible for helping Canadians maintain and improve their health, ensuring that high-quality health services are accessible, and work[ing] to reduce health risks" (Health Canada, 2022a).

With a mandate to provide national leadership for health care and to maximize health promotion and disease prevention strategies, Health Canada is committed to collaborating with the provinces, territories, and Indigenous partners on joint ventures, such as creating policies and financing projects. Health Canada also oversees the transfer of money and tax points to the provinces and territories for health, education, and social programs. The 2017 Health Accord saw the majority of jurisdictions negotiating their own agreements with the federal government for health care funding. Health Canada plays an authoritarian role, ensuring the provinces and territories remain compliant with the *Canada Health Act* and enforcing penalties on those that function outside of the principles within the Act. It is through its control over transfer payments for health care funding that the federal government exerts most of its influence, sometimes referred to as "spending power."

As a care provider, Health Canada is responsible for the health care for the armed forces, veterans, and correctional services; it covers the cost of health services to Royal Canadian Mounted Police (RCMP) members when they have work-related trauma and injuries to their physical or mental health. In 2012, the federal government passed responsibility for all other aspects of the RCMP to the province or territory in which the individuals reside. Care for Indigenous people in Canada is coordinated with Indigenous Services Canada, which is discussed below.

Working with the Interim Federal Health Program (IFHP), Health Canada authorizes temporary basic health care coverage for protected persons, refugee claimants, and resettled refugees who do not qualify for provincial or territorial coverage (Box 2.1). As a result of the war in Ukraine, Canada has temporarily resettled a number of Ukrainians through a newly created pathway called the Canada-Ukraine Authorization for Emergency Travel. In addition, Ukrainians currently in Canada on visitor permits can apply to have their permits extended. Health coverage extended to Ukrainians coming to Canada under this plan varies somewhat with jurisdictions, but individuals must apply for this coverage in the jurisdiction in which they intend to settle. Newfoundland and Labrador, for example, will provide coverage for medical and mental health services as well as coverage for prescription medications. Similar coverage is offered in Ontario and British Columbia upon refugees' arrival (Government of British Columbia, 2022). Many Canadian citizens have opened their homes to welcome Ukrainians and give them the help they need to get settled in Canada.

As a primary source of information for Canadians, Health Canada conducts research projects and provides feedback on policy development. The ministry interacts with equivalent organizations in other nations and with the World Health Organization (WHO) to keep Canadians up to date on health concerns around the world. Health Canada issues travel alerts and warnings for areas where health issues are cause for concern. The ministry collaborates with the PHAC to produce and implement national campaigns for health promotion and disease prevention, such as vaccination, active lifestyle, and anti-smoking campaigns.

### BOX 2.1   Refugee Claimants

The Interim Federal Health Program (IFHP) authorizes (temporary) basic health care coverage for protected persons, refugee claimants, and resettled refugees who do not qualify for provincial or territorial coverage. This supplemental coverage includes limited vision and dental care and medication benefits. Syrian refugees resettled in Canada as part of Operation Syrian Refugees had immediate health coverage and were given resident status upon arrival. In 2021, through a program called the Afghan Resettlement Program, Canada began accepting and resettling Afghan nationals and, in some cases, their families, who had assisted Canadians during the war in Afghanistan. Canada came under heavy criticism because of the inaction in getting Afghan nationals and their families out of the country in the days prior to the withdrawal of the troops and take-over of the country by the Taliban. At the time, Canada pledged to accept 40,000 refugees, but the uptake has been slow, something else for which the federal government has been criticized, leaving thousands of Afghan nationals languishing in their country, fearing for their lives (Immigration, Refugees, and Citizenship Canada, 2022; Walker, 2022).

## Leadership

Health Canada is headed by the Minister of Health and the Ministers of Mental Health and Addictions, appointed by the Prime Minister of Canada (both of whom are elected representatives). These are positions that the prime minister can reassign at any time during the tenure of the party in power. The Minister of Health is responsible for maintaining and improving the health of Canadians, including overseeing more than 20 health-related laws and associated regulations. The federal Minister of Health is responsible for the health portfolio, with the exception of the responsibilities assigned to the Minister of Mental Health and Addictions (Health Canada, 2022a). On occasion, the federal Minister of Health may also be responsible for other portfolios (Nazir & Taha, 2018).

Responsibilities of the Minister of Health include the following:

- Overseeing Health Canada and other agencies within the health portfolio
- Collection and analysis of information carried out under the *Statistics Act*
- Working collaboratively with the provincial and territorial governments

The federal Minister of Health does not routinely become involved in internal matters within the provinces or territories. However, establishing a positive working relationship with the first ministers (i.e., the provincial and territorial ministry heads) and Indigenous leaders is essential for improving Canada's health care system across the country.

The Deputy Minister of Health is an appointed position from the civil service. The Deputy Minister of Health works with the Minister of Health, manages designated operations within the ministry, and may assume duties assigned to the Minister of Health if the minister is temporarily unavailable. Several assistant deputy ministers of health are also appointed from the civil service.

Other agencies, such as the Departmental Secretariat and Chief Public Health Officer, work with the Minister of Health, Deputy Minister of Health, and Associate Deputy Minister of Health. Their primary focus is to provide leadership to the PHAC, whose principal mandate is to manage health promotion and health safety initiatives. This mandate has never been more evident than during the COVID-19 pandemic as the PHAC collaborates with provincial and territorial public health agencies as well as international partners to monitor the status of COVID-19, activate and continuously evaluate safety measures and the management of existing and emerging vaccinations, testing capacity of provinces/territories, and ongoing surveillance of new variants, such as the BA5, thought to be responsible for what was referred to as the seventh pandemic wave in some jurisdictions across Canada in the summer of 2022.

## HEALTH CARE AND INDIGENOUS PEOPLE

Jurisdictional oversight with respect to providing and paying for health care for Indigenous people in Canada is a mosaic. It is often difficult to sort out who is eligible for what services, who provides those services, what those services include, and who pays for them.

The federal, provincial, and territorial governments share certain elements of health care for Indigenous people. For example, there are three similar versions of the federal government's non-insured health plan (NIHP), the dominant plan providing non-insured benefits to certain First Nations and **Inuit** beneficiaries. Indigenous Services Canada's non-insured health benefits are meant for those who are part of Nunavut land claim agreements and the Inuvialuit agreements; the Nunatsiavut government's Non-Insured Health Benefits Program is available to beneficiaries of the Labrador Inuit Land Claim Agreement; and the Nunavik Board of Health and Social Services Insured/Non-Insured Health Benefits Program is available to those who are part of the James Bay and Northern Québec Agreement.

Discussion of the health care services presented below is general in nature and does not address every piece of legislation or organization that provides support and health care services to Indigenous people in Canada.

### Crown-Indigenous Relations and Northern Affairs Canada and Indigenous Services Canada

In 2017, Indigenous and Northern Affairs Canada was dissolved and replaced by two new departments, Crown-Indigenous Relations and Northern Affairs Canada and Indigenous Services Canada, effective June 2019 (Government of Canada, 2022a; Indigenous Services Canada, 2017). Box 2.2 summarizes the division of responsibilities between these two organizations.

---

**BOX 2.2   Division of Responsibilities Between Crown-Indigenous Relations and Northern Affairs Canada and Indigenous Services Canada**

| Crown-Indigenous Relations and Northern Affairs Canada | Indigenous Services Canada |
|---|---|
| Indigenous peoples and communities | Indian Status and status cards |
| Treaties and agreements | Indigenous health |
| Northern Affairs and new Arctic and Northern Policy Framework | Jordan's Principle |
| | Education |
| Recognition of Indigenous rights and self-determination discussions | Water in First Nations communities |
| | First Nations housing |
| New permanent bilateral mechanisms | First Nations community infrastructure |
| Delivering on Truth and Reconciliation Commission calls to action | Social programs |
| | Establishing a new fiscal relationship |
| Residential schools | Emergency management |
| Reconciliation National Inquiry into Missing and Murdered Indigenous Women and Girls | |

Based on Government of Canada. (2022). *Indigenous Services Canada.* https://www.canada.ca/en/indigenous-services-canada.html

Crown-Indigenous Relations and Northern Affairs Canada was established to preserve, promote, and renew relationships across all levels of government and between the federal government and First Nations, Inuit, and Métis peoples.

Indigenous Services Canada (ISC) oversees the delivery of (federally funded) selected health services not covered by provinces or territories to First Nations people living on reserves (Status Indians) and to Inuit communities. In addition, ISC provides Indigenous people with information and resources that are available on the department's government website. This includes current information on Indigenous health, social programs, education, water quality in First Nations communities, non-insured First Nations benefits, and housing.

Health services provided include primary care, health promotion and disease prevention programs, and health education, as well as substance use, mental health, and child development programs. Supplementary benefits, such as dental and vision care, medication coverage, and crisis intervention, are available to those eligible through the Non-Insured Health Benefits (NIHB) program.

ISC also funds or directly provides services for First Nations and Inuit people that supplement those provided by provinces and territories, including primary health care, health promotion, and supplementary health benefits.

It is worth noting that several provinces have partnered with the federal government to facilitate Indigenous autonomy over health care (Indigenous Services Canada, 2021). One of the first was the British Columbia Tripartite Framework, an agreement framework creating a provincewide First Nations Health Authority. This gave First Nations the authority to design, manage, and deliver health care programs to First Nations people in British Columbia (Indigenous Services Canada, 2021). Among its many initiatives, the Authority established the Health Promotion and Prevention Healthy Living Unit supporting First Nations people in the region. In addition to health promotion and disease prevention strategies, the Authority provides ongoing culturally appropriate training for health and parahealth professionals. E-health programs that the Authority has invested in use various electronic technologies such as electronic health records, telehealth capabilities, and Panorama, a software application used nationwide to connect the First Nations Health Authority (FNHA) to other health organizations sharing information and promoting public health initiatives. The FNHA functions under unique governance and accountability guidelines and acts as a resource for Indigenous communities across Canada who want control over their own health care (First Nations Health Authority, 2022).

The long-term goal is to have First Nations and Inuit administer designated funds such that they have autonomy over the design and delivery of their own health care services. The reality is that there is a long way to go to ensure that all Indigenous communities have equitable health care no matter where they live (Blackstock, 2008).

The provision of adequate health care and addressing the glaring inequities in health care (especially in remote communities) remain a challenge. The system is complex, sometimes with jurisdictional disputes over what governmental department or even what government is responsible for paying for selected health services. This can result in disruption, denial, or a delay of services required.

## DID YOU KNOW?

### *Jordan's Principle*

Jordan River Anderson was a little boy from Norway House Cree Nation, who, upon discharge from hospital, required specialized at-home care for a muscular disorder. The government of Manitoba and the federal government argued over who should pay for

Jordan's at-home care for over 2 years, during which time Jordan had to remain in the hospital. Jordan died before he ever returned to his home. He was 5 years old.

Following this tragedy, *Jordan's Principle* was implemented as the result of a private member's bill, which was unanimously passed by parliament in 2007.

If the family of a First Nations child feel they are not receiving the health care services or supplies that child needs, they must contact regional authorities and make a request under Jordan's Principle.

Jordan's Principle initially stated that if there is a disagreement between two governments (e.g., provinces, territories, federal government) or two departments within a government about who should pay for services needed by a Status Indian child—and that service is available to non-Indigenous children in Canada—the government or government department first contacted must pay for those services. That government or government department can subsequently seek reimbursement according to jurisdictional protocol, to ensure that the needs of the child are met without undue delay.

Applications of this principle in the last decade have been controversial, with some cases going to the Human Rights Tribunal. In 2017, the Canadian Human Rights Tribunal issued a ruling that included an expanded and amended definition of Jordan's Principle (Indigenous Services Canada, 2018):

* First Nations children qualify regardless of place of residence—on or off a reserve (the original bill stated the child must be a Status Indian).
* Jordan's Principle is not limited to children with disabilities.
* The services required must be provided and paid for by the department/organization first contacted, *without* conferencing or review of policies or other administrative procedures, to avoid delays in implementing a requested service.
* If a service requested is outside of the standard parameters of services for other children, the department contacted must complete an assessment to ensure that equal culturally appropriate services are provided to that child.

Jordan's Principle may still apply in some situations not involving jurisdictional or interdepartmental payment/service provision disputes. See Box 2.3 for a summary of expanded services under Jordan's Principle.

Source: Assembly of First Nations. (2021, September 29). *The Federal Court of Canada upholds the CHRT's ruling in full*. https://www.afn.ca/the-federal-court-of-canada-upholds-the-chrts-ruling-in-full/

---

**BOX 2.3   Summary of Expanded Services Under Jordan's Principle**

| Health | Social | Education |
|---|---|---|
| Mobility and related equipment | Social worker | School supplies |
| Services from elders | Land-based activities | Tutoring services |
| Assessments and screenings | Respite care (individual or group) | Teaching assistants |
| Medical supplies and equipment | Specialized programs based on cultural beliefs and practices | Psychoeducational assessments |
| Mental health services | Personal support worker | Assistive technology and electronics |

Source: Indigenous Services Canada. (2019, November 21). *Jordan's Principle: Substantive equality principles*. https://www.sac-isc.gc.ca/eng/1583698429175/1583698455266

In addition, systemic racism, which appears to be present throughout the health care system, imposes further inequities in terms of the quality of health care that Indigenous people sometimes receive, compounded by discrimination, an apparent lack of respect, and the abandonment of the duty of care. This situation is illustrated by the death of Joyce Echaquan in September 2020 and the disturbing events leading to her demise. Details of her experience are discussed in Chapter 9. On February 10, 2021, Indigenous Services Canada promised $2 million to Joyce Echaquan's community to advance their work and advocacy for the implementation of Joyce's Principle, a concept that emerged as a result of her death (Box 2.4). The money will also be used for other purposes, including to promote Joyce's Principle to health professionals and to educate Indigenous people about their rights when interfacing with the health care system.

## Métis and Health Care

The Métis population in Canada challenged the federal government in 1982 to gain recognition as a distinct people under the *Indian Act* and therefore have the same rights as "Indians" and the Inuit. Métis communities also wanted to be eligible to receive health care benefits similar to those available to some First Nations. Despite the April 2016 ruling that the federal government had a constitutional responsibility for both Métis and non-Status Indians, little has happened in practical terms of providing health care benefits to either of these population groups (Box 2.5). Some jurisdictions do offer supplementary health benefits to the Métis population living in that province or territory.

---

### BOX 2.4   Joyce's Principal

The intent of Joyce's Principal is to provide guidance that will guarantee Indigenous people equitable access to both social and health services, as well as the right to the "best possible physical, mental, and emotional health."

Source: Indigenous Services Canada. (2021, February 10). *Government of Canada provides $2 million to the Conseil des Atikamekw de Manawan and the Conseil de la Nation Atikamekw for the development of Joyce's Principle*. News Release. https://www.canada.ca/en/indigenous-services-canada/news/2021/02/government-of-canada-provides-2-million-to-the-conseil-des-atikamekw-de-manawan-and-the-conseil-de-la-nation-atikamekw-for-the-development-of-joyce.html

---

### BOX 2.5   Daniels Decision

Daniels Decision describes the outcome of a case that went to the Supreme Court of Canada (*Daniels v. Canada*) regarding the federal government's responsibilities for Métis people and non-Status Indians. On April 14, 2016, after 17 years of jurisdictional wrangling, the Supreme Court ruled that the federal government has a constitutional responsibility for Métis people and non-Status Indians, a decision viewed as a victory for all Indigenous peoples in Canada. This includes an obligation to provide equal access to health care, education, and hunting rights as well as the same programs and services, including non-insured health benefits (NIHB), to Métis people and non-Status Indians living in Canada. Despite the ruling, health coverage for the Métis and non-Status Indians remains fractured.

Much of the federal funding for Métis people is distributed through the Métis National Council, to which some otherwise eligible groups do not belong.

Sources: Congress of Aboriginal Peoples. *Daniels Decision: Daniels v. Canada, a historic Supreme Court ruling*. https://www.abo-peoples.org/en/daniels-decision/; Supreme Court of Canada, *Daniels v. Canada*. 2016 SCC 12, [2016] 1 SCR 99. Case number 35945. https://scc-csc.lexum.com/scc-csc/scc-csc/en/item/15858/index.do

The Health and Wellness Branch of the Métis Nation in Ontario offers programs and health services embracing traditional values and beliefs. They also offer webinars on health and wellness and on mental health, addiction, and gambling awareness (Métis Nation of Ontario, 2022). The Northwest Territory has the Métis Health Benefits Program, paid for by territorial taxes and overseen by Alberta Blue Cross. Benefits closely resemble those offered by the federal government (Saskatchewan Health Authority, 2022). To be eligible, the person must be a self-identified Métis and sign a declaration that they are not registered anywhere as a Status Indian. In addition, the individual must present a letter indicating that they are a member of an Indigenous government or Indigenous organization whose members have (or claim) that they have Indigenous rights in the Northwest Territories affirmed by Section 35 of the *Constitution Act*. Alberta partners with Indigenous people and communities by implementing a program called Indigenous Wellness Core, which provides health benefits for First Nations, Inuit, and Métis people (Government of Northwest Territories, 2021).

Saskatchewan offers a range of health and culturally sensitive services and programs, including the Randall Kinship Centre, Four Directions Community Health Centre in Regina, and Native Counselling services. In addition, the Saskatchewan Métis and Health Services offers a variety of support to Indigenous people navigating the health care system, including connection to elders and others who can facilitate traditional, culturally sensitive support and access to traditional ceremonies (Saskatchewan Health Authority, 2014). Saskatchewan does not offer Métis benefits as such outside of those funded through the federal government.

### The Human Rights Tribunal and Compensation for Indigenous Children and Jordan's Principle

In 2007, a complaint was filed with the Human Rights Tribunal by the First Nations Child and Family Caring Society and the Assembly of First Nations against the federal government claiming that child welfare services provided to First Nations children and families on-reserves did not meet the same standards of care as those received by other children and that they were clearly discriminatory. The Human Rights Tribunal started hearing evidence in 2013 and handed down its decision in January 2016. The tribunal ruled that the federal government had, in fact, discriminated against First Nations children and that the care provided for First Nations on reserves was inadequate, as claimed.

A 2019 tribunal ruling ordered the federal government to pay $40,000 to each eligible person (First Nations Child and Family Caring Society of Canada, 2016). Those eligible to receive compensation included the children's primary guardian (parents, grandparents, or their primary care giver). The federal government challenged this decision. On September 29, 2021, the Supreme Court of Canada upheld the 2019 decision.

The Supreme Court also agreed with the Canadian Human Rights Tribunal that all First Nations children should be eligible for services offered under Jordan's Principle, regardless of their status under the *Indian Act* or where they lived. In addition, a section of the ruling stated that children who did not receive required public services or who experienced a delay in receiving these services (under Jordan's Principle) were also eligible for compensation. This includes the time frame from December 12, 2007—when Jordan's Principle was initially adopted by the House of Commons—to November 2, 2017, when the tribunal ordered Canada to make changes to Jordan's Principle and review some requests that were made previously. Compensation was also extended to children who did not receive an essential public service or faced delays in accessing such services between April 1, 1991 and December 11, 2007.

In January 2022, the federal government and First Nations leaders finally negotiated an agreement-in-principle wherein the government agreed to provide financial compensation to eligible First Nations people. The settlement was for $40 billion, $20 billion of which would be used to reform the children's welfare system, distributed over 5 years (Stefanovich & Boisvert, 2022). The final agreement was signed in July 2022. The final agreement was signed in July 2022. However, in October 2022, a human rights tribunal ruling rejected the historic agreement, claiming that it left some children out and did not guarantee a $40,000 payment for each eligible child and caregiver. This added controversy to the final settlement and the proposed distribution of these funds in 2023. This development complicates the settlement issue.

### Services Provided for Indigenous People in Canada

All Indigenous people, as residents of a province or territory and no matter where they live in Canada or what their legal status is under the *Indian Act*, are eligible for the same health care services as non-Indigenous people—as laid out under the Canadian Constitution and the *Canada Health Act*. Indigenous Services Canada also funds and provides services and designated programs in First Nations and Inuit communities (Indigenous Services Canada, 2021). These benefits are similar to those available to people who have health care coverage through their employer.

Health Canada and the PHAC provide funds for specific services for Indigenous people living in urban settings or in rural and northern settings. There are grants and other monetary contributions available to promote health and to control chronic and infectious diseases and injury.

### Non-insured Health Benefits

Indigenous Services Canada provides non-insured health benefits (NIHB) to eligible First Nations (Status Indians) as well as some Inuit who are registered with and recognized by one of four Inuit land claim organizations (Indigenous Services Canada, 2022). These include regions of Inuvialuit (Northwest Territories and Yukon), Nunavik (in Northern Québec), Nunatsiavut (Labrador) and Nunavut. Box 2.6 provides an overview of NIHBs.

Many jurisdictions are working with Indigenous populations toward establishing health care delivery models that reflect the culture, traditional practices, and needs of individual communities. In some jurisdictions, Indigenous communities have assumed authority for the delivery of health care, including provisions for traditional health care within the structure of provincial and territorial health care systems. Manitoba, Ontario, Prince Edward Island, and Yukon, for example, allow traditional midwives to practice, with exceptions from controls specified under the codes of related regulated health professionals. Ontario has expanded this exemption to include Indigenous traditional healers. In 2019, a tripartite Memorandum of Understanding was signed by the First Nations of Québec and Labrador Health and Social Services Commission, Canada and Québec that committed the partners to work toward a new health and social services governance model.

## DIVISIONS OF HEALTH CANADA

The organizational makeup of Health Canada is complex and sometimes confusing. Although the structure of Health Canada changes frequently (as does the appearance, content, and organization of the Health Canada website), the overall function and responsibilities of each division remain relatively consistent. The role that Health Canada plays in the delivery of health care is largely dependent on its organizational structure and collaborative links with Canada's health portfolio (Fig. 2.1).

### Branches, Offices, and Directorates

The framework itself includes a large number of **branches** and agencies, each with numerous divisions. Some, such as the Departmental Secretariat, oversee the financing, function, and organization of Health Canada. Other divisions are more directly aligned with public initiatives and health care. A selection of these divisions is discussed in this chapter.

## BOX 2.6   Non-Insured Health Benefits: A Brief Overview*

| Benefit | Examples of Benefits |
| --- | --- |
| Medications | Medications supplied are similar to those with other public plans, with exceptions such as some narcotics, cough medicine with codeine, hair growth stimulants, and those available with an independent submission form. |
| Vision | Most routine services, including a person's first pair of glasses (with restrictions on frames and lenses) |
| Dental | Routine dental care, including procedures such as root canals, braces; a predetermination of procedures is necessary |
| Medical Travel | Land, water, air (commercial or charter), land/air ambulance; includes meals/accommodation; may include cost coverage for an escort depending on circumstances; amount paid and for how long varies with region and medical circumstances. See Case Example 2.1. |
| Mental Health | Short-term crisis intervention and counselling and addiction services are provided by NIHB only when no other mental health services are available. These services in the Northwest Territories and Nunavut are covered by the territorial government, not NIHB. Counselling is available for residential school survivors, children, and grandchildren through the Indian Residential Schools Resolution Health Support Program. |

*Note: These examples are not all-inclusive; in addition, exceptions and conditions apply to most benefits.
Source: Based on Indigenous Services Canada. (2021). *Indian Residential Schools Resolution Health Support Program.* https://www.sac-isc.gc.ca/eng/1581971225188/1581971250953

## CASE EXAMPLE 2.1   Travel: Medical Care for W.A.

E.A.'s little brother W.A., age 6, required surgery. His mother was unable to accompany him, so E.A. went as his escort. They were booked on a scheduled flight from their home in Rankin Inlet to Ottawa. W.A. had surgery and was in hospital for 4 days. E.A. stayed in a designated hotel during this time. After W.A. was discharged from hospital, he needed to stay in the city for another week for follow-up, and he stayed with E.A. at the hotel. Accommodations, meals, and travel expenses were covered by the federal government.

### Office of Audit and Evaluation

The Office of Audit and Evaluation is Health Canada's independent internal monitoring system. The Office conducts internal audits and reports to the Deputy Minister of Health. The Office reviews different departments and **bureaus** to ensure that they are operating properly, in accordance with their mandate, and in a cost-effective manner. Working with provinces and territories, the Office of Audit and Evaluation also ensures that government grants are used as intended.

### Chief Financial Officer Branch

The Chief Financial Officer Branch (CFOB) oversees the use of Health Canada's departmental resources and ensures finances are spent efficiently. The Branch also ensures that the

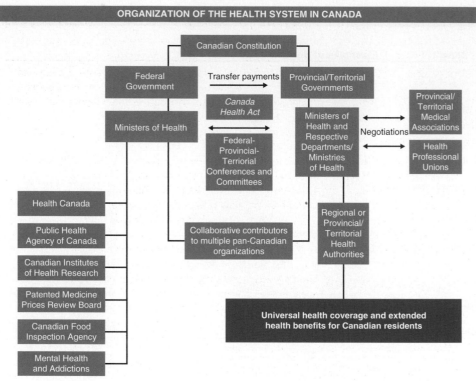

**Fig. 2.1** Organizational chart for Canada's health portfolio. (Source: Adapted from Tikkanen, R. Osborn, R., Mossialos, E., et al. (2020). *International health care system profiles: Canada*. https://www.commonwealthfund.org/international-health-policy-center/countries/canada#:~:text=Canada%20has%20a%20decen tralized%2C%20universal,on%20a%20per%2Dcapita%20basis)

organizational units adhere to government policies and regulations; coordinates risk management; enhances performance measurement and reporting; and monitors the execution of the accountability framework. The CFOB also oversees the financial management of central agencies, including the PHAC.

### Corporate Services Branch

The Corporate Services Branch provides support and services to Health Canada in human resources management, occupational health and safety, emergency and security management, access to information and privacy matters, and information technology.

### Departmental Secretariat

The Departmental Secretariat acts as the link between the executive (appointed) and the political (elected) levels of Health Canada. This executive office clarifies, redirects, or responds to communications from all divisions of Health Canada addressing requests, for example, that fall under the *Access to Information Act* and the *Privacy Act*.

### Healthy Environments and Consumer Safety Branch

The Healthy Environments and Consumer Safety Branch (HECSB) promotes safe and healthy living, work, and recreational environments for Canadians. The HECSB provides information about the safety of various products—for example, toys, smoke detectors, cosmetics, and lifestyle habits—with the goal of helping Canadians make constructive choices (e.g., an active lifestyle, healthy nutritional habits, and avoidance of risky behaviours such as tobacco, drug, and alcohol use). The HECSB is also concerned with and about environmental hazards, such as noise, and contaminants that affect drinking water and air quality indices. The Safety Environment Directorate falls under this branch and collaborates with the federal government in the development of water, air, and climate change initiatives and policies at the national level.

### Natural and Non-prescription Health Products Directorate (NNHPD)

The Natural and Non-prescription Health Products Directorate (NNHPD) evaluates the safety and effectiveness of such products as prescription and non-prescription medications, natural food products, and veterinary drugs before they are introduced to the market. The Health Products and Food Branch also provides information about these products so that Canadians can make their own choices about using and consuming them, in keeping with their individual health and lifestyle philosophies. The following are just some of the offices and directorates that are under the authority of the Health Products and Food Branch (Health Canada, 2022b).

---

**THINKING IT THROUGH**

### *Hand Sanitizer*

During the COVID-19 outbreak, there was initially a high demand for hand and surface sanitizers and not enough product available. In response, Health Canada authorized the temporary use of technical-grade ethanol in alcohol-based sanitizers. Technical-grade ethanol contains impurities not found in pharmaceutical- and food-grade ethanol and is associated with some health hazards, including skin irritation and rashes. The products were introduced to the market on April 15, 2020 and withdrawn in August of the same year. Warnings on the bottles of hand sanitizer included "Adults only, do not use on broken skin or if you are pregnant or breast-feeding" as well as directions to report any adverse reactions to Health Canada.

1. Were you aware of the fact that products containing technical-grade ethanol alcohol were on the market? Have you been reading warnings on bottles of sanitizer? Why or why not?
2. How might Health Canada have made this information more available to the general public?
3. Do you think Health Canada responded appropriately to the shortage of hand sanitizer? Explain your answer.

Sources: Public Health Association of British Columbia. (2020, August 6). *Recall of certain hand sanitizers that contain technical-grade ethanol.* https://phabc.org/recall-of-certain-hand-sanitizers-that-contain-technical-grade-ethanol/; Health Canada. (2022, January 18). *Manufacturers of hand sanitizers and hard-surface disinfectants using technical-grade-ethanol.* https://www.canada.ca/en/health-canada/services/drugs-health-products/natural-non-prescription/legislation-guidelines/covid19-technical-grade-ethanol-hand-sanitizer/manufacturers.html

---

***Biologic and Radiopharmaceutical Drugs Directorate.*** The Biologic and Radiopharmaceutical Drugs Directorate controls the introduction and use of biologic drugs, which are made from plants, microorganisms, or animals, and include vaccines. Sometimes called bio-pharmaceuticals, these medications can be used to treat conditions such as Crohn's disease, ulcerative colitis, multiple sclerosis, rheumatoid arthritis, and diabetes. The directorate also oversees the use of drugs that have radioactive properties—most commonly used to treat cancers. Radioactive materials are also used in some diagnostic tests. This directorate indirectly controls blood and blood products. It also oversees regulations on the use of human tissues and cells, as well as organs for transplants.

***Therapeutic Products Directorate.*** The Therapeutic Products Directorate is responsible for assessing the safety, benefits, and risks of therapeutic medications before they are released for sale in Canada. This is where scientists assess the quality and legitimacy of clinical trials for medications, along with evidence-informed assessments regarding the efficacy and quality of a prescription medication. Physicians apply to this directorate for permission to prescribe medications not on the market when existing therapies have failed (e.g., experimental medications).

For patients with serious, possibly life-threatening health conditions, physicians may seek access to medications that are unavailable in Canada through the Special Access Program (SAP). Access to these medications, if granted, would be on compassionate grounds or in emergency situations after conventional treatments have proven ineffective or are otherwise unavailable.

## DID YOU KNOW?

### *Requests for Drugs for Compassionate Reasons*

The Special Access Program (SAP) is a pathway facilitating physician access to medications that are unavailable for sale in Canada. Physicians may request access for medications for patients with serious or life-threatening conditions on a compassionate or emergency basis and for whom conventional therapies have either failed or are unsuitable. These medications are used for such conditions as blood dyscrasias, autoimmune disorders, and cancer. SAP may also be asked to respond to the need for specific medications during a regional or national health crisis, such as during the COVID-19 pandemic.

Sources: Health Canada. (2022, May 30). *Health Canada's Special Access Programs: Request a drug.* https://www.canada.ca/en/health-canada/services/drugs-health-products/special-access/drugs.html; Health Canada (2005, August 15). *Special Access Programme—Drugs.* https://www.canada.ca/en/health-canada/services/drugs-health-products/special-access/drugs/special-access-programme-drugs.html

## BOX 2.7    The First Ever Food Guide for First Nations, Inuit, and Métis

In April 2007, the first ever national food guide for First Nations, Inuit, and Métis populations, *Eating Well With Canada's Food Guide—First Nations, Inuit and Métis*, was launched in Yellowknife.

Previous versions of the Guide had been tailored to specific regions across Canada, supporting local traditions and food availability. This was the first guide to reflect the needs of Indigenous peoples at a national level. The general guidelines and principles are the same as for everyone, but this guide addresses cultural differences and traditional food choices; for example, bannock as a grain product and traditional meats and wild game. "Snapshots" or short versions of the *Canada's Food Guide* are also produced in a number of Indigenous languages.

See https://www.canada.ca/en/health-canada/services/canada-food-guide/resources/snapshot/languages.html for an interactive *Food Guide* in multiple languages.
Sources: CDA Oasis (2019, February 7). *What's different about Canada's new food guide?* https://oasisdiscussions.ca/2019/02/07/eat-well-live-well-whats-different-about-in-canadas-new-food-guide/; Health Canada. (2019). *Eating well with Canada's food guide—First Nations, Inuit and Métis.* https://www.canada.ca/en/health-canada/services/food-nutrition/reports-publications/eating-well-canada-food-guide-first-nations-inuit-metis.html

***Office of Nutrition Policy and Promotion.*** The Office of Nutrition Policy and Promotion promotes and supports healthy eating through evidence-informed nutrition and dietary guidelines, such as *Canada's Food Guide.* In 2019, the federal government updated *Canada's Food Guide* to encourage Canadians to eat more plant-based protein; replace fruit juices and sugary beverages with water; eat more fruits, vegetables, grains, and legumes; and cook and enjoy meals with family and friends in the home (Health Canada, 2019). (See also Box 2.7 about the first *Food Guide* for First Nations, Inuit, and Métis). The *Food Guide for Indigenous People* was also updated and is available in numerous languages.

***Natural and Non-prescription Health Products Directorate.*** The Natural and Non-prescription Health Products Directorate authorizes which health products containing natural ingredients and which non-prescription medications can be sold in Canada. The health products the directorate regulates include homeopathic medicines, vitamins and minerals, over-the-counter medications, and traditional Chinese medication. The Directorate enforces licensing requirements for natural health products and stipulates packaging and labelling requirements. For example, product packaging must state health claims, ingredients, instructions for use, and potential adverse effects. Natural health product manufacturers must document and report any adverse reactions identified by consumers. Health Canada has the authority to request label changes and to remove any natural health product from the market at any time. If there is a complaint or are complaints about a health product, after investigation, the product may be removed from the market permanently or temporarily until changes are made (if that is the recommendation).

## DID YOU KNOW?

### The Use of Natural Health Products

The use of natural products remains a concern to many health care providers across Canada. Not all consumers realize that a natural product may contain harmful ingredients or interfere with prescription medications. For example, combining a prescription antidepressant (SSRIs, or serotonin reuptake inhibitors) with St. John's wort (an herbal mood elevator used for depression) can cause nausea, vomiting, restlessness, dizziness, and headaches. In addition, when combined with SSRIs, a fatal condition called *serotonin syndrome* can occur if it goes undetected. St. John's wort can also reduce the effectiveness of oral contraceptives (Mayo Clinic, 2022).

Ginseng, another popular herbal medication, can increase blood pressure and should not be taken by someone with hypertension or who is on an antihypertensive medication. Even garlic, when taken with hypoglycemic medications (used by people with diabetes), can cause a drop in blood sugar and, possibly, a **hypoglycemic reaction**.

Reasons why people take natural health and herbal products include to reduce or prevent disease, to maintain health, or for the treatment of an illness. Individuals may take these products as directed by a homeopathic doctor, a medical doctor, and in conjunction with prescribed medications. The best of both worlds is when conventional medical therapies work in tandem with herbal and natural products and alternative care providers. Interestingly, 71% of Canadians have used natural health products such as vitamins and minerals, herbal products, and homeopathic medicines.

***Marketed Health Products Directorate.*** Through the Marketed Health Products Directorate (MHPD), Health Canada collects information about adverse reactions to health products and foods and ensures that the public is aware of any identified risks.

Canadians can report adverse effects of and obtain safety information on health products and medications through online reporting; see Web Resources on Evolve. The Canada Vigilance Program, which is the point of contact for health care providers and consumers, collects and assesses all reports of suspected adverse reactions to health products marketed in Canada (Health Canada, 2022b).

---

### DID YOU KNOW?

#### How Stringent Is the Testing?

All pharmaceutical drugs must undergo rigorous trials and testing before they are approved for use in Canada. On the other hand, Health Canada permits those who manufacture natural health products to make many of the same claims that pharmaceutical companies do (about their products) without the same strict standards, testing, trials, and protocols. As a test, a CBC program created a fictitious children's medicine, submitted it to Health Canada for approval with photocopied documents from an old homeopathic book, and received approval. Watch CBC Marketplace, "How Health Canada Licensed a Fake Children's Remedy as 'Safe and Effective'" (see below). After watching this video, discuss your thoughts and reactions with a classmate or in a small-group setting.

Video: *How Health Canada licensed a fake children's remedy as "safe and effective."* CBC Marketplace. https://www.youtube.com/watch?v=pCADoLKMSFc

---

### Communications and Public Affairs Branch

The Communication and Public Affairs Branch is dedicated to improving the flow of information within Health Canada and with national and regional partners in health care delivery, the media, the general public, and other stakeholders. Offices within this branch include the Ethics and Internal Ombudsman Services (which is a confidential, unbiased resource providing support for Health Canada employees) and the Planning and Operations Division (which provides leadership with respect to human resources, contracts, finances, and strategic planning).

### Strategic Policy Branch

The Strategic Policy Branch (SPB) develops and implements the federal government's health care policies, administering the *Canada Health Act*, creating health protection regulations and legislation, dealing with evolving problems, and authorizing new agencies to report information as required. It aims to promote actionable policies that ensure the delivery of priority-based, cost-effective health care initiatives involving several directorates. The SPB collaborates with numerous professional and research organizations, provincial and territorial ministries, and various program branches of the government's health portfolio.

---

### THINKING IT THROUGH

#### Herbal Medications

A patient, N.R., tells you that they are taking a number of herbal medications, including ones that have estrogen-like effects, and metabolism boosters that they read about on the Internet as combating fatigue and sluggishness. They believe it is unnecessary to tell their primary care provider. How would you respond if you were

1. An administrative assistant?
2. A nurse caring for N.R. in the hospital?
3. If your answers differ, explain why.

### Legal Services Department

The department of Legal Services provides legal services to Health Canada and the PHAC. It is an intermediary through which selected services of the Department of Justice are made available to Health Canada and the PHAC. Legal services include addressing such matters as policy advice, the development of legislative proposals, and litigation support. Legal Services also provides assistance as required to those at the ministry level and senior management, including advice regarding access to information and privacy law, administrative law, and constitutional law.

### The Opioid Response Team

The Opioid Response Team oversees the regulation of drugs and substances under the *Controlled Drugs and Substances Act*. One of the major responsibilities of the Opioid Response Team is to provide a platform for provinces, territories, municipalities, health organizations, health professionals, and other stakeholders to collaborate and produce effective response strategies to the opioid crisis in Canada (as well as other problematic substance use). To achieve this, the team collaborates with numerous other departments and organizations, including the Canadian Institute for Health Information (CIHI), the PHAC, the RCMP, and Correctional Service Canada. Currently the team is collaborating with all jurisdictions to address the upswing in opioid use and related deaths occurring prior to and during the COVID-19 pandemic (Locke, 2022; Public Health Agency of Canada [PHAC], 2019a). During the first year of the pandemic, Statistics Canada reported an increase in apparent opioid toxicity deaths of 95% compared to the previous year (Government of Canada, 2022b).

Several factors may have contributed to the increase in the overdose crisis during the pandemic, including the increase in the supply of toxic and contaminated drugs; increased anxiety, stress, and feelings of isolation; and decreased access to services that individuals using drugs depend on (see Chapter 10).

### Pest Management Regulatory Agency

The Pest Management Regulatory Agency regulates the use of pesticides in Canada to ensure minimum harm to both human health and the environment. Pesticides that are sanctioned for use by this department are reviewed and re-evaluated on a 15-year cycle. Through this agency, Health Canada addresses any situations of noncompliance with regulatory standards. The agency collaborates with provinces and territories as well as stakeholders at an international level, including the United States Environmental Protection Agency, the North American Free Trade Agreement Technical Working Group, and the Organization for Economic Co-operation and Development, to ensure the continued development of related policies and regulations.

### Controlled Substances and Cannabis Branch

The Controlled Substances and Cannabis Branch works to ensure the appropriate and legal distribution and use of controlled substances, lessoning the negative impact of improper and illegal use of these drugs on Canadians. It is important to note that the *Controlled Drug and Substances Act* operates under the mandates of several pieces of federal legislation and international conventions.

Several cannabis directorates deal with compliance, licensing and medical access, or strategic policy to oversee the safe and legal production, use, and distribution of cannabis in Canada. Responsibilities include creating and enforcing policies and regulations regarding medical as well as recreational cannabis use as mandated by law. Control over what edible products can be sold, and where, is also a responsibility of these directorates. A Government of Canada website provides comprehensive information about cannabis, including its uses and forms, health effects and risks, and the laws and regulations that control its distribution in the provinces and territories (Government of Canada, 2022c).

## AGENCIES MAKING UP CANADA'S HEALTH PORTFOLIO

Several independent agencies within Canada's health portfolio collaborate on various levels and report directly to the Minister of Health. The functions of some of these agencies are described below.

### Canadian Food Inspection Agency (CFIA)

The CFIA's highest priority is the mitigation of food safety risks in order to protect Canadians' health and safety. The agency collaborates with industry, consumers, federal, provincial, and municipal organizations and intergovernmental and nongovernmental organizations to protect Canadians from preventable health risks related to food, plants, and zoonotic diseases. The agency ensures safe, sustainable access to animal and plant resources, invokes food recalls and animal alerts (diseases in animals entering the food chain), and provides a forum for the public to report food labelling or safety concerns.

The CFIA is Canada's largest science-based regulatory agency, employing well over 1200 scientists in numerous departments with specific responsibilities, including diagnosing problems within the food chain and surveillance actives. The Charlottetown Laboratory in Prince Edward Island, for example, monitors for diseases in plants and soil pathogens and oversees the safety of both imported and exported plant products. The National Centre for Foreign Animal Disease, in Winnipeg, Manitoba, is a secure laboratory that provides state-of-the-art expertise and technologies to prevent, detect, control, and report on existing and emerging diseases. This facility also serves as reference laboratory for the World Organisation for Animal Health (WOAH) for classical swine fever and avian influenza. Saskatoon is home to a laboratory that tests animal feed for parasites and drugs that may have been given to animals.

### Canadian Institutes of Health Research (CIHR)

The CIHR directs and funds research across Canada, including initiatives concerning social, cultural, and environmental factors that affect population health. CIHR distributes research funding based on priority and need, expanding research as required, and recruiting and training research scientists. CIHR is also responsible for ensuring that the research information gathered and analyzed is used properly—for example, to craft policies or to generate products and services for which a need has been determined.

The CIHR operates 13 research institutes nationwide (Box 2.8) with a multimillion-dollar funding budget. More than 10,000 scientists and researchers in various hospitals, universities, and research institutes are involved with the agency. Targeted, ongoing, health-based research projects include those related to biomedical research, clinical science, and health care systems and services (Canadian Institutes of Health Research, 2022).

### Patented Medicine Prices Review Board (PMPRB)

The PMPRB is a "watch" agency that monitors the prices of **patented medicines** to ensure fairness to both manufacturer and consumer. A risk-based framework allows the PMPRB to assess patented medicines that have the greatest potential for overpricing. This assessment is based on two factors: (1) the medication's benefit to the consumer and (2) the impact of a medication's cost on value and affordability. This process results in an improved assessment of a medication's impact on population health—for example, that of newer, more expensive medications used by an aging population, many of whom are on a limited income.

---

**BOX 2.8  Canadian Institutes of Health Research Across Canada**

Aging
Cancer Research
Circulatory and Respiratory Health
Gender and Health
Genetics
Health Services and Policy Research
Human Development, Child and Youth Health
Indigenous Peoples' Health
Infection and Immunity
Musculoskeletal Health and Arthritis
Neurosciences, Mental Health, and Addiction
Nutrition, Metabolism, and Diabetes
Population and Public Health

---

Source: Canadian Institutes of Health Research. (2015). *CIHR institutes.* http://www.cihr-irsc.gc.ca/e/9466.html#a

If a manufacturer is thought to be overcharging for a medication, the review board first offers the manufacturer an opportunity to voluntarily adjust its pricing. If the company refuses, a judicial hearing may take place, with a binding federal court decision resulting.

The PMPRB also monitors ongoing trends in the sales, price, and distribution of patented medicines and drug products. This board operates independently of other organizations within Health Canada that deal with product safety and inspection.

The PMPRB is not involved with the pricing of generic medications, which are traditionally significantly less expensive than brand-name drugs. The amount that provinces and territories spend on generic medications fluctuates dramatically. An agreement among jurisdictions to buy some generic medications in bulk has reduced prices for selected medications.

---

**THINKING IT THROUGH**

*Patent Protection for Drugs*

Billions of dollars are spent annually on research, development, and clinical trials to test the safety and effectiveness of new medications. Patent protection allows 20 years for pharmaceutical firms to make a profit on medications they have brought to market. Companies that produce generic medications are able to produce generic versions of brand-name medications only after a patent expires, so they can bring cheaper, generic brands of patented medications to the market.

1. What do you think is the ideal length of time for patent protection and why?
2. If the patent protection time for new medications were shortened, how do you think the pharmaceutical companies might react (what actions might they take)?
3. Do you think that the pharmaceutical companies who developed the vaccines against the coronavirus should dispense with patent protection for these vaccines? Why or why not?

---

## Public Health Agency of Canada (PHAC)

Senior leadership of the PHAC includes the Minister of Health, the Minister of Mental Health, the Chief Public Health Officer, the President, and the Executive Vice President of the PHAC. There are 10 branches under the umbrella of the PHAC, including the Health Security and

Regional Operations Branch, Emergency Management Branch, and the National Microbiology Laboratory Branch (located in Winnipeg).

This organization plays a central role in all population health promotion research, policy, and program development. The PHAC works with other organizations within Canada's health portfolio as well as with provinces and territories and other stakeholders to prevent injury and reduce the incidence of chronic diseases. The agency promotes health by motivating Canadians to adopt healthy lifestyles and reduce risk-related behaviours. The PHAC also responds to national and international public health emergencies and infectious disease outbreaks, most recently the COVID-19 pandemic.

In terms of "health watch" activities, the PHAC responds to food recalls, food poisonings, and other risks and outbreaks; tracks outbreaks of seasonal flu, measles, and other infectious illnesses; and recommends corrective and preventive measures.

The PHAC organizes, posts, and updates online information regarding health issues. This includes travel warnings related to disease outbreaks and information about vaccinations (e.g., influenza and COVID-19). The PHAC plays a significant role in keeping Canadians informed about issues related to the COVID-19 pandemic. This includes monitoring the COVID-19 epidemiological indicators in order to promptly detect and communicate emerging trends of concern (e.g., variants that mutate as COVID-19 infections continue to spread). The Chief Public Health Officer makes periodic public announcements informing Canadians of emerging risks and trends and recommending safety measures.

## Other Organizations Working With Health Canada

Health Canada collaborates with other Canadian agencies and organizations in a variety of matters involving the health of Canadians. This includes the exchange of information, policies, and best practices involving almost every aspect of health care.

### Canadian Agency for Drugs and Technologies in Health (CADTH)

The CADTH was created as a result of collaborative effort by the federal, provincial, and territorial governments in 1989. It is a nonprofit, independent organization that provides relevant authorities, stakeholders, and decision makers with research data to enable making objective, evidence-informed decisions about the medications, diagnostic tests, and medical, dental, and surgical devices used within the Canadian health care system. The CADTH works with a variety of health technology assessment organizations across Canada to evaluate technical devices at any point during its use. For example, after Health Canada has reviewed a medication for consideration in Canada's public drug programs and cancer agencies, the CADTH conducts a reimbursement review to determine the medication's clinical and cost-effectiveness relative to others, avoiding duplication. Once a medication is approved, public drug plans across Canada (except Québec) decide if they will cover the cost of the medication.

### Accreditation Canada/Health Standards Organization (HSO)

Accreditation Canada is a nonprofit organization that conducts on-site, organization-specific, third-party assessments of health care, social, and diagnostic services and entire health care systems (Accreditation Canada, n.d.). Benchmark standards are tailored to comparable organizations (e.g., a diagnostic facility would be expected to uphold standards of care that differ from those of a long-term care facility).

Participation in the accreditation process is voluntary in some jurisdictions and mandatory in others. The assessment process is, for the most part, on a 4-year cycle to ensure that required and recommended standards of care and practice are maintained.

Formed in 2017 and accredited later that year by the Standards Council of Canada, the nonprofit Health Standards Organization (HSO) develops assessment programs and standards of care for use by health care, diagnostic, and social services. HSO is the only standards development organization in Canada that focuses on developing standards of care for health and social services. Accreditation Canada uses HSO tools in their accreditation and evaluation processes.

Development of HSO standards is based on the latest research and global evidence. Reviews of the standards are conducted through processes that include consultation with the individuals who use the services as well as those who provide them.

## The Canadian Institute for Health Information (CIHI)

The CIHI works closely with the Canadian Institutes of Health Research and Statistics Canada to gather and assimilate information from hospitals, clinics, long-term care facilities, and other health care facilities about Canada's health care system and the health of Canadians. The data provide valuable and comprehensive information to plan, organize, and implement policies and strategies that improve the performance of the health care system across Canada (see Chapter 6).

Funded by the federal, provincial, and territorial governments, the CIHI reports to an independent board of directors that represents government health departments, regional health authorities, hospitals, and health-sector leaders across the country. The CIHI maps the patterns of health care in Canada by working with 28 national and provincial information systems (databases) to gather data about the costing and delivery of health care services and the supply and distribution of health care providers. The organization produces an annual report of general information and several specific reports. Information gathered by the CIHI is used to initiate and advance improvements in the quality and delivery of health care, system performance, and population health strategies nationwide.

## Public Safety Canada

Public Safety Canada is the federal government department responsible for public safety, emergency management, and emergency preparedness as well as national security. The departments of health in all provinces and territories collaborate with Public Safety Canada when addressing national and global threats, from health and natural hazards to terrorism and cyberattacks.

## Statistics Canada

Statistics Canada is a branch of the federal government whose primary purpose is to gather and publish accurate statistics on almost every aspect of life in Canada. Statistics Canada is used extensively by all levels of government as well as agencies involved in public health and population health initiatives.

Every 5 years, in the first and sixth years of every decade, Statistics Canada conducts a national census, sent to one in five households. By law, participating households must complete this census. In 2010, amid much controversy, the federal government replaced the long-form census with a voluntary short National Household Survey. In 2011, a short mandatory census was also sent to one in three households (to which two questions on language had been added). The long-form census was reinstated in 2016 and sent to one in four households and now can be completed online. In the new census, questions about income were eliminated, and Statistics Canada was given permission to access Revenue Canada files to obtain information on personal income and benefits files. Questions about religion were eliminated. The most recent national census was in 2021. Information from this census is being released in stages up until the fall of 2022. The information from the census is important and used in a number of ways that are advantageous for businesses, communities, and individuals. For example, it is used in addressing the needs of a community, such as transportation needs, choosing the location of schools, and assessing the health care needs of cities or regions within a city. The information is also used by Statistics Canada for statistical purposes (e.g., immigration, population growth, population density, hospitalizations, and trends in health and illness).

## GLOBAL ORGANIZATIONS WORKING WITH HEALTH CANADA

For the federal government to provide leadership, advice, and direction on health care issues on a national front, it needs to interact regularly with global organizations, such as the World Health Organization (WHO), the Pan American Health Organization (PAHO), and the US Centers for Disease Control and Prevention (CDC). These organizations issue warnings and advisories about regional and global health threats, including Zika virus disease and Lyme disease, which have spread through the Americas in the last decades. Lyme disease, for example, is present in most regions in Canada. Lyme disease is often not diagnosed promptly, which can result in serious and long-term health problems for individuals.

### World Health Organization (WHO)

As the United Nations (UN) authority on health issues, the WHO provides leadership in health matters on a global level. The organization spearheads global research, provides technical support to members, monitors and assesses health trends, and sets standards within the fields of health and medicine. The WHO recommends policies and actions regarding population health initiatives. It is also instrumental in gathering information and statistics on health matters, coordinating responses to global health threats, and developing guidelines to help countries prevent the spread of infectious diseases (e.g., COVID-19).

As of 2021, a total of 194 countries composed the membership of the WHO. Each member country of the UN may become a member of the WHO by accepting its constitution. Countries outside the UN may be admitted as members if their applications are approved by a majority vote of the World Health Assembly. Jurisdictions without responsibility for their international affairs (regions within a country, for example) may become associate members if approved. The WHO Member States are grouped into six regions: African Region, Region of the Americas, South-East Asia Region, European Region, Eastern Mediterranean Region, and Western Pacific Region. Each region has a regional office covering specific Member States.

The WHO collects data and provides the international community with advice and direction on a wide variety of health topics, including air quality and environmental health, diabetes, obesity, cardiovascular health, mental health, and vaccines and immunization (including travel recommendations). The WHO also provides technical support in countries, for example, by assisting with the development of strategic plans for the medical, nursing, and midwifery professions.

The WHO, like Canada and many other countries, stresses the important role of social determinants of health (see Chapter 6) in influencing an individual's opportunity to live a healthy life, the risk factors for acquiring illnesses (physical and mental), and their impact on life expectancy.

### DID YOU KNOW?

#### Canada and the World Health Organization

Canada has a long history of collaboration with the World Health Organization (WHO), having worked for decades with the WHO in worldwide polio immunization, tuberculosis treatments, and other international health concerns. Many Canadians would also have become aware of the work of this intergovernmental organization during the SARS pandemic of 2003 and, most recently, the COVID-19 pandemic. The WHO has also monitored and shared information about monkeypox, which, in July 2022, the WHO declared to be a public health emergency of international concern (see Chapter 10).

## Pan American Health Organization (PAHO)

The Pan American Health Organization (PAHO) aims to improve health and living standards in the Americas. This international public health agency serves as the Regional Office for the Americas of the WHO. Member countries include the 35 nations that compose the Americas. Because many member states lack basic health care, clean drinking water, and adequate sanitation, one of PAHO's main priorities is to promote current, effective, and community-based primary health care strategies.

## Centers for Disease Control and Prevention (CDC)

Canada works closely with the Centers for Disease Control and Prevention (CDC), a US federal agency based in Atlanta, Georgia, that is responsible for disease prevention, control, and management on a global level. The CDC collaborates with Canadian agencies, sharing information, research outcomes, and surveillance initiatives regarding national and international health threats.

## Organisation for Economic Co-Operation and Development (OECD)

The Organisation for Economic Co-operation and Development (OECD) consists of 38 member countries (including Canada) that adhere to the principles of democracy and a free market economy. Through this organization, governments compare policy experiences and seek answers to common problems (Government of Canada, 2021). The organization, among other things, measures the quality of medical care in member countries and rates health outcomes. For example, a report called OECD Health Statistics 2021 is an extensive health database offering detailed sources of comparable health statistics on a variety of health topics and health care systems inclusive of all OECD countries. It is an essential tool for comparative, evidence-informed analyses.

---

### DID YOU KNOW?

#### *The Commonwealth Fund International Health Policy Survey*

The Commonwealth Fund International Health Policy survey provides annual comparable information from 11 countries on selected aspects of each country's health care system. These countries include Australia, Canada, France, Germany, the Netherlands, New Zealand, Norway, Sweden, Switzerland, the United Kingdom, and the United States.

The Commonwealth Fund is an American-based nonprofit private organization that leads the development of the surveys. Information used in the reports is gathered from the OECD and the WHO as well as the survey data. Areas measured include continuity of care, patient experience, health promotion and disease prevention, access to health care, and equity and health outcomes (71 areas are measured in total).

In the report released in August 2021, Canada's health care system placed second from the bottom (ahead of the United States). Canada placed tenth in equity and health care outcomes, ninth in access to care, seventh in administrative efficiency, and fourth in care process.

Sources: Neustaeter, B. (2021, August 4). *Canada's health system ranked second last among 11 countries: Report.* CTV News. https://www.ctvnews.ca/health/canada-s-health-system-ranked-second-last-among-11-countries-report-1.5533045#:~:text=CANADA'S%20RANKING,%2C%20New%20Zealand%2C%20and%20Norway; Tollinsky, N. (2021, September 30). Canada's healthcare system scores poorly against peers. *Canadian Healthcare Technology.* https://www.canhealth.com/2021/09/30/canadas-healthcare-system-scores-poorly-against-peers/#:~:text=The%20Commonwealth%20Fund's%202021%20report,was%20at%20the%20very%20bottom; Canadian Institute for Health Information. (n.d.) *Commonwealth Fund metadata.* https://www.cihi.ca/en/commonwealth-fund-metadata

## COVID-19 AND SEASONAL INFLUENZA: A CLOSER LOOK

### Seasonal Influenza

Influenza is a respiratory infection caused by the influenza virus types A, B, or C. Types A and B are responsible for most of the infections. H1N1 is a subtype of influenza A (also known as the "swine flu"), which, in 2009 was declared a pandemic by the WHO. Type C causes milder symptoms. Flu season in Canada and other regions of the northern hemisphere typically lasts from October until early spring; the exact timing varies somewhat, as does the seriousness of the infection. Most vulnerable to this infection are children under the age of 5, adults over 65 years old, those with comorbidities, and immunocompromised individuals.

All Canadians are offered the influenza vaccine each year. The influenza vaccine, available for types A and B only, is updated yearly. WHO experts meet twice a year (in February or March, and September) to review data from surveillance, laboratory, and clinical studies, analyze information from the WHO Global Influenza Surveillance and Response System, and decide about the formula for the next influenza vaccine.

The winter of 2020−2021 saw fewer cases of influenza and even of the common cold. This was attributed to the public health measures put into place to mitigate the spread of COVID-19, particularly the wearing of face masks, frequent handwashing, and physical distancing. Conversely, the 2022−2023 influenza season started earlier, with increased case numbers along with an upswing in COVID-19 cases, as well as the respiratory syncytial virus (RSV) which affected children in particular (Government of Canada, 2022d, 2022e).

### DID YOU KNOW?

#### High-Dose Vaccine

Older persons are advised to get a high-dose vaccine (brand name Fluzone High-Dose) that contains four times the amount of antigen of the regular flu shot. This vaccine has been shown to stimulate a higher immune response. It is recommended because, as we age, our immune system weakens and does not respond as effectively to the standard dose of influenza vaccination. Some jurisdictions run out of this vaccine early in the season, prompting older persons to seek their vaccines as soon as they are available.

Source: Centers for Disease Control and Prevention. (2021, August 26). *Influenza (flu). Adults 65 & over.* https://www.cdc.gov/flu/highrisk/65over.htm

### Protocols for Epidemics and Pandemics

In the event of an outbreak or epidemic (or pandemic), surveillance, containment, and treatment strategies must follow guidelines determined by all levels of government, as well as by regional public health authorities working with other stakeholders such as physicians, hospitals, or long-term care facilities.

### Influenza Preparedness in Canada

Outbreaks of influenza are recurrent but unpredictable events that can have serious effects on global and national economies, as well as on the health of populations. The WHO is responsible for monitoring the threat of potential global influenza and issues appropriate alerts based on specific criteria, as outlined in the WHO guidance document, *Pandemic Influenza Risk Management,* which was updated in 2017−2018 over the previous (2013) guidance to include improved alignment with pertinent United Nations procedures for emergency management as well as strategies for the use of available vaccines at the beginning of a pandemic

(WHO, 2017). The guidance informs and harmonizes national and international pandemic responses (not just for influenza).

In Canada, the *Canadian Pandemic Influenza Preparedness: Planning Guidance for the Health Sector* (CPIP) is a guidance put together by policy experts from the federal, provincial, and territorial governments in the event of an influenza pandemic (PHAC, 2019b). Updates and improvements are made to this guidance as they become available. For example, significant changes were made after the 2006 **severe acute respiratory syndrome (SARS)** pandemic, and again after the 2009 H1N1 pandemic, the first true test of this version of the guidance, when valuable lessons were learned about communication, surveillance, tracking methodologies, containment, and treatment as a result of these events. The latest update was made in 2020. Appendix B of this document provides guidance for pandemic strategies and planning for influenza outbreaks for First Nations communities and tribal councils, as well as for public health departments, regional health authorities, and the provinces (PHAC, 2021).

New additions to the guidance emphasize that each level of government, when deemed necessary, must adjust risk management strategies based on the unique needs of any given region or community. The CPIP encourages a "take what you need" approach to its recommendations, recognizing that the most effective way to manage a national health emergency must consider the situation in each community, and that each community—and individuals within those communities—has different needs.

## DID YOU KNOW?

### *Understanding the Terms*

The differences between a disease outbreak, an epidemic, and a pandemic are outlined as follows:

*Outbreak:* A flare-up of an infectious disease, either globally or within a specific region, or as a localized event (e.g., the seasonal flu/influenza in a long-term care facility or on a floor in an acute care hospital).

*Epidemic:* An epidemic occurs when the incidence of an infectious disease rises (usually suddenly) above the average or expected number of cases within a specific geographic area. An epidemic typically involves more serious health outcomes that affect both healthy individuals and those considered vulnerable (e.g., the very young or older people, those with chronic health problems, and those who have compromised immune systems).

*Pandemic:* A sustained, worldwide transmission of an infectious disease (e.g., the influenza A [H1N1] 2009 pandemic and COVID-19). The severity of disease and its mortality rate are not defining characteristics of a pandemic.

## COVID-19

The federal government led the way, with the recommendations from the WHO, in laying out specific protocols for Canada to follow once COVID-19 was declared a pandemic. Provinces and territories, working with local public health authorities that followed jurisdictional guidelines, fell into step, and adapted rules and regulations at municipal levels. The federal government has six main areas of responsibility with respect to managing the pandemic nationally:

- Protecting the health of Canadians, and collaborating with jurisdictional governments and Indigenous community leaders to ensure Canadians have the latest information on all aspects of the pandemic (current issues, vaccinations, protocols and guidelines, etc.)

- Providing travel advice, in collaboration with the WHO (including information about border closures and openings), and restrictions (e.g., in July 2022 after a brief hiatus, random testing for international travellers was reinstated at major airports across Canada and use of the ArriveCAN app remained in place)
- Supporting research into protocols and securing vaccines, ensuring their viability (e.g., proper storage), and organizing distribution of vaccines across the country
- Managing the health needs of Indigenous communities, members of the Canadian Armed Forces, people in federal institutions, and consular staff abroad
- Activating federal, provincial, and territorial agencies, when required, to respond in a collaborative manner to public health threats at various levels (e.g., Federal/Provincial/Territorial Public Health Response Plan for Biological Events)
- Working with all jurisdictions to ensure that the federal government maintains all services under its jurisdiction while working within the confines of public health and government restrictions (Fig. 2.2)

### Federal Government's Responsibilities Contributing to International COVID-19 Response

Canada, as with other countries, has international as well as national obligations when global threats related to an infectious outbreak arises. The following summarizes Canada's responsibilities with respect to the COVID-19 pandemic:

- Working with the G7 health and finance ministers in collaborating on COVID-19-related issues and searching for evidenced-informed solutions to evolving issues affecting the health and wellness of their population groups
- Contributing financial aid to the WHO to assist vulnerable population groups. This includes providing vaccines through an international organization called *COVAX* (Box 2.9). Canada and other nations have fallen behind their commitments to lower- and middle-income countries to distribute the number of vaccines necessary to vaccinate their populations (Government of Canada, 2022f).
- Donating personal protective equipment (PPE), diagnostic tests (for COVID-19), and therapeutic medications

## SUMMARY

2.1 Health Canada has a wide variety of responsibilities, not the least of which is collaborating with various departments in the health portfolio as well as with international partners. This is in addition to playing an authoritarian role, ensuring the provinces and territories remain compliant with the *Canada Health Act* and enforcing penalties on those that function outside of the principles within the Act. As a care provider, Health Canada is responsible for the health care for the armed forces, veterans, and correctional services; it covers the cost of health services to RCMP members when they have work-related trauma and injuries to their physical or mental health. Health Canada also coordinates care for other population groups, including refugee claimants and defined groups of Indigenous people in Canada.

2.2 Responsibilities for health care for Indigenous people are shared among the federal, provincial, and territorial governments (most programs are delivered in collaboration with Indigenous Services Canada). Health care for Indigenous people is a mosaic at best. It is sometimes difficult to work out who is eligible for what services, what those services are, and what level of government provides and pays for them. For example, there are three similar versions of the federal government's Non-Insured Health Plan (NIHP), the dominant plan providing non-insured benefits to certain First Nations and Inuit beneficiaries. The Métis population in Canada challenged the federal government in 1982 to

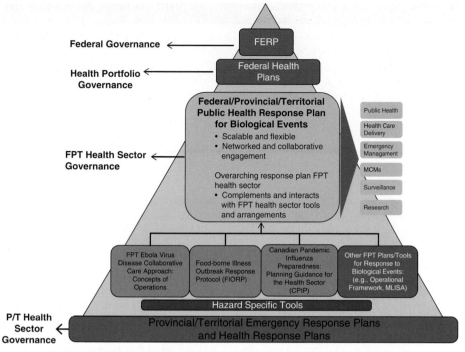

**Fig. 2.2** The hierarchy of emergency response plans at all levels of government.

1. At the top of the pyramid is the Federal Emergency Response Plan (FERP), which describes the federal governance structure that all federal departments are to activate when faced with any defined hazard emergency response.

2. The second tier shows the federal health plans, which illustrate the fact that federal health plans such as the Health Portfolio Emergency Response Plan (which details the steps to be followed in an emergency situation) must be aligned with the FERP.

3. The third tier of the pyramid is the Federal, Provincial Territorial Public Health Response Plan for Biological Events. This plan describes the federal/provincial/territorial (FPT) health sector's governance structure. Activities that will be facilitated by this response plan include public health, health care delivery, emergency management, medical countermeasures, surveillance, and research.

4. At this level of the pyramid (supporting the Federal/Provincial/Territorial Public Health Response Plan for Biological Events) are jurisdictional plans and procedures used by the related health sectors for a variety of possible hazards, such as responses for an Ebola virus disease outbreak, bloodborne illnesses, and the Canadian Pandemic Influenza Preparedness Planning and Response Guidance.

5. At the fifth tier of the pyramid are hazard-specific tools, which are meant to illustrate additional plans for specific hazards not included in the illustration.

6. At the bottom of the pyramid are Provincial/Territorial Emergency Response Plans and Health Response Plans. As required by legislation, all jurisdictions in Canada and ministries of health maintain emergency response plans. These plans describe provincial/territorial (P/T) health sector governance.

(Source: Government of Canada. (2017). *Federal/Provincial/Territorial Public Health Response Plan for Biological Events*. https://www.canada.ca/en/public-health/services/emergency-preparedness/public-health-response-plan-biological-events.html#s4-2-7. Appendix L, Figure 3.)

---

### BOX 2.9  COVAX: An Explanation

Access to COVID-19 Tools (ACT) Accelerator is a global collaboration with the aim of providing accelerated access to tests, equipment, vaccines, and medicines to treat the coronavirus. The focus of the COVAX pillar of ACT is to provide access to vaccines, irrespective of price. Jointly managed by the Coalition for Epidemic Preparedness Innovations, the World Health Organization, and Gavi (an international organization working with public and private sectors whose mandate is to provide access to vaccines to children in developing countries), COVAX partners with organizations such as UNICEF to assist with the delivery of vaccines and products.

Source: Based on Gavi. (n.d.). *What is COVAX?* https://www.gavi.org/covax-facility

---

gain recognition as a distinct people under the *Indian Act* and therefore have the same rights as "Indians" and Inuit, and to be eligible to receive health care benefits similar to those available to some First Nations. Despite the April 2016 ruling that the federal government has a constitutional responsibility for both Métis and non-Status Indians, little has happened in practical terms of providing health care benefits to either of these population groups.

2.3 Health Canada's organizational structure includes a large number of branches and agencies, each with numerous divisions. These branches, offices, and bureaus have specific obligations and some are split into functional divisions within the same general category of responsibilities. For example, the Natural and Non-prescription Health Products Directorate evaluates the safety and effectiveness of such products as prescription and non-prescription medications, natural food products, and veterinary drugs before they are introduced to the market. Subdivisions of this Directorate include the Biologic and Radio-pharmaceutical Drugs Directorate, the Therapeutic Products Directorate, and the Natural and Non-prescription Health Products Directorate. These separate directorates are all interconnected and within the same general category.

2.4 Several autonomous agencies work collaboratively with Health Canada, reporting directly to the Minister of Health. These agencies include the Public Health Agency of Canada (PHAC), the Canadian Institutes of Health Research (CIHR), the Hazardous Materials Information Review Commission, and the Patented Medicine Prices Review Board. The PHAC plays a significant role in health promotion and disease prevention initiatives; tracks outbreaks of seasonal influenza, tuberculosis, measles, and other illnesses; and recommends corrective and preventive measures. The PHAC has been instrumental in overseeing Canada's response to the COVID-19 pandemic.

2.5 Health Canada is active on an international level, working with several organizations to improve health at both a national and an international level. The World Health Organization (WHO), a key player in such initiatives, provides leadership on health matters globally. The WHO recognizes health threats, as it did for the coronavirus, and initializes pandemic alerts in response to information gathered. The Pan-American Health Organization aims to improve health and living standards in the Americas. The Organisation for Economic Co-operation and Development measures the quality of medical care in member countries and rates health outcomes.

2.6 Flu season in Canada and other regions of the Northern hemisphere typically lasts from October until early spring; the exact timing varies somewhat, as does the seriousness of the infection. Most vulnerable to this infection, as well as others such as the coronavirus and its variants, are children under the age of 5 years, adults over 65 years old, those with comorbidities, and immunocompromised and unvaccinated individuals. All Canadians are offered the influenza vaccine each year. The influenza vaccine, available for types A and B only, is updated yearly. By March 2022, three doses of the COVID-19 vaccine(s) had been offered to all individuals living in Canada, with a fourth to selected population groups. The WHO has an updated guidance that informs and harmonizes national and international pandemic responses. Canada has a national pandemic response plan, as do provinces and territories responding appropriately at a regional level to any such threat.

## REVIEW QUESTIONS

1. What are the primary responsibilities of the Minister of Health?
2. What population groups does the federal government provide health services for?
3. What was the funding for Joyce's Principle used for?
4. Discuss the benefits provided by the Non-Insured Health Benefits Program.
5. What is Jordan's Principle, and what benefits does this principle offer Indigenous children under the expanded services?
6. What are the responsibilities of the Natural and Non-prescription Health Products Directorate?
7. How do the functions and responsibilities of the Canadian Institute of Health Information and the Canadian Institute of Health Research differ?
8. Identify two international organizations that Health Canada works with and briefly list their functions.
9. How often is a census done in Canada, and what is the information gathered used for?
10. What is the difference between Fluzone and regular influenza vaccine?
11. Explain the differences between a disease outbreak, an epidemic, and a pandemic.
12. What is COVAX?

## REFERENCES

Accreditation Canada. (n.d.). *Qmentum Accreditation Program*. https://accreditation.ca/qmentum-accreditation/.

Blackstock, C. (2008). Jordan's Principle: Editorial update. *Paediatrics and Child Health, 13*(7), 589—590.

Canadian Institutes of Health Research. (2022). *Research in priority areas*. https://cihr-irsc.gc.ca/e/50077.html.

First Nations Child and Family Caring Society of Canada. (2016). *Victory for first nations children. Canadian human rights tribunal finds discrimination against first nations children living on-reserve. Information sheet.* https://fncaringsociety.com/sites/default/files/Information%20Sheet%20re%20CHRT%20Decision.pdf.

First Nations Health Authority. (2022). *About the FNHA*. https://www.fnha.ca/about/fnha-overview.

Government of British Columbia. (2022). *Welcoming Ukraine*. https://www2.gov.bc.ca/gov/content/tourism-immigration/ukraine/welcome#healthcare.

Government of Canada. (2021). *Canada and the organisation for economic Cooperation and development (OECD)*. https://www.international.gc.ca/world-monde/international_relations-relations_internationales/oecd-ocde/index.aspx?lang=eng.

Government of Canada. (2022a). *Crown-Indigenous Relations and Northern Affairs Canada*. https://www.canada.ca/en/crown-indigenous-relations-northern-affairs.html.

Government of Canada. (2022b). *Opioid- and stimulant-related harms in Canada*. https://health-infobase.canada.ca/substance-related-harms/opioids-stimulants/.

Government of Canada. (2022c). *Cannabis*. https://www.canada.ca/en/health-canada/services/drugs-medication/cannabis.html.

Government of Canada. (2022d). *FluWatch report: October 2, 2022 to October 15, 2022 (weeks 40–41)*. https://www.canada.ca/en/public-health/services/publications/diseases-conditions/fluwatch/2021-2022/weeks-40-41-october-2-october-15-2022.html.

Government of Canada. (2022e). *COVID-19 epidemiology update*. https://health-infobase.canada.ca/covid-19/.

Government of Canada. (2022f). *Canada's aid and development assistance in response to the COVID-19 pandemic*. https://www.international.gc.ca/world-monde/issues_development-enjeux_developpement/global_health-sante_mondiale/response_covid-19_reponse.aspx?lang=eng.

Government of Northwest Territories. (2021). *Métis health benefits program*. Alberta Blue Cross. https://www.hss.gov.nt.ca/sites/hss/files/resources/metis-health-benefits.pdf.

Health Canada. (2017). *Health portfolio*. https://www.canada.ca/en/health-canada/corporate/health-portfolio.html.

Health Canada. (2019). *Canada's food guide*. https://food-guide.canada.ca/en/.

Health Canada. (2022a). *Health Canada*. https://www.canada.ca/en/health-canada.html.

Health Canada. (2022b). *Health products and food branch*. https://www.canada.ca/en/health-canada/corporate/about-health-canada/branches-agencies/health-products-food-branch.html.

Immigration, Refugees, and Citizenship Canada. (2022, March 30). *Canada marks 10,000 arrivals of Afghan refugees*. https://www.canada.ca/en/immigration-refugees-citizenship/news/2022/03/canada-marks-10000-arrivals-of-afghan-refugees.html.

Indigenous Services Canada. (2017, December 4). *Government of Canada moving forward with departmental changes needed to renew the relationship with Indigenous peoples*. https://www.canada.ca/en/indigenous-services-canada/news/2017/12/government_of_canadamovingforwardwithdepartmentalchangesneededto.html.

Indigenous Services Canada. (2018). *Definition of Jordan's principle from the Canadian human rights tribunal*. https://www.sac-isc.gc.ca/eng/1583700168284/1583700212289.

Indigenous Services Canada. (2021). *Indigenous health care in Canada*. https://www.sac-isc.gc.ca/eng/1626810177053/1626810219482.

Indigenous Services Canada. (2022). *Inuit client eligibility for non-insured health benefits*. https://www.sac-isc.gc.ca/eng/1585310583552/1585310609830.

Locke, G. (2022, January 9). *2021 deadliest-ever year for drug overdose deaths in British Columbia. World Socialist Website*. https://www.wsws.org/en/articles/2022/01/09/opio-j09.html.

Mayo Clinic. (2022). *Serotonin syndrome*. https://www.mayoclinic.org/diseases-conditions/serotonin-syndrome/symptoms-causes/syc-20354758.

Métis Nation of Ontario. (2022). *Healing & wellness*. https://www.metisnation.org/programs-and-services/healing-wellness/.

Nazir, T., & Taha, N. (2018). Pharmacy health system in Canada: An adoptable model for advanced clinical and pharmaceutical care. *Journal of Applied Pharmacology, 10*, 6–14. https://doi.org/10.21065/19204159/10.06

Public Health Agency of Canada (PHAC). (2019a). *Updated numbers on opioid-related overdose deaths in Canada*. https://www.canada.ca/en/public-health/news/2019/04/updated-numbers-on-opioid-related-overdose-deaths-in-canada.html.

Public Health Agency of Canada (PHAC). (2019b). *Canadian pandemic influenza preparedness: Planning guidance for the health sector*. https://www.canada.ca/en/public-health/services/flu-influenza/canadian-pandemic-influenza-preparedness-planning-guidance-health-sector.html.

Public Health Agency of Canada (PHAC). (2021). *On-reserve First Nations communities: Canadian pandemic influenza preparedness: Planning guidance for the health sector*. https://www.canada.ca/en/public-health/services/flu-influenza/canadian-pandemic-influenza-preparedness-planning-guidance-health-sector/influenza-pandemic-planning-considerations-in-on-reserve-first-nations-communities.html.

Saskatchewan Health Authority. (2014). *First Nations and Métis health service: Our service*. https://www.saskatoonhealthregion.ca/locations_services/Services/fnmh/service/Pages/What-We-Do.aspx.

Saskatchewan Health Authority. (2022). *First nations and Métis health: Programs and services*. https://www.rqhealth.ca/department/native-health/first-nations-and-metis-health-programs-and-services.

Stefanovich, O., & Boisvert, N. (2022). *Ottawa releases early details of landmark $40B First Nations child welfare agreement.* CBC News. https://www.cbc.ca/news/politics/first-nations-child-welfare-agreements-in-principle-1.6302636.

Walker, M. (2022). *March 16). Afghan interpreters voice frustrations over delays in bringing families to Canada.* CTV News. https://toronto.ctvnews.ca/afghan-interpreters-voice-frustrations-over-delays-in-bringing-families-to-canada-1.5822611.

World Health Organization. (2017). *Pandemic influenza risk management: A WHO guide to inform and harmonize national and international pandemic preparedness and response.* https://apps.who.int/iris/handle/10665/259893.

# 3

# The Role of Provincial and Territorial Governments in Health Care

## LEARNING OUTCOMES

3.1 Discuss the common elements of health care delivery among provinces and territories.
3.2 Outline the differences and similarities between regional and single health authorities.
3.3 Explain how provinces and territories finance health care services.
3.4 Discuss the particulars of public and private health insurance in Canada.
3.5 Describe what hospital and health care services are insured under public health plans.
3.6 Explain the prevalence of drug and dental plans in Canada.

## KEY TERMS

| | | |
|---|---|---|
| Copayment | Enhanced services | Rationalization |
| Deductible | Formulary list | Regionalization |
| Dispensing fee | Longitudinal care | |
| Drug identification number (DIN) | | |

Chapter 3 provides an overview of the structure of the provincial and territorial health care systems, emphasizing the common elements among them and outlining significant differences. It is important to note that although details of how each jurisdiction funds and implements specific health care services cannot be covered here, the chapter will give you a general understanding and overview of how each province and territory manages its own health care system within and outside of the confines of the *Canada Health Act*. You will note that most health care services rendered across Canada are similar; differences are related to how some services are delivered and variations in those publicly funded outside of the *Canada Health Act* (e.g., pharmacare, home care, community and long-term care, and supplemental benefits).

This chapter follows three families—two who are new to Canada, and one moving from one province to another—as they interface with the health care system within their respective provinces to meet their health care needs. The families will be discussed in the Case Examples: the J family in British Columbia (Case Example 3.1), the W family in New Brunswick (Case Example 3.2), and the L-O family, who moved from Saskatchewan to Ontario (Case Example 3.3).

---

**CASE EXAMPLE 3.1 The J Family**

J.J. is a Canadian citizen, born in Vancouver. He moved to Germany with his mother and father when he was very young. He has been back to Canada frequently for holidays and to visit relatives. On February 20, J.J. (now 40 years old) and his family returned to live in Canada, landing in Vancouver, British Columbia. J.J.'s family includes his wife, A.J., age 36 (who is expecting twins), and their three children: E.J., age 16; L.J., age 10; and C.J., age 3. Although somewhat familiar with Canada, J.J. has no idea how to apply for health coverage, which documents he needs and where to obtain them, and how to find a family doctor. He is even unsure which services specifically are covered under British Columbia's medical care plan.

---

**CASE EXAMPLE 3.2 The W Family**

The W family applied for immigrant status 2 years prior to their arrival and were accepted 6 months ago. Q.W., age 36, and his wife, L.W., age 35, arrived in New Brunswick on January 15 with their two children: a son, H.W., age 10, and a daughter, N.W., age 6. Q.W., a doctor, would like to certify as a physician in New Brunswick when they are settled and financially stable, but he realizes this will take time and money. L.W. is an architect who also would like to return to school. At this time their funds are limited. The family has no outstanding health problems.

---

**CASE EXAMPLE 3.3 The L-O Family**

C.L. and his partner, K.O., are moving from Saskatchewan to Ontario. C.L. was transferred by his engineering company. K.O., a respiratory therapist, plans to look for work when they get settled in Toronto. They have one son, R.L-O, who is 15 years old.

---

## PROVINCIAL AND TERRITORIAL HEALTH CARE PLANS

### Division of Powers

Both Canadians and non-Canadians often ask, "Does Canada have a national health insurance plan?" The answer is no. Canada has universal health care implemented by 13 single-payer insurance plans, each administered and operated by a province (10) or a territory (3). A national plan would mean there would be one plan across the country administered by one organization (e.g., the federal government). Universal health care, on the other hand, means that all eligible citizens of a particular country have insured health coverage, which can be achieved through a variety of health care plans in each province or territory. There are basic similarities with each plan, but each province and territory is free to deliver health care in a manner that best suits the health care needs of residents within each jurisdiction. As mentioned in Chapter 1, these programs are frequently referred to collectively as *medicare*.

Although the federal government works in partnership with the provinces and territories to deliver health care, the provinces and territories maintain the bulk of the responsibility for its delivery. Under the *Constitution Act* (Box 3.1), provincial and territorial governments oversee

> **BOX 3.1**   **The *Constitution Act*: A Clarification**
>
> The original *British North America Act* of 1867 became the *Constitution Act* in 1982, when Britain surrendered the power to make Canada's laws, including its Constitution. Among other things, the *Constitution Act* outlines the division of health care responsibilities.

matters relating to the personal health of their populations—the promotion of good health, preventive care, health maintenance, and the diagnosis and treatment of health problems. As noted in Chapter 1, to receive continued federal funding for health care, provinces and territories must abide by the principles and conditions of the *Canada Health Act* which obliges them to operate a health insurance plan that covers hospital care and medically necessary treatment for eligible residents. The Act is not concerned with the specifics of additional public or private health care delivery (unless private services contravene the principles and conditions of the Act). For example, the *Canada Health Act* does not address home care, long-term care, or coverage of diagnostic services. Each province and territory controls which supplementary services are covered and how they are delivered.

### Structure of Provincial/Territorial Health Care: An Overview

Within each provincial and territorial government there is a ministry or department of health that is assigned to managing health care. The health ministries or departments oversee a variety of subdivisions, branches, agencies, and programs that assume responsibilities for various matters and types of health care. Ministries also work with other service partners in the community—some government-funded, others private or nonprofit, and others a combination of government and private initiatives.

Each ministry is headed by an elected Member of Parliament appointed by the premier to the position of Minister of Health (MOH). Typically, a government also appoints a Deputy Minister of Health (sometimes more than one), who is (as in the federal government) not an elected Member of Parliament. One or more associate deputy ministers and a management committee may also be assigned. Ultimately responsible for the health care system in the province or territory, the MOH has numerous organizations within the ministry reporting to them. These organizations provide leadership, direction, and support to service delivery partners, which include provincial/territorial (centralized) single health authorities, regional health authorities, regional councils, physicians, public health authorities, and other health care providers. A good example is the collaboration between the MOH and public health authorities in each jurisdiction during the pandemic. The direction and oversight provided by public health have been invaluable in guiding provinces and territories through the pandemic, and continue to do so.

One of the ministries' greatest responsibilities is implementing and regulating the provincial or territorial health insurance plan—that is, overseeing hospital and medical care. In some jurisdictions this responsibility belongs to a single authority. In others, two administrative bodies share the duty—one handles hospitals and other health care facilities; the other, medical care. For example, in British Columbia the Medical Services Commission administers the medical care plan. The government, through the Ministry of Health Services, administers hospital services under the *Hospital Insurance Act*, reimbursing facilities for the medically necessary services they provide. But in Prince Edward Island, Health PEI administers both the hospital and medical services plans. The provincial and territorial ministries must also oversee the negotiation of salaries and other policies with physicians' professional associations (e.g., the Ontario Medical Association, the British Columbia Medical Association). Committees are typically created to manage these negotiations.

All provinces and territories provide three general categories of health care—primary, secondary, and tertiary. Some also provide quaternary care. The interaction between these categories is illustrated in Fig. 3.1. Bear in mind that because all jurisdictions are currently strategizing to improve the efficacy and delivery of healthcare, modifications of these healthcare services are likely to occur.

*Primary care* refers to "first contact" services to which the public has direct access. Traditionally a person would go to see a primary care provider, who for the most part is a family physician or a nurse practitioner, for medical advice. However, with an interprofessional team approach to primary care that may vary, enabling individuals to contact a variety of providers for initial treatment (in addition to a physician or nurse practitioner), ranging from a chiropractor, physiotherapist, nutritionist, counsellor, or psychologist. Primary care facilities include the provider's office or facility, a variety of clinics (walk-in, rapid access, ambulatory care), and the emergency department. If a patient's primary care provider cannot manage the patient's health issue or feels the patient needs more in-depth, specialized assessments, they will refer the patient to a specialist who provides secondary care.

*Secondary care* occurs when a patient is sent to see a specialist (seeking a consultation), which usually requires a referral (e.g., from a physician, nurse practitioner, or midwife). The referring physician is required to send a detailed (consultation) report about the patient to the

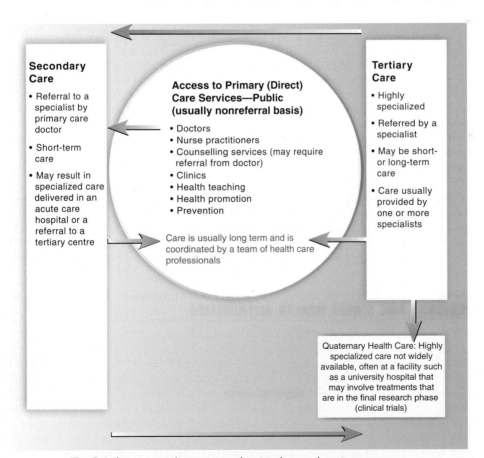

**Fig. 3.1** Access to primary, secondary, tertiary, and quaternary care.

CASE EXAMPLE 3.4   **Mr. A.B.: Levels of Care**

Mr. A.B., who lives in Saskatoon, went to see his family doctor about persistent headaches. After a couple of weeks the headaches got worse, which prompted his doctor to order magnetic resonance imaging (MRI). The MRI revealed a growth in his brain—*primary care.* The family doctor referred Mr. A.B. to a neurologist—*secondary care.* Following further investigation, the neurologist concluded that Mr. A.B. had a malignant tumour, which might need surgery. The neurologist referred him to a neurosurgeon in the Department of Neurosurgery at the University of Saskatchewan—*tertiary care.* After a highly specialized surgery with unfavourable results, the neurosurgeon consulted with another specialist who was running clinical trials in neurosurgical oncology for a new procedure that was combined with other interventions—*quaternary care.*

specialist, concerning the reason for the referral, including lab and diagnostic tests. A specialist assists the primary care provider to diagnose a patient's health problem and orders the appropriate treatment, but the specialist's involvement is usually short term. Secondary care may involve admission to a general hospital or referral to a highly specialized facility, which provides tertiary care.

Highly specialized *tertiary care* also requires a referral. A cancer centre or cardiology centre, for example, would provide tertiary care. Other examples include facilities that specialize in treating burn patients, neurosurgery, complex mental health, and palliative care. In a tertiary care setting, the patient may receive care from the referring specialist or from another specialist (or both). Once care is considered complete, the patient may be sent back to the referring specialist, who will then discharge the patient back to their primary care provider, usually a family doctor. Alternatively, the tertiary care centre itself may refer the patient back to the family doctor.

Finally, *quaternary care* is an extension of tertiary care and even more specialized, sometimes involving experimental procedures. Hospitals that do research (often linked with universities) may provide this level of care. Case Example 3.4 shows how each level of care works in a practical scenario.

Although ultimately accountable for all aspects of health care, the provincial or territorial ministry or department of health assigns responsibilities to various departments. The most common method of delivering primary, secondary, and tertiary/quaternary care initially was under a regional model using organizations commonly called *regional health authorities* (RHAs). This is slowly changing, with many jurisdictions moving back to one centralized health authority.

## REGIONAL AND SINGLE HEALTH AUTHORITIES

In the early 1990s, because of the rising cost of health care and the increasing demand for services in a variety of settings, many governments conducted public forums, reviews, and other studies to determine a way to improve health care delivery. There was a concurrence across provinces through the political leadership, and a commitment was made to a nation-wide or pan-Canadian agenda. **Regionalization** was the first significant coordinated pan-Canadian reform. The conclusion: to decentralize decisions about health care issues through regionalization (Box 3.2), a concept of assessing the need for specific types of care and delivering that care which is best suited to a population group within a given geographic area. Four desired goals for implementing a regionalized approach were shared by all provinces and

---

**BOX 3.2 Regional Health Authorities: A Definition**

Regional health authorities (RHAs) are autonomous health care organizations responsible for health care administration in a defined geographic region within a province or territory. Through appointed or elected boards of governance, RHAs manage the funding and/or delivery of community and institutional health care services within their regions. RHAs are sometimes referred to as *Local Health Authorities*. Ontario's (now remodelled) regional entities were referred to as *Local Health Integration Networks*.

---

territories. The first was to amalgamate health care services over a broad continuum of care, the second was to stress health promotion and disease prevention, the third to involve the public, and the last to implement appropriate and effective governance. Governance of RHAs varies. They are typically overseen by a board. In some regions, the provincial government appoints the board members; in others, board members comprise a mix of elected and appointed people from a variety of backgrounds. The RHAs in provinces and territories across Canada differ in terms of size, structure, responsibility, and name.

The desired effects of regionalization on primary care include designing care within a community that provides individuals with the type and level of care best suited within the region; for example, there may be a need for primary care services more suited to an older population, or care more tailored to a culturally diverse demographic. Regional authorities are responsible for funding services, facilities and sometimes health professionals within their catchment area. A physician working up north, for example, may be assigned a funding mechanism called a *global budget*: A family doctor decides to practice in rural Newfoundland and Labrador. They accept a contract to work in a designated area for 2 years and are paid by the government of Newfoundland and Labrador.

## Single Health Authorities

Although initially all the provinces and territories adopted the regionalized approach to health care delivery, in the past few years several jurisdictions have moved back to a single health authority (Box 3.3). The decision to move back to a centralized health care delivery system was made for various reasons (somewhat different for each jurisdiction), including the desire to create more distance from all the bureaucratic "red tape" and layered services and make services more cohesive and easier to access. It is important to note that no formal evidence-informed studies have determined which model works best.

## Rationalization and Centralization of Health Services

Most jurisdictions have adopted a centralized approach to delivering health care services as another way to reduce costs and improve the quality and continuity of patient care. This has led to the **rationalization** (or centralizing) of health services within communities—particularly in hospitals. Larger hospitals were merged under one administrative body offering specialized services at different sites or campuses. In other communities, one hospital may act as a regional centre for cancer, for example, whereas another would act as the regional centre for cardiac or maternal-child services. For example, Women's College Hospital in Toronto transitioned from an acute care hospital to an ambulatory centre specializing in women's health. Amalgamating hospitals and redistributing services resulted in the closure of a number of smaller hospitals across the country. Rural areas often allocated services normally found in a larger acute care hospital to smaller hospitals in surrounding towns in order to justify keeping them open. For

**BOX 3.3   Jurisdictions With Either Regional Health Authorities or a Single Health Authority**

| Regional Health Authority (RHA) | Single Health Authority |
| --- | --- |
| British Columbia: 5 RHAs, First Nations Health Authority | Alberta: Alberta Health Authority |
| Manitoba: 5 RHAs | Saskatchewan: Saskatchewan Health Authority |
| Nova Scotia: 2 RHAs | Ontario: Ontario Health |
| Newfoundland and Labrador: 4 RHAs | Nova Scotia: Nova Scotia Health Authority |
| New Brunswick: 2 RHAs | Prince Edward Island: Prince Edward Island Health Authority |
| | Nunavut: Nunavut Health Region (service in 25 communities) |
| | Yukon: Yukon Health Region |
| | Northwest Terrirorites: NWT Health and Social Services Authority |
| | Québec: Ministère de la Santé et des Services sociaux, which oversees health care in the province, sharing responsibilities with health and social services networks |

instance, some rehabilitation services moved to one community hospital, while certain types of surgeries (e.g., cataract surgery) moved to another location.

## PROVINCIAL AND TERRITORIAL APPROACHES TO THE DELIVERY OF PRIMARY CARE

The basic hierarchical structure of each jurisdiction is briefly described here, as well as a summary of the various primary care organizations each province and territory uses in the delivery of primary care services. All jurisdictions have a range of clinics (ambulatory care, walk-in, urgent care), which are also discussed in Chapter 5.

### British Columbia

In British Columbia, the Ministry of Health works collaboratively with a provincial health authority, five regional authorities, and First Nations Health Authority to deliver health care in the province. The Ministry of Health establishes performance and evaluation guidelines for health care delivery and performance outcomes. The RHAs oversee the funding, planning, and delivery of customized care required in their geographic areas. Another regional authority, the Provincial Health Services Authority, collaborates with the five RHAs to implement provincial programs (Office of the Auditor General of British Columbia, n.d.).

The RHAs also manage community health councils (CHCs), which offer a variety of services throughout the province, including primary care clinics, health promotion, addictions services, home care, community mental health services, and specialized services, such as assistance for new immigrants, support for new mothers, and youth health drop-in centres. The range of services each CHC offers reflects the needs of the community it serves.

The First Nations Health Authority, as discussed in Chapter 2, has assumed responsibility for delivering culturally safe and appropriate health care programs and services to First

---

**BOX 3.4  2021–2022 Goals for the First Nations Health Authority**

1. Augment First Nations existing health governance.
2. Continue to support the BC First Nations Perspective on Health and Wellness.
3. Promote excellence in current programs and services.
4. Continue to manage the organization effectively, improving the health of First Nations people.

---

Source: Based on First Nations Health Authority. (2021, June 10). *The FNHA Summary Service Plan: An operational plan for the fiscal year 2021/2022.* https://www.fnha.ca/about/news-and-events/news/the-first-nations-health-authority-releases-2021-22-summary-service-plan

Nations people in the province (formerly overseen by Health Canada's First Nations Inuit Health Branch—Pacific Region). The FNHA issues an annual health services summary plan describing the organizations goals and objectives (Box 3.4).

### Primary Care

Primary care in British Columbia is undergoing a transition to primary care networks with the goal of having over 40 in place by approximately 2024. These networks will become patients' medical home (PMH) as in other jurisdictions.

*Primary care networks.* Stakeholders along with Indigenous leaders collaborating with the Ministry of Health have helped to develop the framework for primary care networks in British Columbia. Elders will be available to offer Indigenous people support, leadership, and traditional knowledge; this will ensure that facilities will continue with the delivery of culturally safe and individualized care to Indigenous people.

As with other primary health care organizations, these networks offer a full range of primary care services delivered by an interprofessional team and operate with expanded hours (see Chapter 5).

*Urgent and primary care centres.* As an alternative to the emergency department (ED), British Columbia's Urgent and Primary Care Centres (UPCCs) offer access to those needing same-day appointments requiring urgent and non-urgent health care. Most centres have diagnostic equipment, the type of which varies with the centre. These centres have expanded hours including weekends and statutory holidays.

---

**THINKING IT THROUGH**

### What Does Primary Care Mean to You?

Primary care is the first point of contact a person makes with the health care system, typically a family physician or a nurse practitioner. Would you view any of the following as primary care providers? Why or why not?

1. You visit a pharmacist for your influenza and COVID-19 vaccinations.
2. A paramedic attends to you in an ambulance after an accident.
3. You visit a dietitian, a social worker, a psychologist, or a chiropractor or physiotherapist.

---

### Alberta

In 1994, the Government of Alberta passed legislation, the *Regional Health Authorities Act,* to abolish nearly 200 existing local hospital and public health boards and replace them with 17 RHAs. In 2004, the 17 RHAs were reduced to 9, with the cancer, mental health, and addiction boards continuing.

In 2008, the Government of Alberta reduced the nine RHAs to one agency called the Alberta Health Services Board. The original Alberta Health Services Board was disbanded by the provincial government (over financial disputes) and reintroduced in 2017. The board is responsible for the governance of Alberta Health Services (AHS), working collaboratively with Alberta Health. The board also assumed responsibility of the Alberta Mental Health Board, the Alberta Cancer Board, and the Alberta Alcohol and Drug Abuse Commission. The responsibilities of this governance model is to strengthen Alberta's approach to managing health care services, including surgical access, long-term care, chronic disease management, addiction and mental health services, and primary care access.

### Primary Care

Primary care is delivered through three models in Alberta, all delivering team-based interprofessional primary health services, led by a physician or a nurse practitioner (Government of Alberta, 2022). These primary care models are also referred to as a "patient's medical home"—a place meeting the patient's health care needs either directly or through referral (e.g., for specialized care or for mental health and/or social support), while maintaining continuity of care. The three models are primary care networks, community health centres, and family care clinics.

*Primary care networks.* Primary care networks are the most common primary care delivery model in the province. The networks were formed as the result of a partnership between AHS and groups of primary care and family physicians (approximately 84% of primary care physicians in the province serving about 3.8 million people). The province has provided funding for the Primary Care Network Nurse Practitioner Support Program, which supports using the expertise of nurse practitioners in the primary care setting, closing gaps in related care services (Government of Alberta, 2021).

*Family care clinics.* Family care clinics provide direct access to a variety of nonemergency services to underserviced areas in Alberta. Family care clinics are frequently managed by a nurse practitioner and, as with primary care networks, include an interprofessional team of health professionals. Individuals can see any team member without a physician's referral (e.g., counsellor, dietitian, podiatrist).

*Community health centres.* Community health centres provide primary care services with social and other community-based programs, including preventive care, health promotion, well baby and child services, immunizations, communicable disease control, and school health services. Such centres are more active in serving populations that are vulnerable, including refugees and immigrants, homeless people, members of the LGBTQ2S community, as well as Indigenous people in the province (this setting is described in more detail in Chapter 5).

*Strategic clinical networks.* Strategic clinical networks focus on improving health in specific areas, including maternal-child care, cardiac care, cancer care, mental health, and critical care programs.

### Saskatchewan

The delivery of health care in Saskatchewan is overseen by the Saskatchewan Health Authority (SHA), which is the largest organization in the province. Established in 2017, the SHA replaces 12 RHAs.

### Primary Care

In 2016, building on the recommendations of a government-sponsored advisory panel, the SHA moved forward with the recommendation to promote team-based primary health care in the province. This was accomplished through collaborative efforts by the Ministry of Health, the SHA, and the Saskatchewan Medical Association. The model adopted for delivering primary care was in the form of primary care networks with the goal of improving the delivery of health care services at a local level, tailored to the needs of each community (Saskatchewan Health Authority, 2021). Information is provided to health care teams working within each network to help define the type of care that best suits each region. This information includes demographic information, such as age groups (e.g., a younger or older population base, or a mix), and the prevalence of certain types of chronic diseases (e.g., diabetes, heart disease, chronic obstructive pulmonary disease [COPD]). It may be determined that a community needs emphasis on health promotion and disease prevention relating to such concerns as obesity, smoking, or hypertension. The move to health networks will have little impact on patients, some of whom may have no idea what network they belong to (that is how seamless the transition across the province is supposed to be). Organizing the networks is described as being "internal," with the SHA working behind the scenes with physicians' practices, stakeholders, and community partners to implement the improvements in primary care. Patients will have the flexibility to move between networks to receive care. Congruent with the primary care network model, interprofessional teams with community partners will coordinate care at numerous levels, from primary care providers, pharmacists, public health, and First Nations services to community and home care services, to residential and long-term care. Fig. 3.2 demonstrates the interconnectivity and inclusivity of all aspects of health care services provided by health networks.

## Manitoba

Currently, Manitoba has five RHAs. Each is overseen by a board of directors headed by a chairperson reporting ultimately to the Ministry of Health. The RHAs along with community partners assess and prioritize community needs ranging from primary care to long-term, home, and community care, as well as public health services. Many regions are divided into smaller geographic sections called *Community Areas* (CAs), which are made up of two to four geographic areas called *Neighborhood Clusters* (Winnipeg Regional Health Authority, 2022). Each region is profiled at designated intervals by the CA to determine the specific health needs of that area. These assessments are related to newer primary care initiatives.

### Primary Care

The government of Manitoba is reshaping the delivery of primary care through home clinics and My Health Teams, working collaboratively to deliver patient-centred care to patients within their own community.

*Home clinics.* A home clinic is where the patient's primary care provider (either a family physician or a nurse practitioner, or both) is located. Home clinics must be registered with Manitoba Health and Seniors Care (Manitoba Health, n.d.; Shared Health Manitoba, 2022a). A patient's medical records are located at the person's home clinic. Individuals are advised to confirm which home clinic they belong to as well as their primary care provider. Once that decision is made, patients must register with their clinic of choice. Patients can still see other providers (e.g., at a walk-in clinic) with no penalty. Through electronic health record systems, their medical information will be sent to their home clinic if they receive care elsewhere. The provider a person chooses will provide the person with centralized care (also called **longitudinal care**), from physical examinations to caring for common medical issues, to providing health teaching and preventative care.

*My Home Team.* A My Home Team is a collaboration between regional health authorities, fee-for-service primary care practices, and community organizations. The My Home Team collectively and collaboratively plans, develops, and provides enhanced primary care services for a specific community area or population group. My Home Teams share common and

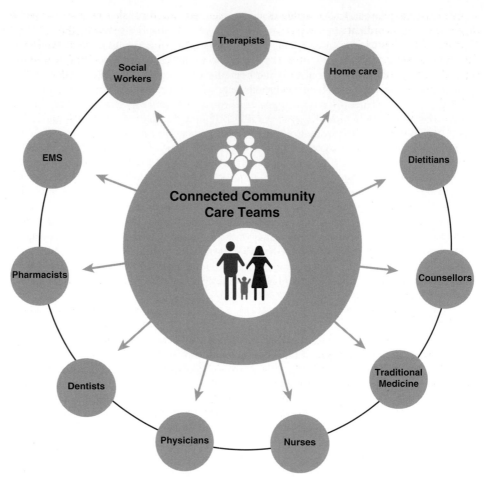

**Fig. 3.2** Health networks: Connected Care Strategy. *EMS,* Emergency medical service. (Source: Saskatchewan Health Authority. (n.d.). *Health networks in Saskatchewan* (p. 18). https://www. saskhealthauthority.ca/sites/default/files/2021-04/Presentation-2019-09-TBC-HealthNetworksPhysician-v01.pdf)

standardized resources, information, and responsibilities, providing primary care services to their collective patients in a timely, efficient manner (Manitoba Health, n.d.; Winnipeg Regional Health Authority, 2022).

The structure of and services offered by each team are determined by the needs of the population the team serves. This includes expanded hours, mobile and outreach services, as well as mental health support and group counselling sessions. In addition, the teams will organize public health and home care services. Note that as these teams are still being developed, they will not all be able to offer a full range of services until they become more established.

***Shared health in Manitoba.*** Shared Health Manitoba was established as a result of recommendations from a Provincial Clinical and Preventive Services Planning Report in 2015 (the Peachey Report) (Peachy, 2017) and a KPMG Sustainability and Innovation Report, submitted in 2017 (KPMG, 2017).

In Manitoba, Shared Health facilitates patient-centred care through strategies focused on organizing and coordinating integrated preventive care across the primary care spectrum (Friesen, 2017; Shared Health Manitoba, 2022b). Through patient-centred care, services are delivered to communities in response to the health needs of each community in addition to supporting a centralized administrative structure.

## Ontario

In Ontario, the Ministry of Health and the Ministry of Long-Term Care collectively remain responsible and accountable for publicly funded health care in the province (Government of Ontario, 2022). Until 2019, 14 corporations called *Local Health Integration Networks* (LHINs) were responsible for implementing health care services for designated regions across Ontario; they were based on a population health/health promotion approach. These nonprofit organizations, responsible to and funded by the Ministry, operated within the scope of agreements negotiated with the Ministry. The function and responsibilities of the LHINs were similar to those of RHAs in that they were directly responsible for organizations ranging from hospitals, community support service organizations, and mental health services, to primary care, and community access centres (the point of entry for Ontarians to apply for home care and admission to long-term care facilities).

In early 2019, the Ontario government (under the *Peoples Health Care Act 2019*) implemented sweeping changes to the structure of the provincial health care system. Health agencies and organizations were rolled into a single "super" agency called *Ontario Health*. Ontario Health is headed by a CEO and a board of directors. The 14 LHINs were reduced to 5 to accommodate transition of funding and responsibilities to Ontario Health and ultimately integration into Ontario Health Teams (Team Dapasoft, 2019).

Ontario Health Teams (slowly replacing LHINs), which numbered 52 in January 2023, are made up of a number of local providers such as hospitals, primary care organizations, home care agencies, and mental health agencies (Government of Ontario, 2019). To form a Health Team, candidates must apply to the Ministry for the designation. If accepted, they receive an integrated funding envelope and enter into an agreement of accountability with the Ministry. Each team is responsible for a smaller geographic area than the LHINs were; they are able to provide more focused and individualized health services to smaller communities. The end goal is to have approximately 50 teams across Ontario when the program reaches maturity. Other changes are ongoing. For example, in 2021 the Ministry transferred the Trillium Gift of Life Network and nonprofit care from the LHINs to Ontario Health.

Modernizing and improving home and community care services in the province is one of the Ministry's priorities, also addressing challenges that surfaced during the COVID-19 pandemic (Ontario Ministry of Health and Ministry of Long-Term Care, 2021). In 2021, the government resumed the transfer of home and community care services to Ontario Health, which was delayed because of the pandemic. The transition remains in progress and will take time in order to minimize disruption of services. LHINs, until the transition is complete, will operate under a new name: Home and Community Care Services, and will function in much the same way until the LHINs are phased out and the organization's transition to Ontario Health Teams is complete.

### Primary Care

Currently, primary care in Ontario is delivered through a number of different primary care organization models. There are more similarities than differences in how health care is delivered by any of these models. They all deliver care using an interprofessional team-based approach. Major differences are related to specific responsibilities of team members, mix of

---

**BOX 3.5   Aboriginal Health Access Centres in Ontario**

Fashioned after community health centres, Aboriginal Health Access Centres are community-based and community-led primary care organizations. They provide a range of primary care services that combine traditional healing, cultural programs, health promotion, and community development programs as well as social services to Indigenous communities. Other services include addiction counselling, traditional healing practices (instead of Western medicine), mental health support, and youth employment.

Source: Based on Alliance for Healthier Communities. (n.d.) *Aboriginal Health Access Centres.* https://www.allianceon.org/aboriginal-health-access-centres#main-content

---

health professionals on the team, remuneration, and administrative management. Primary care enrollment models and Community Health Centres are discussed in more detail in Chapter 5.

As of January 2022 there were 297 organizations across Ontario that provide primary health care services in interprofessional team-based care (187 Family Health Teams [FHTs], 75 Community Health Centres (CHCs), 25 Nurse Practitioner-Led Clinics (NPLCs), and 10 Aboriginal Health Access Centres (AHACs) (Box 3.5), and there are now other new Interdisciplinary Indigenous Primary Care Teams (M. Perrin, personal communication, November 26, 2021).

At present, Ontario Health Teams will not affect models of primary care delivery. The goal at maturity of Ontario Health Teams will be a single fiscal and clinical accountability. As yet, it is unclear how this will impact Ontario Health Insurance Plan (OHIP) billing providers that do not currently have accountability agreements with the Ministry of Health/Ontario Health.

In primary care, FHTs, NPLCs, and AHACs have accountability agreements with the Ministry of Health (Primary Health Care Branch) and the CHCs have multiservice accountability agreements with Ontario Health (formerly with LHINs).

***Indigenous primary health centres.*** Indigenous Health Care Centres were introduced in Ontario in 2021. They are culturally based, Indigenous-informed health care organizations with the goal of providing Indigenous people across Ontario with culturally safe and unbiased primary care services. Services are based on a health and wellness needs-based approach to care. These centres are "status" neutral, supporting Indigenous people on and off reserves. Membership includes AHACs, Aboriginal Community Health Centres (ACHCs), other Indigenous-governed providers, and partnering Indigenous health researchers and scholars (Indigenous Primary Health Care Council, n.d.).

---

**DID YOU KNOW?**

***A Course in Culturally Safe and Appropriate Care***

The Indigenous Primary Care Health Council has created a learning opportunity called Foundations of Indigenous Cultural Safety. The course is for individuals working in health care teaching the importance of providing care to Indigenous people that is both culturally appropriate and safe. The course is 3 hours in length and available online through the Indigenous Primary Care Health Council (https://www.iphcc.ca/ontario-ics-program/). British Columbia also has a cultural safety course available for health care providers called the San'yas Indigenous Cultural Safety Training Program (https://sanyas.ca/).

## Québec

The Québec Health and Social Services System is comprised of two management levels, the Ministère de la Santé et des Services sociaux, which oversee health care in the province, sharing responsibilities with health and social services networks. These are spread over 18 health regions. The goal is to both maintain and improve the health of the population in each region using a population-based approach. This is accomplished through improved access to a wide range of integrated health and social services.

Integrated health and social services centres (CISSS) and integrated university health and social services centres (CIUSSS) lie at the heart of local networks collaborating with numerous agencies and organizations to meet the health and psychosocial needs of Québec residents. They include different types of establishments such as hospitals, local community service centres (e.g., family medical groups and medical clinics), residential and long-term care centres (CHSLDs), youth centres, rehabilitation centres (for those with either physical or intellectual disabilities), centres for individuals suffering from substance use disorders, as well as communication organizations. Of note, CIUSSS centres are located in a health region where a university offers a full undergraduate medical program or operates a centre designated as a university institute in the social field.

These networks provide comprehensive, accessible health care services to the populations in their region by, at least in part, constructing service agreements with partners and stakeholders within their local service region. University centres ensure seamless access to primary, secondary, and tertiary care and adequate follow-up for the populations they serve.

Primary care is offered through various primary care delivery models. These include medical groups, which are groups of primary care doctors who work with other health and social service professionals (Government of Québec, 2022). If a patient's doctor is unavailable, they can see another doctor within the group.

In the university family medical group, supervised care may be rendered by family medical residents, interns, and students, as well as students from other health-related disciplines.

Medical clinics and local community services centres offer a range of services on-site, in schools, or in workplaces. Services range from wound care and dressing changes, vaccinations (e.g., influenza, COVID-19, or childhood immunizations), and psychosocial services to preventive care programs and chronic disease management (Government of Québec, n.d.)

The organizations work with interprofessional teams of health professionals. Patients who are not registered at a clinic (or whose doctor is unavailable) can usually get an appointment at a super clinic. These clinics offer a variety of primary care health services for all but urgent health matters.

For psychosocial support, patients can contact their local community service centre (CLSC), which offers the patient individual assessments and referral services for complaints of a social or psychological nature. A psychosocial worker can be accessed at most centres without an appointment during the day and evenings during the week and at specific locations on weekends.

## New Brunswick

The Department of Health in New Brunswick is responsible for all health care in the province, including overseeing the funding, planning, and delivery of selected health care services through the province's two regional health authorities, Vitalité Health Network and Horizon Health Network (Government of New Brunswick, n.d.) A board of directors oversees the operation of each RHA. These RHAs are responsible for hospital services, community health centre services, home and community care services, most public health services, mental health and addictions services, and some tertiary services such as cardiac care and neurosurgery. The Department of Health retains responsibilities for other services such as long-term care and

Ambulance New Brunswick. New Brunswick has also created FacilicorpNB, which is responsible for designated nonclinical services such as health information services and material management (FacilicorpNB, 2015).

### Primary Care

Primary care physicians in New Brunswick practice independently or as a member of a primary care organization called a *Family Health Team* (present in other jurisdictions). The first Family Health Team was introduced in New Brunswick a decade ago. Primary care organizations in New Brunswick, like those in other jurisdictions, rely significantly on nurse practitioners to provide primary care as there is a shortage of primary care doctors in the province. In 2018, Family Medicine New Brunswick introduced a new concept for group practices and clinics operated by a group of doctors, and by 2021 had eight clinics operating in the province. These medical clinics offer after-hour care and a new compensation model and have a focus on recruiting young family physicians. The blended payment model (used in other jurisdictions) is a mix of capitation-based funding and fee-for-service along with additional remuneration if a physician works evenings and weekends. New Brunswick also has a number of community centres.

## Nova Scotia

In 2015, the nine previous district health authorities were merged into one—the Nova Scotia Health Authority (NSHA). Health services are organized through four regions. The NSHA also works with the Izaak Walton Killam (IWK) Health Centre, an independent women's and children's tertiary care hospital, to plan and deliver primary care, community health, and acute care. The new single authority is also responsible for Nova Scotia's Cancer Care Program (Government of Nova Scotia, n.d.).

### Primary Care

Currently, family physicians in independent practice provide care to the majority of Nova Scotia residents. The province has introduced primary care teams, often adding nurse practitioners and other health professionals to an existing practice. Teams include primary care physicians, registered nurses, licensed practical nurses, social workers, and dietitians (Nova Scotia Health Authority, 2021, 2022). There is a shortage of doctors in Nova Scotia (as in other jurisdictions) and the government continues to actively recruit both doctors and nurse practitioners.

## Prince Edward Island

The Department of Health and Wellness in Prince Edward Island (PEI) established Health PEI in 2010 to promote the concept of a "one island" health care system. The island formerly delivered health care under a regionalized delivery model. Health PEI is overseen by a board of directors who are appointed by the Minister of Health and Wellness. Health PEI consists of two divisions: frontline services and systems supports. Frontline services comprise community hospitals and primary health care, including five primary health care networks, home and long-term care, and mental health and addictions services. Systems supports include responsibility for financial services, the management of health information, medical affairs (e.g., residency programs, tissue and organ donation), and corporate development and innovation.

### Primary Care

Primary care in PEI is delivered for the most part through five primary care networks involving health centres (Government of Prince Edward Island, n.d.). The province also has emergency centres offering extended hours for patients as an alternative to going to the ED. In

PEI, a patient's care within an established primary care network is referred to as the patient's medical home (Prince Edward Island College of Family Physicians, 2019).

## Newfoundland and Labrador

The Department of Health and Community Services in Newfoundland and Labrador delivers provincial health care through four RHAs, which are responsible for health promotion and disease prevention initiatives, family and rehabilitation services, addictions and mental health, public health, ambulance services, and both acute and long-term care. Also operating under this department are numerous divisions with unique roles and responsibilities (e.g., Memorial University Medical School, the Newfoundland and Labrador Centre for Health Information Services, the Department of Health and Wellness, and the Medical Services Division). The Department of Health and Wellness provides leadership, policies, planning, and direction for the delivery of health care in the province. In addition, the department oversees health-related legislation and finances. The Medical Services Division is responsible for the delivery of medical, pharmaceutical, and dental services in the province. The RHAs have the authority to grant hospital privileges to qualified doctors.

### Primary Care

In Newfoundland and Labrador, physicians work as independent practitioners or are employed by RHAs working in primary health care teams. The structure and function of primary health care teams are more fluid than in other jurisdictions, with team members and services designed to meet the unique geographic challenges of rural regions within the province. The government's primary health care framework initiative, called *Healthy People, Healthy Families, Healthy Communities (2015–2025),* aims to improve the delivery of primary care services in the province (Department of Health and Community Services, 2014) with four goals in mind. The first is to engage individuals and families to assume responsibility for their own health care (including prevention); the second is to provide a primary care team for every resident in the province; the third is to ensure care is accessible and comprehensive; and lastly, the fourth is to ensure that all services are connected across the health care spectrum. The primary care framework also takes the socioeconomic determinants of health into consideration in developing strategies to improve the health of the province's residents (recognizing the tremendous impact these determinants have on the health of both individuals and population groups).

Providing adequate health care to those living in more remote communities remains a challenge. Physician turnover is high and attracting doctors to the area is difficult. Care is provided through smaller centres staffed by a variety of health professionals, often nurses, nurse practitioners, or both. Doctors visit remote communities on a rotational basis. As within the territories, more remote communities are connected through the use of virtual appointments, phone appointments, and other information technologies.

## Northern Regions

In northern regions, primary care physicians usually practise in larger centres as part of a primary care team working in a hospital or clinic. Physicians visit isolated community health centres on a rotational basis. Nurse practitioners and registered nurses provide most primary care services for population groups within and around their communities.

## Northwest Territories

In 2016, six of the Health and Social Services Authorities were merged into one body—the Northwest Territories Health and Social Services Authority (Practice NWT, n.d.). In 2022, the population in the territory was 45 504 (World Population Review, 2022). The overriding goal was to improve the coordination and delivery of health services with input from residents in the territory. There are two remaining health authorities. The Hay River Health and Social Services Authority will continue to deliver care in its jurisdiction with its own management board, whereas the Tł ļchǫ Community Services Agency will deliver care under the *Hospital Insurance and Health and Social Services Act.*

In the Northwest Territories, Yellowknife, Inuvik, Hay River, and Fort Smith are the largest communities with hospitals or health centres. Stanton Territorial Hospital and two primary health care clinics are located in Yellowknife. The hospital in Inuvik has 50 beds offering acute care, rehabilitation, as well as long-term care services. There are nine physicians who visit surrounding communities. Hay River Health Authority has a facility with 19 acute care beds and 25 long-term care beds and assisted living. Other services include diagnostic capabilities such as ultrasound and mammography. There are nine long-term care facilities in the Northwest Territory (Canadian Institute of Health Information [CIHI], 2021).

## Yukon

The vast territory of Yukon consists of fewer people than most midsized towns elsewhere in Canada, with a population of approximately 38,640. This population is expected to grow to 43,000 by 2025. By that time, it is estimated that 18% of the population will be 65 years of age and older, while the portion of those under 25 will decrease to 25%. The majority of Yukon's population (75%) lives in Whitehorse and the surrounding area. The biggest challenge is providing health care to the rest of the surrounding population.

The territory does not have RHAs or similar organizations. The Department of Health and Social Services (DHSS) manages and delivers all components of health care through the following divisions: Health Services, Social Services, Continuing Care, and Corporate Services. The Health Services division is responsible for community nursing and community health programs, including the community health centres, which deliver frontline care. The Continuing Care branch oversees residential and home care in addition to day care and palliative care programs. The territory has three hospitals in Whitehorse (56 beds), Dawson City, and Watson Lake, each with 6 beds (Yukon Hospital Corporation, 2021). The Whitehorse hospital offers a full range of services and access to specialists. The hospital has an MRI scanner and a chemotherapy suite. Primary care is offered at the hospitals as well as at community health centres and nursing stations located in smaller communities. These are primarily staffed by registered nurses and nurse practitioners, most of whom rotate into the community on a 4- to 6-month time frame. The territory has four long-term care facilities located in Whitehorse and one in Dawson City (Government of Yukon, 2022).

## Nunavut

Nunavut spans one-fifth of Canada's land mass and has 25 communities spread across three regions—Baffin, Kivalliq, and Kitikmeot. Approximately 85% of the territory's population of roughly 32,000 people are Inuit. In Nunavut, the Department of Health is responsible for the delivery of health care as well as policy development and legislation governing the health care system. As with the other northern regions, primary care is provided by registered nurses, nurse practitioners, and visiting physicians—with widespread use of videoconferencing. Nunavut has approximately 22 community health centres and 3 regional health centres: Cambridge Bay, Rankin Inlet, and the Qikiqtani General Hospital in Iqaluit.

Iqaluit has a family practice clinic and is the only hospital in Nunavut. Ottawa is the main referral centre. Health care funding is centrally managed and distributed, with a significant portion of expenses going toward medical travel and out-of-territory treatments as a result of shortfalls in infrastructure such as diagnostic and service capabilities. Prompt, equitable access to health care services is more difficult in Canada's territories (Box 3.6).

> **BOX 3.6  Accessibility of Health Care for Indigenous Peoples in Canada's North**
>
> Accessibility to services refers to the reasonable access to health care services relative to where that person or persons live. Geographic location impacts heavily how accessible health care services are. Indigenous people in the territories (primarily Inuit) and First Nations people living in remote northern regions of some of Canada's provinces have access to only basic health care services. Otherwise, individuals must be transported out of their communities (often hundreds of kilometres) to larger centres for treatment, such as for surgery, cancer treatments, even to have a baby. Individuals often must travel alone and cope with their health issues without the support of friends and family members. Some health problems can be dealt with at larger regional hospitals, such as in Yellowknife, Whitehorse, or Iqaluit. If those hospitals cannot treat the individual, they must be flown to hospitals or treatment centres in larger cities such as Ottawa, Winnipeg, or Edmonton.

Continuing care services include two continuing care centres, three long-term care facilities, and a facility for children with disabilities. These beds are continually full, requiring people to be moved out of their communities and sometimes out of their territory for suitable accommodation (Government of Nunavut, 2015). A 2015 continuing care needs assessment in Nunavut estimates that as many as 72 beds will be required by 2035. There is a new facility planned for Rankin Inlet projected to provide varying levels of care, as well as assisted living and residential care (Nunavut Department of Health, n.d.). Long-term care facilities in all of the territories have moved to a homelike, traditional family-oriented model.

## WHO PAYS FOR HEALTH CARE? PROVINCIAL AND TERRITORIAL ROLES

Each province and territory has a method (e.g., premiums, payroll tax, general revenues) of financing health care services not covered by federal funding. Private and volunteer organizations provide significant revenue for specific services or hospitals. For example, when a community hospital builds a new wing, a government grant usually covers part of the expense, while volunteer groups and municipal governments frequently make up the balance. A formal building campaign, often launched by the hospital undergoing the expansion, provides a conduit for donations.

### Health Care Premiums

Each province and territory determines how health care will be paid for, which until recently included health premiums in both Ontario and British Columbia. In 2020, the Government of British Columbia eliminated health care premiums in favour of an Employee Health Tax to help to pay for health care in the province. Ontario is the only jurisdiction in Canada that charges its residents health care premiums.

Premiums are paid for through the provinces' personal income tax system. Premiums, in most cases, are automatically deducted from an employee's pay, or a person's pension if the individual's taxable income is over $20,000 annually (Government of Ontario, 2021). Those individuals making less than that do not pay anything.

Statis Indians in Ontario must pay premiums if income they earn off a reserve exceeds $20,000, which is taxable income. They do not have to pay premiums based on income earned on a reserve (where their income is not taxable). Ontario offers premium assistance for those who need it, and premiums are income based.

Premiums paid for private health insurance are tax deductible, but those paid to the province of Ontario are not. The payment of premiums and other tax revenues do not contravene the *Canada Health Act* as long as residents are not denied medically necessary services because of an inability to pay.

### Payroll Tax

Some jurisdictions, including British Columbia, Manitoba, Ontario, Québec, and Newfoundland and Labrador, levy a payroll tax. This is a tax collected from employers that specifically raises funds for health care that may extend to education and social services. This is also referred to as a *dedicated tax*. The amount paid depends on many factors. Newfoundland and Labrador have a Health and Post Secondary Education (payroll) tax wherein a 2% tax is payable by employers whose annual remuneration is over a predetermined exemption threshold (Government of Newfoundland and Labrador, n.d.). This threshold was raised in January 2019 from $2 million to $2.3 million. The Ontario government also raised their Education and Health Tax (EHT) exemption for 2020 from $490,000 to $1 million because of "special circumstances" caused by COVID-19 in the province (Rotfleisch, 2021). Saskatchewan's EHT is applied at a rate of 6% on selected goods and services. Employers with a payroll below a certain amount may be exempt; others may pay a reduced amount based on their salary or wage payout.

### Other Sources of Funds

In addition to federal funding (discussed in Chapter 4), provincial, territorial, and municipal governments provide some funds for services such as preventive health measures, medical- and hospital-based services (both inpatient and outpatient), treatment of chronic diseases, home and community and rehabilitation care, and long-term care.

Provincial and territorial health ministries fund and regulate hospitals. They may also contribute financially to community health organizations, services delivered by certain health care providers (other than physicians), and teaching and research institutions.

### Distribution of Funds

Precisely how finances are organized and administered varies among the provinces and territories. In some provinces, for example, the ministry responsible for health care may directly manage hospital and medical insurance, cardiology, and cancer care. Other provinces or territories may establish separate public organizations to oversee and finance these services. Currently, governments in jurisdictions with RHAs provide funding envelopes, at least in part, to their RHA. RHAs in turn finance hospitals and health care services within their regions depending on each area's particular needs. For example, an RHA responsible for hiring community nurses would contract with private nursing agencies to provide care in a certain region. The mix of nurses is also considered (e.g., registered nurses [RNs], licensed practical nurses [LPNs]/registered practical nurses [RPNs], personal support workers [PSWs]). Managing its own funds, each nursing agency would then hire the nurses to deliver care. In jurisdictions with single health authorities, funding is distributed directly to local organizations depending on the structure and function of the model of health care delivery the jurisdiction has adopted.

In some jurisdictions, other ministries provide funds for additional health care—related services. For example, the Ministry of Labour might oversee occupational health matters, and the Ministry of Community and Social Services might provide services (e.g., counselling, group homes, special education) for those with specific health issues, such as learning and physical disabilities.

The provinces and territories also allocate funds to supplementary benefits (e.g., medical supplies, prescription medications, hearing aids). In jurisdictions with a regionalized framework these funds, most commonly distributed through the RHAs, finance regional facilities and services.

During the COVID-19 pandemic, the federal government provided (and continues to provide) funding to all provinces to assist with expenses related to the pandemic, including vaccinations. For example, in July 2021 the federal government allocated $5 billion distributed evenly per capita across all jurisdictions to support vaccination campaigns (Department of Finance Canada, 2021). Provinces and territories are responsible for vaccination rollouts for their own residents.

## PRIVATE AND PUBLIC HEALTH INSURANCE

Third-party health insurance plays a significant role in offsetting the costs of services not covered by provincial and territorial health services. Approximately 60% of Canadians carry private health insurance, provided either through group employment benefits or purchased personally. Group employment benefits cover the employee and their families and dependents for a selection of goods and services deemed not medically necessary, such as vision and dental care, physiotherapy, chiropractic visits, private nursing services, assistive devices, and enhanced medical services (e.g., private or semi-private hospital room). Note that some of these goods and services usually have conditions attached, such as age, income, and some health conditions. Getting private health insurance is not always straightforward; insurance companies, for the most part, require individuals to be in good health. Individuals with high risk factors or pre-existing conditions may be refused private coverage, have restrictions on their insurance policy, or pay significantly more for coverage.

The 40% of Canadians who do not have private health insurance include those who are unemployed, underemployed, or self-employed (all risk factors when considering the socioeconomic determinants of health). Lack of drug coverage appears to be the greatest hardship. For a number of years now, the federal government has been considering the concept of universal pharmacare.

All jurisdictions do offer certain population groups free (sometimes limited) prescription drug coverage, again, usually based on such criteria as age (e.g., those over the age of 65), income, or the overwhelming cost of some drugs deemed medically necessary, which are sometimes called *catastrophic drug expenses* (e.g., biologics).

### Provincial Insurance Plans
#### Eligibility
All of the following criteria must be met for a person to be eligible for provincial or territorial health insurance:
- Canadian citizenship or permanent resident status
- Resident of the province or territory in which they are seeking health coverage
- Physically residing in that jurisdiction for at least 5 months of the year (this criterion varies slightly among jurisdictions)
  Babies born in a given province or territory are insured from birth in most circumstances.
  People with study or work permits, issued under the federal *Immigration and Refugee Protection Act*, may be considered residents for a designated time frame. Permanent residents are not subject to any time frames; a person granted permanent residency has almost all of the same rights and privileges as a Canadian citizen (they cannot vote or hold public office).

Refugee claimants (asylum seekers), protected persons, or convention refugees have limited coverage under the federal government until such time as they are granted permission to remain in Canada.

Terms and conditions for insuring other population groups can be obtained from the provincial or territorial health websites. No Canadian can be denied medically necessary hospital or physician care under any circumstances.

## Application for Coverage

Documents required for provincial or territorial health insurance are similar. Usually, a citizen of Canada must present proof of that citizenship, proof of residency in a particular province or territory, and further (or supporting) proof of personal identification (all original documents). To prove citizenship, a birth certificate, passport, citizenship or Canadian residency card, or similar documentation is required. To show provincial/territorial residency, an income tax assessment, a child tax benefit statement, or a utility or property tax bill is acceptable. Proof of personal identification requires something with a photo ID, such as an employee ID card or a driver's licence. In each province and territory, newcomers must apply to the ministry or department of health for health insurance coverage. The application process and documentation required can vary. Specific instructions for applying for health care coverage can be found on the individual websites of the provincial and territorial health departments. The application processes of British Columbia, New Brunswick, and Ontario are illustrated here as our three families, the J Family (Case Example 3.1(a), the W Family (Case Example 3.2(a), and the L-O family (Case Example 3.3(a)) apply for provincial health coverage.

Documents required by anyone moving to Canada (not previously a Canadian citizen) include Canadian Immigration identification records (or a permanent resident document and record of landing, e.g., entry stamp on passports, or a single journey document). Syrian refugees who resettled in Canada between November 2015 and 2016 were granted residency

---

### CASE EXAMPLE 3.1(A)   The J Family: Applying for Health Coverage in British Columbia

The J family must apply for health care immediately upon arrival in British Columbia. They have several means of obtaining application forms, the easiest of which is to download them from the Medical Services Plan (MSP) website. This family can also call a toll-free number to be connected to the nearest Service B.C. Centre for assistance. Forms can be completed online (the information will be saved on the computer until the form is submitted in case completion takes a couple of days). In addition, a forms-by-fax service is available from the provincial government 24 hours a day, 7 days a week. Coverage begins *3 months* after arrival and showing proof of residency in the province.

To complete MSP enrollment and obtain a Photo BC Services Card, the J family must go to an Insurance Corporation of BC driver's licensing office (effective January 2018). The family must bring several documents, including two pieces of identification such as immigration documents and passports. Since J.J. was born in Canada, he would need to bring his birth certificate. Parents J.J. and A.J. must sign a declaration that they now live in British Columbia and have their picture taken. They must bring documentation for their children E.J. , L.J., and C.J. as well. J.J. wondered about private insurance instead of the MSP and was told that enrollment in the public plan was mandatory, but he could apply for private, supplemental insurance if he wished. Because the J family are immigrating to Canada, they did know that they had the option of arranging private insurance to cover the 3-month wait time.

### CASE EXAMPLE 3.2(A)   The W Family: Applying for Health Coverage in New Brunswick

Q.W. and L.W. may only submit their own application forms for health coverage when they arrive in New Brunswick. The three children can be added to their parents' form (as for all children under the age of 19 in all jurisdictions). Forms can be downloaded and brought to a Service New Brunswick office or completed and sent electronically. Application forms are not to be mailed. Required original documents must be submitted with the application form. These documents include a copy of all Canadian Immigration identification records, an entry stamp on passports, proof of personal identification (e.g., birth certificate or a baptism certificate), and proof of residency (rental or lease agreement). Once their application has been reviewed and the family is considered eligible, they will be issued a letter of confirmation, which will verify the start date of their health coverage (on or close to the confirmation date). Remember that New Brunswick has eliminated the wait period except for Canadians moving from another province or territory in accordance with the reciprocal agreement. It takes up to 8 weeks for their New Brunswick Medical Card to arrive—via mail—until then they use a temporary paper document with a health number.

### CASE EXAMPLE 3.3(A)   The L-O Family: Applying for Health Coverage in Ontario

C.L-O., K.L-O., and their son R.L-O. have moved from Saskatchewan to Ontario, arriving on February 14. Because they are moving from another province their coverage would begin on the first day of the third month after their arrival, which would be May 1 (the balance of the month in which they moved, plus 2 months). However, the family's health coverage from Saskatchewan will cover them until Ontario Health Insurance Plan (OHIP) takes over in accordance with the reciprocal agreement. To apply, they need proof of Canadian citizenship (e.g., birth certificate or passport), personal ID (e.g., driver's license), and proof of residency in Ontario (e.g., utility bill, rental agreement). They can apply for coverage online or fill out a hard copy of the application form and bring it to a Service Ontario centre. Their photo ID OHIP cards will be mailed to them. Their son, R.L-O., who is 15, will also automatically receive comprehensive coverage for prescription medications until his twenty-fifth birthday. R.L-O. will also be covered for medications under OHIP+ until he turns 25, as long as he is not covered by a private insurance plan. It is worth noting that had they moved from out of the country they would have had to wait a full 3 months.

status upon landing, so they would include these documents when applying for health care coverage in the province or territory where they plan to live. Individuals coming to Canada from Ukraine will be granted permission to live and work in Canada for up to 3 years, but not immediate permanent residency status.

Under the *Canada Health Act*, as indicated in the three case studies, the waiting period for health coverage is not to exceed 3 months; therefore, all provinces and territories must comply, although there are some variations. For the most part, coverage will begin on the first day of the third month after a person or family has moved permanently to a jurisdiction. Other regions will require the person or family to wait a full 3 months (the balance of the month in which they arrived plus 3 more full months) as noted in British Columbia (see Case 3.1[a], the J Family in New Brunswick) (see Case 3.2[a], The W Family) has removed the condition of having to wait 3 months for most newcomers.

Under the reciprocal agreement (Box 3.7), health card holders qualify for health care services anywhere in Canada (other than Québec), barring some exceptions; for example, people may not seek elective surgery in another province or seek a service that is uninsured in their province or territory of origin.

## Health Cards

Once an application is approved, the Ministry or Department of Health issues the applicant a health card, identified by a number for the province or territory in which they reside. Some jurisdictions assign a number to a whole family, and later when the children reach a certain age, issue the children an individual health number. Other jurisdictions issue a personal health

---

### BOX 3.7   Reciprocal Agreement

The reciprocal agreement supports the principle of health insurance portability (see Chapter 1) among the provinces and territories. Through the agreement, a person's province of origin will pay for required health services in another province or territory at the rates imposed by the host province/territory. This interprovincial agreement is not mandatory. For example, Québec has not signed this agreement.

As a result of this agreement, Canadians, for the most part, will not face point-of-service charges for medically required hospital and physician services when they travel within Canada. In most cases, a person can receive care in a host province by simply presenting their health card, and the patient's province of origin will pay the host province for services delivery. If you receive health care services in Québec, for example, for a respiratory tract infection, you would have to pay up front for the service and at the rate charged for that service in Québec (instead of the amount paid in your province of origin). You can submit the receipt for the service to the Ministry of Health in your province of origin for reimbursement. See Case Example 3.5.

Source: Based on Health Canada. (2007). *Health care system—Canada Health Act.*

---

### CASE EXAMPLE 3.5   M.K. and Reciprocal Agreements

M.K., a 20-year-old resident of New Brunswick, is visiting friends in Saskatchewan. While there, M.K. developed a severe and persistent sore throat and paid a visit to a local doctor. The cost of the visit in Saskatchewan was $45. The cost of the same service in New Brunswick where M.K. lives is only $35. The doctor's office (in Saskatchewan) submitted a bill to the New Brunswick health plan through reciprocal billing. The New Brunswick health plan will pay the $45 to the Saskatchewan doctor even though the service in that province is $10 less. M.K. pays nothing out-of-pocket for the visit.

Now consider the situation if M.K. is from Québec. If the fee for the same doctor's visit is $35 in Québec, the Québec health plan will pay only $35 to the doctor in Saskatchewan (where the cost was $45), and M.K. will have to pay $10 out-of-pocket at point-of-service. Québec does not honor the host province's or territory's fee schedule if it is higher than its own. However, M.K. could retrieve their money from the Saskatchewan government by submitting their invoice to the provincial health plan.

number to each person. In Ontario, for example, babies are issued an individual health number at birth.

Almost without exception, health care facilities require individuals to present their health cards at the point of service. If the health card does not contain a picture, the person may also be asked for photo ID (e.g., a driver's licence) with a current address. (In many jurisdictions, only providers of provincially or territorially funded health care can ask a person to produce a valid health card; the card itself should never be used for identification purposes.)

Exceptions include British Columbia, where the photo ID card is structured for such purposes. In that province, anyone can replace their existing care-card with a Photo BC Services card. Rather than having two cards (a care card and a driver's license), a person can have the information on the two cards combined into one card.

Health cards are usually electronically validated each time they are presented at point of care. If an "invalid" message appears (e.g., if the card has expired or was reported lost, or if an unreported address change has since occurred), the cardholder may be asked to pay for the service they are seeking. After finding the health card or renewing an invalid one, the person can submit the receipt for the service they paid for to the Ministry for reimbursement. In smaller centres where care providers know the patients, they may make exceptions or not require the person to show their card at each visit. In the same situation, if a health card comes up as invalid and is invalid, the doctor's office may not submit the fee for service until the patient returns with a valid card (not charging the person for the visit).

An invalid health card is much like an expired credit card. Most jurisdictions send a notice to the card-holder well in advance of the expiry date. This date may also show up on the computer when it is validated—if so, the administrative assistant is likely to let the patient know if the card is about to expire.

---

### DID YOU KNOW?

#### *The Use of 'X' as a Choice Regarding Gender Identification*

Since 2016, Ontario has issued health cards that do not identify a person's gender. As of 2017, individuals can put an "X" in the space for their gender on their driver's licence and passports. This is to ensure inclusivity and respect for those who want to remain gender neutral, and also those who have been marginalized with respect to gender identity and nonbinary residents. In 2017, Yukon, Northwest Territory, Nunavut, and Newfoundland and Labrador followed suit, with Alberta and Saskatchewan in 2018, Nova Scotia and New Brunswick in 2019, Manitoba in 2020, and Prince Edward Island in 2021 also adopting this practice.

British Columbia issues each baby a health card with "U" as the gender marker, when requested by the parents; they want the child to decide for themselves what gender to identify with, or even to remain gender neutral.

These changes required amendments to the *Vital Statistics Act* in each jurisdiction. In addition, in all jurisdictions, trans individuals can change their gender without having to have sex-reassignment surgery, which was not always the case.

In 2019 the federal government adjusted legislation enabling Canadians to mark "X" (related to gender) on Canadian identification documents, which include passports, citizenship certificates, and permanent resident cards.

### Health Card Fraud

Health card fraud occurs when a person uses another person's health card to seek medically insured services, when a nonresident of a province/territory falsifies information to obtain or retain a health card, or when a person continues to use health services in a jurisdiction where they are no longer an eligible resident. Health card fraud is a significant problem across Canada, resulting in an enormous cost—in the millions of dollars—to the provinces and territories. It is virtually impossible to detect fraudulent use of older health cards that have no special security features or photo identification. Ontario's old red and white health cards were no longer accepted after July 2020, necessitating individuals to transfer to the more secure photo ID health card. Most jurisdictions now have photo identification health cards for those over a certain age—usually 15 or 16—and increased security measures to protect the information on the cards, such as a holographic topcoat and hidden ultraviolet ink printing that can be viewed only under ultraviolet light. These cards must be renewed at designated intervals, unlike the older-style cards that never expired. Some cards also require signatures. A magnetic strip on the health card contains coded information, such as the holder's name and address. The Manitoba Health and Services Card (also called a registration certificate) was updated in June 2021 and is a paper document with a nine-digit lifetime number (issued to a family or an individual person). The card also has a six-digit personal or family registration number. There is no photo ID.

Lost cards must be reported immediately, as must changes of one's address or name. All provinces and territories have a protocol to follow for lost or misplaced health cards. As soon as a card is reported lost or missing, it is invalid. When the user applies for a new card, they will be issued a temporary document to use until the new card arrives. Often a hole will be punched in the invalid card to signify it can no longer be used. A person convicted of health card fraud under section 380 of the Criminal Code of Canada can be fined thousands of dollars and face prison time.

### Insured and Uninsured Services

Provincial and territorial governments are responsible for administering the health care insurance plan in their jurisdictions. They must decide on a multitude of things, including the need for different types of hospital beds (e.g., acute care, rehabilitation, and long-term care), the mix of professional health care staff, and the structure of the system that will best serve various regions within the province or territory. In addition, the jurisdictional governments approve hospital budgets and negotiate physicians' fees with medical associations.

Under the *Canada Health Act*, medically necessary hospital and medical services are insured everywhere in Canada, in addition to in-hospital care (see Chapter 1). The *Canada Health Act* does not include long-term care, residential and rehabilitation facilities, or home and community care services. These services are under provincial/territorial legislation; as a result, the consistency across the country regarding services offered, the cost of services to the individual, and how they are managed—publicly or privately owned, profit or nonprofit—varies.

All jurisdictions provide supplementary benefits and services outside of the *Canada Health Act*. The governments then determine eligibility guidelines for specific services, funding formulas, and the length of time these services will be insured. Supplementary benefits include health care services such as optometric, dental, physiotherapy, or chiropractic care. In all provinces and territories dental surgery is covered if it must be done in a hospital (e.g., facial or dental fractures, tumours, reconstructive surgery, and other medically necessary reasons). Prior approval is usually required for procedures other than regular dental assessments and care (e.g., fillings).

All provinces and territories provide specific services (e.g., eye care, dental care, drug benefits) to certain population groups, such as those receiving income assistance or guaranteed income supplements and disabled persons. Many jurisdictions also provide some of these services to children of low-income families. Note that there are some differences among jurisdictions in terms of services provided and to which groups.

## Private Health

Despite some strictly private clinics in Canada being perceived as illegal under the principles of the *Canada Health Act*, numerous such clinics and services exist across the country. Some circumvent the legal principles of the Act largely by offering services not technically considered medically necessary (see Chapter 8). For example, private clinics may provide patients with a wide range of diagnostic tests (noted as preventive screening). A good example is when pregnant people want an ultrasound to view their developing baby and sometimes to find out if they are having a boy or a girl (this is outside of any diagnostic imaging that may be ordered by their doctor, which would be covered under the public plan).

### Eligibility to Private Clinics

Private clinics can legally offer (private) services to certain population groups, including Workers' Compensation cases, Federal Government employees, federal inmates, and members of the RCMP, and to anyone living outside of Canada or who lives outside of the province in which the service is being performed. J.J., for example, who lives in British Columbia, could not legally have an elective knee replacement privately in British Columbia, but he could in Alberta because he is not a resident of that province (of course, he would have to pay for the procedure). How private clinics are able to function within legal frameworks is discussed in Chapter 8. There are some "grey" areas that push the boundaries of what is legal.

### Private–Public Partnerships

Private clinics often work in a private/public partnership with the public system in addition to offering completely private services to eligible patients. This occurs when the government in a province or territory contracts selected services, ranging from minor surgical procedures (cataract surgery, for example, or a hernia repair) to laboratory and diagnostic or surgical facilities, usually at no cost to the patient. This is often done to reduce wait times in the public system, as is currently the case as many jurisdictions attempt to "catch up" from the delays incurred during the COVID-19 pandemic.

### Licensing of Private Clinics

Private clinics charge substantial fees to individuals using their services for procedures such as shoulder, wrist, knee, and hip surgery. There are numerous clinics offering these procedures across the country, but most are not allowed to keep a patient overnight. Shoulder and wrist repairs are most often day surgeries. Hip and knee arthroplasties are increasingly being done as day surgeries, but only for patients in good health otherwise, those who are usually younger, and those with the resources to be able to manage at home when discharged the day of the surgery. This is a challenge for individuals who travel out of their province of origin or from out of the country for surgery. As previously mentioned, Québec has more private health care facilities than in other jurisdictions (the types of private clinics operating in Québec with respect to the law is addressed in detail in Chapter 8, as well as the legality of private clinics in British Columbia).

Each jurisdiction that operates private clinics does so under province-specific legislation. Canadian Surgical Solutions is a private clinic in Calgary that is owned by Centric Health and is one of several private clinics across Canada that offers a selection of surgical procedures. The facility is accredited by the College of Physicians of Alberta under the Non-Hospital Surgical Facilities Accreditation to perform inpatient-stay surgical procedures and day-stay procedures. Surgeons at this clinic work in both the public and private system (which is not allowed in Québec). Another example is Gateway Surgery in Calgary, where knee and hip arthroplasties are performed in addition to other services. A person seeking hip surgery must have an initial consultation, which costs $450 +GST. The cost of a hip replacement (2022) is $29,500 +GST (personal correspondence with J. Carson, Surgical Booking Coordinator, Gateway Surgery). This includes all surgical costs, an overnight stay at the facility after the surgery, and all postoperative follow-up appointments, but not travel or accommodation costs. Patients are asked to stay one or two nights in a hotel following discharge from the clinic. Upon returning home, postoperative checkups can be done virtually, and patients can go to their primary care provider for wound assessments, removal of clips or sutures, and other postoperative needs, which for Canadians is covered by the public plan in the province or territory they live in. Follow-up physiotherapy is usually the financial responsibility of the patient.

### Private Clinics and Preventive Care

A number of private clinics offer "wellness" services, which concentrate on healthy lifestyles, illness prevention, and health promotion. These include what are sometimes called "boutique" private clinics operating across the country offering a bundle of public and privately funded services described as a *personalized and comprehensive lifestyle health plan.*

Such groups (e.g., the Copeman Healthcare Centres in Vancouver, Calgary, and Edmonton) charge an enrollment fee and an annual membership fee. For a price (e.g., $40,000) a person can enroll in the "elite" program at Copeman, wherein patients receive the guarantee of prompt access to an impressive team of health care professionals, including primary care providers, dietitians, psychologists, and specialists, along with an array of other services. These may include consultations with a dietitian, genetic analyses, pharmacogenetics, supportive and lifestyle coaching, and strategy planning sessions. Despite the fact that members pay an annual fee, the clinics still charge the provincial plan for a good portion of their services, including office visits and some laboratory and diagnostic tests (Husni et al., 2017).

Fees are generally tax deductible, and many of the services are covered by third-party insurance. Critics of this type of private health care point out that these fees are well out of reach of the average Canadian family.

Other services that Canadians often pay for privately include counselling, physiotherapy, sports medicine, travel health assessments, genetic testing, and pharmacogenomics testing. The emergence of these private clinics raises many concerns (Box 3.8).

### Counselling

Across Canada, counselling and psychotherapy services are woefully underfunded, particularly in the presence of a rising need for mental health services exacerbated by the COVID-19 pandemic. Canadians (of all ages) have been negatively affected by pandemic-related rules and restrictions, including social isolation, stresses related to home-schooling children, working at home, job disruption or dismissal, and financial worries.

Most primary care organizations will offer limited counselling sessions as part of the basket of preventive and supportive initiatives available to patients enrolled or registered with that particular group. Otherwise, private insurance (if a person has a plan) will cover a limited number of sessions. Insurance plans frequently require a counsellor or psychologist to have a certain level of education (usually a PhD), restricting prepaid access to a large number of mental health professionals. Out-of-pocket expenses for an hour of counselling or psychotherapy can be upwards of $100. During the pandemic, many Canadians have found "wellness coaches" online and turned to them for support. Wellness coaches receive a certificate after

---

BOX 3.8 **The Presence of Private Clinics**

Significant concerns exist across Canada about private clinics. At the forefront lies the worry that the availability of private clinics will lengthen wait times for those using the public system because private clinics use the services of physicians and other health care providers who also work in the public system. Some believe that doctors' time in the public system will be lessened; others argue that physicians working in the private sector do so on their own time, thus not interfering with services offered in the public system. For example, in Canada, a surgeon may have only 2 days of operating room time (in the public system) available to them per week, leaving 3 days a week during which they cannot perform surgical procedures. On such days, the surgeon can see patients in a private clinic, performing procedures, thus shortening the wait times in the public system.

**Enhanced Services**

Another concern is that patients paying for **enhanced services** will unfairly move to the top of wait lists because of the additional revenue for the clinic or hospital. For example, in many jurisdictions, a patient having a hip replacement in the public system will receive offers of "upgrades" to a superior product for the replacement part used in the procedure (e.g., titanium), which generates revenue for the hospital.

A private clinic performing cataract surgery for the public system can "bundle" an uninsured laser surgery with the insured cataract surgery. The patient paying for the laser portion of the procedure could be bumped up the list, while someone wanting routine cataract surgery continues to wait.

To what extent a two-tier system will develop in Canada is anyone's guess. The availability of private clinics and services suggests that, in one form or another, a two-tiered system will continue to exist.

---

completing an online program of various length, some of which can take up to 8 months to complete and may or may not have a practical component. Increasingly, psychologists, social workers, and others with educational backgrounds in counselling offer private virtual sessions, which are almost always paid for out-of-pocket.

## INSURED AND UNINSURED HOSPITAL AND MEDICAL SERVICES

### Hospital Services

In the hospital setting insured services for inpatients include standard hospital accommodation, meals, certain medications (in some regions, patients are asked to bring their own medications), operating room and delivery room services, anaesthetic facilities, diagnostic and laboratory services, routine medical and surgical supplies used for hospitalized patients, routine nursing care, and certain rehabilitative services (e.g., physiotherapy received in the hospital, which varies with jurisdiction). Provincial and territorial plans do not cover private nursing care unless ordered by a doctor, at which point the care becomes medically necessary and is covered. Note that the cost of a private room may be covered by the provincial or territorial plan under some circumstances (e.g., for patients who have infectious diseases such as COVID-19 requiring isolation or for compassionate reasons).

Insured outpatient hospital services include emergency treatment, day surgery, diagnostic and radiological procedures at a hospital or at private diagnostic centres (e.g., outpatient cancer or orthopedic clinics). In addition, most jurisdictions insure physiotherapy, occupational therapy, and respiratory therapy services for a limited period if deemed medically necessary.

## Medical Services

Under the *Canada Health Act*, medically necessary care provided by a medical doctor (i.e., primary care provider or specialist) is an insured service. Rules also govern insured services provided by a specialist. For instance, in most provinces and territories, a doctor must refer a patient to a specialist; the patient may see the specialist again for the same problem within a calendar year. After that, or for a new symptom or complaint, the primary care provider or nurse practitioner must provide another referral. In most jurisdictions, when a patient requests the opinion of a second specialist, the provincial or territorial plan will pay for that visit if the family doctor provides another referral request. After receiving a second opinion, however, the patient would usually have to pay for further consultations even if referred by their primary care provider.

Each province and territory generates its own list of insured services, which is reviewed periodically by the Ministry or Department of Health and the province's or territory's medical association. At this time, some services may be delisted, and others added. Since "medically necessary" is subjective, services vary from one jurisdiction to another. Ontario's provincial plan no longer covers what used to be called an *annual checkup* but now recommends a less extensive assessment, called a *periodic health review* or *visit*, limited to one visit per patient per 12-month period. British Columbia and several other jurisdictions do not cover an annual health exam; rather, the extent of an examination is complaint-driven. Another example involves differences in coverage for cochlear implants and related maintenance, which vary among jurisdictions.

Physicians, especially in primary care groups, may choose to offer a selection of services to their patients that are deemed not medically necessary by their provincial or territorial health care plan. Because primary care groups offer team-based care, these services can include dietary counselling, podiatry services, grief counselling, access to psychotherapy sessions, and a range of preventive care services.

For other noninsured services (e.g., third-party physical examinations required for a work-related driver's license), physicians may bill patients directly, or they may bill a third party—an insurance company, the Workplace Safety Insurance Board (WSIB), or an employer or other payer. The amount a doctor charges for uninsured services depends on guidelines set by the governing medical association (Box 3.9).

---

### THINKING IT THROUGH

#### *Block Payments*

Primary care providers (as well as specialists) are required to inform patients of the price of any procedure, assessment, or treatment *not* covered by their provincial or territorial plan before any uninsured service is carried out. Patients typically pay out-of-pocket each time an uninsured service is performed. Some doctors, however, offer patients an alternative called a *block payment plan*, whereby patients pay a flat fee for selected (uninsured) services over a predetermined time frame, usually not less than 3 months. Examples of such services include medicals for employment or camp, return-to-school or return-to-work notes, and travel immunizations. The physician must not refuse services and must not show preferential treatment to patients who pay block fees.

1. If you had a treatment provided by a doctor, learning afterward that the service was uninsured and that you were required to pay for it, what would you do?

THINKING IT THROUGH—CONT'D

2. Would you be more likely to opt for a block payment plan or a pay-as-you-go plan for uninsured services?
3. If you considered a block fee payment plan, what questions would you have for your provider?

---

## BOX 3.9  Uninsured (Chargeable) Versus Insured Physician Services

| Uninsured Services | Insured Services |
|---|---|
| • Telephone prescription renewal | • Visit to a doctor and prescription written in the office |
| • Travel advice | • Advice or counselling regarding health issues |
| • Missed appointments | • No charge if notice given for missed appointments |
| • Form completion (e.g., passport, driver or pilot fitness test) | • Visit to the doctor and a diagnosis of an illness keeping patient home |
| • Back-to-work or back-to-school note | • Doctor sending pertinent records to a specialist |
| • Faxing or transfer of medical records | • Breast reduction because heavy breasts were causing back and shoulder problems |
| • Nonmedical tuberculosis (TB) skin testing | • Routine childhood vaccinations |
| • TB testing due to possible exposure | • Advice given on a primary care group Telehealth line |
| • Cosmetic procedures (e.g., breast reduction) | |
| • Uninsured vaccinations | |
| • Telephone advice (dependent on practice guidelines) | |

Note: Services that are uninsured vary; many primary care organizations or groups offer "bundled" services, which may include travel advice, counselling (e.g., smoking cessation, dietetics, and grief), prescription renewals, and telephone advice. These groups also may offer wart clinics (wart removal has historically been an uninsured procedure). Third-party physical assessments, certain vaccinations, and completion of most insurance forms often remain uninsured in primary care groups.

## Ambulance Services

In most jurisdictions, land and air ambulance services are either under regional management, and costs are shared with the provincial or territorial government, or these services are delivered privately through performance-based contracts. Because ambulance services are not addressed in the *Canada Health Act*, provinces and territories can establish their own guidelines, including fee schedules for these services.

People using an ambulance even for medically necessary reasons may be responsible for a **copayment** (Case Example 3.1(b) The J Family). However, fees are not usually charged for transportation between hospitals—whether the destination hospital is within a short distance, in another part of the province, in another province altogether, or outside of the country—as long as the transfer is for medically necessary reasons (Case Example 3.1(c) The J Family).

### CASE EXAMPLE 3.1(B)   The J Family: J.J. Seeking Medical Care

While tobogganing with his children, J.J. fell and broke his ankle. He was transported by ambulance to the local hospital for treatment. J.J. was responsible for a copayment of $80 for the ambulance service.

### CASE EXAMPLE 3.1(C)   The J Family: A.J. Delivers Her Twins

When A.J. went into labour with her twins 8 weeks before her due date, her husband brought her to St. Paul's Hospital in Vancouver. The obstetrician determined that delivery was inevitable and contacted bed management (called *patient flow* in some jurisdictions) to find two beds in a neonatal intensive care unit (NICU) for the babies when they were born. The BC Patient Transfer Network (BCPTN) coordinates services in the province to ensure patients get the type of bed and care they will need. The response was that there were no NICU beds available in the province. The BCPTN found space for the babies and A.J. in the Regina Regional Hospital, which is the tertiary centre for neonatal services for southern Saskatchewan. A.J. was transported by air ambulance to Regina where she delivered two small but generally healthy baby girls who required ventilation and supportive care for well over a week. Ten days later, A.J. and her babies were returned to Vancouver General Hospital. The British Columbia medical services plan covered the entire cost of the round-trip air ambulance because the province was unable to meet A.J.'s medically necessary needs at home—as outlined in the *Canada Health Act*. All required care was also paid for by the British Columbia medical service plan.

Interfacility transfers (e.g., from one long-term care facility to another) usually require a copayment. Most jurisdictions either reduce or eliminate the copayment for low-income individuals and families.

Copayments (also sometimes called *user fees* or *service fees*) vary, and all jurisdictions exempt some people from them, including individuals in long-term care facilities or on provincial or territorial subsidized programs. Ambulance services are sometimes used to transport individuals from one location to another when ambulance services are not actually medically required (e.g., the patient is medically stable but does need varying amounts of assistance). There are numerous "patient transport" options becoming more available that are being used for transporting suitable patients instead of using an ambulance.

### Coverage for Non-physician Providers

Services provided by midwives and nurse practitioners are insured by public health plans, although remuneration formulas differ. In all jurisdictions, optometrists are paid by public plans for services rendered under certain conditions such as the age of the patient and the presence of an eye condition requiring medically necessary care. Glasses are not covered. Services rendered by other non-physician providers (e.g., chiropractic, massage therapy, podiatry, nonsurgical dental services, counselling [other than by a psychiatrist], and physiotherapy) may be partially covered by the province or territory, covered by private insurance, or paid for by the patient.

## Continuing Care Health Care Services

Continuing care includes home, long-term, and community care services, although continuing care is often used synonymously with long-term care.

### Long-Term Care

Long-term care facilities (see Chapter 1) include 24/7 accommodation, including meals, nursing and medical care, and as well as other services to individuals no longer able to live on their own. These facilities offer residents more comprehensive care than retirement homes provide. Long-term care facilities may be owned and operated by private corporations (either profit or nonprofit), municipal councils, churches, or ethnic, cultural, or community groups. These facilities are overseen by one or more pieces of legislation. The province or territory sets standards of care in long-term care facilities and performs regular inspections to ensure these standards are met. Long-term care facilities are encouraged to seek accreditation through Accreditation Canada (see Chapter 2). Funding is discussed in Chapter 4.

### Assisted Living

The Assisted Living Program provides assistance for Indigenous people at home, in group homes, as well as institutional care for eligible low-income persons to keep them independent within their communities for as long as possible (Indigenous Services Canada, 2021).

### Home and Community Care

Home and community care are separate entities, although they share similar objectives and one often supports the other. Both types of care contribute to a person's independence by providing services that allow them to manage at home with either short-term or long-term support. Both home and community care are publicly funded, although the funding formulas vary with each jurisdiction in terms of how much is paid for what services, for how long, and for whom (eligibility criteria). These services are available to individuals of all ages. The point of entry for community or home care services are usually through a case worker or intake coordinator from a community services agency who will assess the persons need and level of care required.

*Home care.* Required services are provided by a range of health professionals, assigned in accordance with the person's needs and may include registered nurses, licensed/registered practical nurses, personal support workers, physiotherapists, or an occupational therapist. The person's care plan is overseen by a case manager or the equivalent, and the care plan is adjusted as necessary. The number of hours of care a person is given varies but is often deemed insufficient by the patient and their family. A person can purchase additional hours of care if available within the community and if they can afford to pay for it. If home care cannot provide all of the services a person needs, the organization will seek out community services to help with the provision of care. Often volunteers, family, and friends provide care where gaps in care exist.

Current challenges facing home as well as long-term care include a shortage of human health resources, long before the COVID-19 pandemic. Many care providers (including registered nurses, registered practical nurses, and personal support workers) left the profession during the pandemic (because of, for example, working conditions, remuneration, or burnout). For a period of time, in some regions those individuals who were not vaccinated were either suspended or were terminated, but more recently that criterion was abandoned by many organizations in jurisdictions across the country.

*Community care.* Community care offers individuals a variety of services within their community other than care in the home. This could include transportation a person may need, for example, to a doctor's appointment, for diagnostic tests, or to go grocery shopping. Other community services include day care programs, adult day care, and food provision such as meals-on-wheels. Meals-on-wheels is run by volunteers; recipients of the meals are required to pay a modest amount for the meals they receive.

Other home and community-based programs include the following:

- *Respite care* offers short-term relief for family members who are looking after someone who is sick or disabled in the home. Respite care can occur in the home, during a limited stay at a long-term care facility, or at an adult day care program.
- *Assisted living* accommodation usually involves living arrangements that allow a person the privacy of their own living space but offers meals, housekeeping, and other supports as required. Some jurisdictions require an eligible person to be medically and physically stable and able to move independently or with minimal assistance. A person in assisted living might have, for example, a physical disability, a mental health diagnosis, or mild dementia.
- *Group homes* allow adults with disabilities to live in a group environment, usually a house that provides the person with personal care and supervision. In some jurisdictions (e.g., in Saskatchewan), the person or their family are asked to pay a base fee for the accommodation while the government pays for support staff.
- *Palliative care*: *Palliative* refers to relieving a patient's symptom without dealing with the cause of the pain (or the patient's diagnosis). A patient does not have to be in an end-of-life situation to receive palliative care. Thus, palliative care comprises specialized care for individuals who have a serious or life-threatening illness. It is meant to support individuals through an illness or end-of-life situation, improving their quality of life. Services provided include pain and symptom management, emotional support, and counselling for the patient as well as for their loved ones. For individuals receiving end-of-life care, the wishes of the patient are followed as closely as possible. For example, the patient may want comfort measures only, refusing interventions, nutrition, intravenous therapy, or even oxygen therapy. Sometimes a palliative patient will reach a point in their journey where they request conscious sedation or medical assistance in dying (see Chapter 9).
- *Hospice care* is provided in a homelike setting for individuals not expected to recover from an illness or medical condition and facing an end-of-life situation. A hospice is an alternative for those unable or unwilling to die at home or in another health care facility such as a hospital. Individuals are cared for by a team of health professionals who specialize in various aspects of care required. Physicians and nurses manage pain and symptom control, while other health professionals offer grief counselling and provide emotional support to the patient and their family. When a community or region builds a hospice, funding is often from multiple sources ranging from community resources to municipal and provincial governments. Hospice services include support for the family as well as the person who is palliative. Palliative and hospice services are covered by provincial/territorial health plans.
- *Conscious or palliative sedation* refers to the use of sedative medications to control or alleviate severe pain and intolerable suffering on the part of the patient when a person is close to the end of their life (in the terminal stages of an incurable illness). Palliative sedation is only initiated if the patient requests it (or the person who has power of attorney for personal care on behalf of a cognitively impaired patient ). Sedation is carefully monitored to keep the patient in a state of diminished awareness and in a sleeplike state. Palliative sedation is usually only given in a hospice, hospital, or long-term care setting where the sedation therapy can be continuously monitored (Cherny, 2022).
- *Medical Assistance in Dying* is provided in accordance with the law and paid for by provincial and territorial governments (see Chapters 7, 8, and 10).

## Continuing Care for First Nations and Inuit Peoples

Status Indians and Inuit living on reserves typically have access to home and community care services funded by provincial/territorial and federal programs—for example, those provided by the First Nations and Inuit Home and Community Care (FNIHCC) program, as well as or in addition to the Assisted Living Program through Indigenous Services Canada.

The National and Inuit Home and Community Program funds and develops home care and community programs for Indigenous people living in First Nations and Inuit communities (Indigenous Services Canada, 2016). There is no age restriction. Individuals with disabilities, chronic illnesses (e.g., diabetes, heart disease), acute illnesses and elders requiring care can apply if they meet eligibility criteria.

Eligibility is restricted to First Nations people who live on reserves, in a community north of the sixtieth parallel, or in an Inuit community; the individual's needs must be assessed by continuing care services and require one or more of the services offered. The program offers both nursing and personal care and support, depending on the individual's needs. This includes respite care as well as care (for a predetermined time frame) for individuals who cannot be left at home. Across Canada, non-Status Indians living off reserves have the same access as non-Indigenous Canadians have to home care and community services. As with other publicly funded services outside of the *Canada Health Act*, what amenities are offered vary within jurisdictions. Some bands fund services accessible to those within their own community, others do not.

## Assistive Devices and Medical Products

Those in need of but unable to afford health care products and assistive devices—mobility devices (e.g., wheelchairs, walkers, motorized carts), prosthetic devices (e.g., postmastectomy products, artificial limbs), bathing and toileting aids, and hospital beds and accessories—can receive supplemental coverage; however, the coverage for such items varies across Canada. In most jurisdictions, patients able to pay are responsible for a portion of the cost of selected assistive devices. For those that cannot pay, the cost is absorbed by the public plan. For example, Alberta offers two income-based programs: the Alberta Aids to Daily Living (AADL) and the Dental Assistance for Seniors programs. The AADL offers financial support to eligible patients.

## DRUG PLANS AND THE COST OF MEDICATIONS

Medications consume a huge portion of the health care dollars spent across Canada, second only to hospital spending. The immensity of this expenditure stems in part from the use of newer, more expensive medications and an aging population with chronic diseases and multiple health problems who are prescribed an astonishing array of medications. More detail about drug costing is discussed in Chapter 4.

As mentioned earlier in the chapter, all provinces and territories across Canada offer publicly funded prescription medication programs (often called *pharmacare*). Criteria will vary among jurisdictions, but generally this includes individuals on social assistance, anyone who must make payments that are disproportionate to their income, and individuals over the age of 65. In the province of Manitoba pharmacare is strictly based on household income regardless of age. For example, individuals over 65 must pay for private insurance for medications or pay up to the required amount based on income. For anyone on the welfare system all medications are fully covered.

In Québec, every permanent resident must have prescription drug insurance. They can obtain the insurance through private plans or through employee benefits packages. Alternatively, a person can obtain insurance through RAMQ's Public Prescription Drug Insurance Plan.

As discussed previously, an estimated 60–70% of working Canadians have some type of private or employer-sponsored insurance plan with drug benefits. However, many jobs available now are contract positions with no benefits; in addition, a number of Canadians are changing jobs more frequently than in the past. These trends mean that the security of having employer-subsidized benefits are limited or nonexistent, leaving more Canadians in the position of having to buy private health insurance, or rely on the public system if they cannot afford the cost or their prescription medications (or they go without them).

### Deductibles and Dispensing Fees

Most private drug plans are fairly comprehensive, but public plans insure only certain medications. Both publicly funded drug benefit packages and private insurance plans have copayments or **deductibles** (usually percentage based) that beneficiaries pay, depending on their income and medication costs. As a rule, jurisdictions require the family or individual to pay a predetermined deductible for prescription medications. Once the deductible is reached, the public plan will pay a percentage of the beneficiary's eligible medication costs. Some jurisdictions also set a maximum amount, or a "cap," that the family or person must pay, after which point the plan will cover the costs.

Private insurance plans also require beneficiaries to pay **dispensing fees** themselves. For individuals on a public drug plan, the dispensing fee is either calculated as a percentage of the prescription cost or set at a flat rate, depending on the plan.

### Drug Plans, Formulary and Nonformulary Drugs

To qualify for provincial or territorial drug benefits, an individual must first apply for assistance. Primary care providers and sometimes pharmacists can assist an individual to navigate their way to the appropriate organization where they can get more information and fill out an application. Provinces/territories also provide that information online.

Some plans (both private and public) will cover only medications prescribed from a **formulary list**. Formulary lists, although they include hundreds of medications, have some limitations, containing for the most part generic versions of more frequently used medications. Some brand-name drugs may be covered, but only if there is not a less expensive alternative. Combination drugs and time-release drugs, for example, are more expensive. Most "lifestyle drugs" are not covered, such as drugs used for erectile dysfunction, drugs to treat obesity, to prevent hair loss, and also cosmetic drugs. Some antibiotics and inhalers used for asthma are excluded. The general thought is that there are less expensive drugs available that will be effective. However, most plans will cover a nonformulary drug if the generic drug does not produce the desired therapeutic effect or causes adverse effects (Case Example 3.2(b) The W Family). Providers prescribing the medication must seek approval to prescribe a nonformulary

---

### CASE EXAMPLE 3.2(B)    The W Family: Q.W. and Nonformulary Drugs

Q.W. is receiving assistance through pharmacare because he does not yet have a job. He has developed an irregular heartbeat, and his doctor put him on Aspirin for its anticoagulant effects. Within days, Q.W. developed a pain in his stomach and other gastrointestinal (GI) symptoms. The doctor decides that the Aspirin is causing the GI upset and wants to switch him to clopidogrel bisulfate (Plavix)—another medication to prevent clots. This medication is on a limited use list (LU) on the New Brunswick drug formulary list. The doctor fills out a special request form so that pharmacare will cover the drug. The doctor must note the **drug identification number (DIN)** and explain the situation before the request is considered and potentially approved.

drug. Nonformulary drugs also are likely to include high-cost drugs or drugs with a high potential for misuse. Many private insurance plans offer an "open access" plan that will insure all prescription medications approved by Health Canada that are prescribed on an outpatient basis. Drugs are constantly being added to the formulary list; for example, new medications used to prevent blood clotting (anticoagulants).

## Limited Use Drugs

Each formulary includes a limited use (LU) list, which lists drugs deemed unsuitable or too expensive to be on the formulary list. These drugs may, however, have therapeutic benefits in special circumstances—for example, an antibiotic that can treat resistant bacteria.

Some medications are not on either the formulary or the LU list. The prescribing provider must seek special permission to have these drugs covered by a publicly funded drug benefit plan. Some biologics that are used to treat inflammatory diseases (e.g., inflammatory bowel disease and rheumatoid arthritis) require special permission. Medications used to treat the following conditions (in no particular order) were the costliest: cancer treatment (neoplastic agents), antineovascularization medications (e.g., for the wet form of macular degeneration), anti-inflammatory drugs, antivirals (for hepatitis C), and protein pump inhibitors (for gastric problems).

---

### THINKING IT THROUGH

#### *The Cost of Prescription Drugs*

A growing number of Canadians cannot afford the out-of-pocket cost of some prescription medications—many choosing not to fill prescriptions. Medications for some individuals cost up to or more than $100,000 per year for one person, and the person may be required to take the medication for the rest of their life.

1. Do you think the public system should cover the cost of all medications, no matter the price?
2. What provisions are there in your jurisdiction to assist individuals who can't afford the cost of their medications?
3. Are there any provisions to assist individuals "caught in the middle" (those who do not qualify for provincial medication assistance because of their income, but who still cannot afford the cost of their medications)?
4. What do you think are the risks and benefits of a national pharmacare plan? Should everyone be eligible even if cost is not a barrier?

---

## SUMMARY

3.1 Universal health care, means that all eligible citizens of a particular country have insured health coverage, which can be achieved through a variety of health care plans in each province or territory. In Canada, adherence to the principles and conditions of the *Canada Health Act* binds the provinces and territories to a set of predetermined obligations for health care delivery. Each Ministry of Health is overseen by a Minister of Health and one or more deputy ministers. Medically necessary care is delivered on four levels: primary, secondary, tertiary, and quaternary care.

3.2   Jurisdictions delivering health care through regional health organizations or authorities do so using a decentralized framework administered through regional health authorities or a single health authority wherein the Ministry of Health is responsible for the overall manner in which health care is delivered. Either way, these health authorities assess the type and mix of services appropriate for a geographic area and support services that meet the needs of that region (e.g., the region may have an older population and need more long-term care and community services; another may need more primary care services). Evidence-informed studies have determined which model works best.

3.3   The manner in which primary health care services are delivered among provinces and territories has many similarities. Most jurisdictions have moved (or are in the process of moving) to delivering care through primary care groups based on a interprofessional team approach. Primary care networks, primary care teams, community health centres, and a variety of clinics are some of the models being used. There are nurse practitioner—led clinics in most jurisdictions, particularly in rural and more remote regions. Most delivery models offer extended hours, health promotion and disease prevention initiatives, as well as access to virtual and telephone visits. Care is more centralized, offering individuals longitudinal care that is patient-focused and individualized. Health care in the territories is delivered by nurse practitioners and visiting physicians. All too often, individuals have to leave their communities to receive health care services unavailable close to where they live, sometimes travelling thousands of kilometres.

3.4   Payment for health care services is provided in part by the federal government. The largest cash transfer is the Canada Health transfer. A blend of taxes at the provincial and territorial level makes up the rest. Only Ontario requires its residents to pay health care premiums. Volunteer organizations across the country contribute significantly to covering the cost of some services (e.g., hospice) and equipment (e.g., CT scanners).

3.5   All those eligible for health care in each jurisdiction receive hospital and medical care deemed medically necessary. Dental care is included only if it is dental surgery done in a hospital (then regarded as medically necessary surgery). Health care deemed medically necessary is somewhat subjective, although most insured services are similar across Canada. For newcomers to Canada and individuals moving from one jurisdiction to another, wait times (usually no more than 3 months) or other criteria apply. Private clinics delivering health care are fairly prevalent across Canada, delivering health care to eligible individuals. In addition, health authorities in most jurisdictions contract out health services to private clinics, mostly minor surgeries and diagnostic procedures.

3.6   Coverage for hospital services for inpatients includes standard hospital accommodation, meals, medications, operating room and delivery room services, diagnostic and laboratory services, routine nursing care, physician care, and supplies required for patient interventions. Midwifery services are also paid for whether the baby is born at home or in the hospital. Care by other providers varies with jurisdiction. Long-term care is covered across Canada, with the costs to the patient and exemptions determined by each province and territory. Home and community care services are also paid for by provincial/territorial health plans, but with varying limits imposed by each jurisdiction.

3.7   Spending on medications is second only to hospital expenditures. All jurisdictions have a drug plan for individuals who meet specified criteria—for example, those receiving financial assistance, those with medication costs disproportionate to their income, disabled persons, and older persons. Almost everyone, including those with private drug insurance, must pay a deductible for prescribed medications.

| TABLE 3.1 | Primary Care Organizations by Province |
|---|---|
| **Province/ Territory** | **Primary Care Organizations** |
| British Columbia | • Delivered through urgent and primary care centres (UPCCs)<br>• Family health networks where elders are available to offer Indigenous people support, leadership, and traditional knowledge |
| Alberta | • Team-based interprofessional primary health services led by a physician or nurse practitioner<br>• Delivered through three models: primary care networks, community health centres, and family care clinics |
| Manitoba | • Delivered through home clinics and My Health Teams, delivering patient-centred care to patients within their own community<br>• Collaboration between regional health authorities, fee-for-service primary care practices, and community organizations |
| Saskatchewan | • Primary care networks with interprofessional health teams<br>• Health care is delivered on the basis of the needs of each community<br>• Health care teams (working with primary care networks) provide each network with information to help the network tailor care to community needs. This includes demographics (age) and statistics regarding the prevalence of chronic diseases within a community. |
| Ontario | • Delivered through family health teams, family health networks, family health groups, family health organizations, and community health centres. Aboriginal health access centres and Indigenous primary health care teams<br>• Interprofessional teams that provide in-person care, home visits, the ability to book online appointments, virtual appointments, and phone visits |
| Québec | • Delivered through medical groups, the University Family Medical Group, medical clinics, and local community services centres<br>• Multidisciplinary teams deliver services in a variety of settings, and patients who are not registered at a clinic (or whose doctor is unavailable) can be seen at "super" clinics that offer a variety of primary health services for all but urgent health matters. |
| New Brunswick | • Primary care physicians practice independently or as a member of a family health team and rely heavily on nurse practitioners because of the shortage of family physicians.<br>• Established in 2018, new group practice clinics offer after-hour care, a new compensation model, and focus on recruiting young family physicians. |
| Nova Scotia | • Family physicians in independent practice provide care to the majority of Nova Scotians.<br>• Primary care teams are a new development and often include nurse practitioners, registered nurses, licensed practical nurses, social workers, and dietitians. There is also a shortage of doctors in Nova Scotia. |
| Prince Edward Island | • Delivered through five primary care networks and provided by primary care physicians and health centres |

*Continued*

| TABLE 3.1 | Primary Care Organizations by Province—cont'd |
|---|---|
| **Province/ Territory** | **Primary Care Organizations** |
| Newfoundland and Labrador | • Delivered by independent practitioners or primary health care teams<br>• The structure and function of primary health care teams is fluid, with team members and services being designed to meet the unique geographic challenges of rural regions in the province |
| Northern Regions | • Delivered by primary care physicians practising in larger centres as part of a primary care team in a hospital or clinic<br>• Physicians visit isolated community health centres on a rotational basis and nurse practitioners and registered nurses provide most primary care services. |
| Northwest Territories | • Delivered by primary care physicians in communities with hospitals and health centres<br>• Physicians also visit surrounding communities |
| Yukon | • Delivered primarily by nurses and nurse practitioners in hospitals, community health centres, and nursing stations in smaller communities<br>• Nurses and nurse practitioners rotate into communities on a 4- to 6-month time frame |
| Nunavut | • Delivered by nurses, nurse practitioners, and visiting physicians in community health centres and regional health centres with widespread use of videoconferencing<br>• Ottawa is the main referral centre, and funding is centrally managed and distributed, with a significant portion going toward medical travel and out-of-territory treatments |

## REVIEW QUESTIONS

1. How would you respond if someone asked you if Canada had a national health care plan?
2. What are the differences among primary, secondary, tertiary, and quaternary care? Give an example of each. Identify a secondary, tertiary, and a quaternary care facility in your region.
3. What were the four common objectives prompting some jurisdictions to adopt a regionalized approach to health care?
   a. Why are some jurisdictions moving back to a central health authority framework?
   b. Does your province or territory use a regionalized or centralized approach to managing health care? In your opinion, is it effective? Why or why not?
4. What happens if a primary care provider prescribes a medication for a patient on a subsidized provincial/territorial drug plan and that drug is not listed on the provincial/territorial formulary of available drugs?
5. Does charging health care premiums contravene the principles of the *Canada Health Act*? Why or why not?
6. What is the purpose of the 3-month wait period in most provinces before a person can become eligible for health care, and who is exempt? Explain your answer.
7. What is the purpose of the reciprocal agreement and how does it benefit Canadians?

8. What types of private health care are available in your jurisdiction?
   a. Are their policies and procedures compliant with the principles of the *Canada Health Act?*
   b. Do you feel that a "two-tiered" health care system could work in Canada without compromising our universal health care plan? What would be the benefits and drawbacks?

## REFERENCES

Canadian Institute of Health Information (CIHI). (2021). *Long-term care homes in Canada: How many and who owns them?* https://www.cihi.ca/en/long-term-care-homes-in-canada-how-many-and-who-owns-them#:~:text=Northwest%20Territories%20has%20a%20total,%3B%20100%25%20are%20publicly%20owned.

Cherny, N. (2022). *Palliative sedation.* UpToDate https://www.uptodate.com/contents/palliative-sedation.

Department of Finance Canada. (2021, July 14). *Federal government delivers $5 billion in pandemic support to provinces and territories for vaccines and health care.* https://www.canada.ca/en/department-finance/news/2021/07/federal-government-delivers-5-billion-in-pandemic-support-to-provinces-and-territories-for-vaccines-and-health-care.html.

Department of Health and Community Services. (2014). *Healthy people. Healthy families, healthy communities: A primary health care framework for Newfoundland and labrador, 2015–2025.* https://www.gov.nl.ca/hcs/files/publications-phc-framework-update-nov26.pdf.

FacilicorpNB. (2015, Summer). *InfoEvolution, newsletter of FacilicorpNB.* http://facilicorpnb.ca/files/Info_Evolution_summer_2015.pdf.

Friesen, C. (2017, July, 3). *New provincial health organization announced.* MySteinbach. https://www.mysteinbach.ca/news/1555/new-provincial-health-organization-announced/.

Government of Alberta. (2021). *Primary network nurse practitioner support program: Program information.* Version 2. https://open.alberta.ca/publications/primary-care-network-nurse-practitioner-support-program-version-2#summary.

Government of Alberta. (2022). *Primary health care.* https://www.alberta.ca/primary-health-care.aspx.

Government of New Brunswick. (n.d.). Regional health authorities. https://www2.gnb.ca/content/gnb/en/services/services_renderer.9435.Regional_Health_Authorities.html#:~:text=see%20Related%20Links.-,Description,and%20most%20Public%20Health%20Services.

Government of Newfoundland and Labrador. (n.d.). Health and post-secondary education tax (payroll tax). *Department of Finance.* https://www.gov.nl.ca/fin/tax-programs-incentives/business/education/.

Government of Nova Scotia. (n.d.). Department of Health and Wellness. https://beta.novascotia.ca/government/health-and-wellness.

Government of Nunavut. (2015). *Continuing care in Nunavut 2015 to 2035.* https://assembly.nu.ca/sites/default/files/TD%2078-4(3)%20EN%20Continuing%20Care%20in%20Nunavvut,%202015%20to%202035_0.pdf.

Government of Ontario. (2019). *Ontario health teams: Guidance for health care providers and organizations.* https://health.gov.on.ca/en/pro/programs/connectedcare/oht/docs/guidance_doc_en.pdf.

Government of Ontario. (2021). *Health premium.* https://www.ontario.ca/page/health-premium.

Government of Ontario. (2022). *Ministry of long-term care.* https://www.ontario.ca/page/ministry-long-term-care.

Government of Prince Edward Island. (n.d.) Backgrounder: Primary care. https://www.gov.pe.ca/photos/original/hw_speechback8.pdf.

Government of Québec. (n.d.). *CLSC—local community services centre.* https://www.santeestrie.qc.ca/en/care-services/general-services/services-communautaires-clsc.

Government of Québec. (2022). *Primary care health and social services.* https://www.quebec.ca/en/health/health-system-and-services/service-organization/primary-care-health-and-social-services.

Government of Yukon. (2022). *Find information on long-term care in Yukon.* https://yukon.ca/en/health-and-wellness/care-services/find-information-long-term-care-yukon.

Husni, S., Khan, Z., MacMillan, R., et al. (2017). *Canada should not allow two-tiered practicing for medically necessary services [web log comment].* https://www.ivey.uwo.ca/healthinnovation/blog/2017/7/canada-should-not-allow-two-tiered-practicing-for- medically-necessary-services/.

Indigenous Primary Health Care Council. (n.d.). About the IPHCC. https://www.iphcc.ca/about/about-the-iphcc/.

Indigenous Services Canada. (2016). *First Nations and Inuit home and community care.* Government of Canada. https://www.sac-isc.gc.ca/eng/1582550638699/1582550666787.

Indigenous Services Canada. (2021, June 8). *Assisted living national program guidelines, 2019 to 2020.* Government of Canada. https://www.sac-isc.gc.ca/eng/1557149461181/1557149488566#chp2.

KPMG. (2017). *The road ahead: The KPMG survey of corporate responsibility reporting,* 2017 https://assets.kpmg/content/dam/kpmg/be/pdf/2017/kpmg-survey-of-corporate-responsibility-reporting-2017.pdf.

Manitoba Health. (n.d.). Home clinics and My Health Teams. https://www.gov.mb.ca/health/primarycare/homeclinic/.

Nova Scotia Health Authority. (2021, October 30). *Collaborative family practice teams.* https://cfpt.nshealth.ca/.

Nova Scotia Health Authority. (2022). *About primary health care.* https://www.nshealth.ca/about-primary-health-care.

Nunavut Department of Health. (n.d.) Long-term care centre: Rankin Inlet. https://gov.nu.ca/information/long-term-care-centre-rankin-inlet.

Office of the Auditor General of British Columbia. (n.d.). Health authority: Overview. https://www.bcauditor.com/online/pubs/775/782.

Ontario Ministry of Health and Ministry of Long-Term Care. (2021). *Connected care update. Health system integration update: Modernizing the delivery of home and community care while maintaining stability of services.* https://www.health.gov.on.ca/en/news/connectedcare/2021/CC_20210317.aspx.

Peachy, D. (2017). *Provincial clinical and preventive services planning for Manitoba: Doing things different and better. Submitted to deputy minister, ministry of health, Seniors, and active living.* https://www.gov.mb.ca/health/documents/pcpsp.pdf.

Practice NWT. (n.d.) The NWT Health and Social Services System. https://www.practicenwt.ca/en/nwt-health-and-social-services-system.

Prince Edward Island College of Family Physicians. (2019). *Patient's medical home implementation kit.* https://patientsmedicalhome.ca/files/uploads/PMH2019_ImplementKit_PEI.pdf.

Rotfleisch, D. (2021). *Canada; Ontario employer health tax (EHT): Canadian tax lawyer's guidance.* Mondaq. https://www.mondaq.com/canada/tax-authorities/1070274/ontario-employer-health-tax-eht-canadian-tax-lawyer39s-guidance.

Saskatchewan Health Authority. (2021). *Health networks in saskatchewan.* https://www.saskhealthauthority.ca/our-organization/our-direction/team-based-care/health-networks-saskatchewan.

Shared Health Manitoba. (2022a). *Home clinics.* https://sharedhealthmb.ca/services/digital-health/home-clinics/.

Shared Health Manitoba. (2022b). *Shared health.* https://sharedhealthmb.ca/.

Team Dapasoft. (2019, November 19). *14 LHINs reorganized into 5 transitional regions in Ontario.* News: Health IT. https://www.dapasoft.com/14-lhins-reorganized-ontario/.

Winnipeg Regional Health Authority. (2022). *Community area profiles.* https://wrha.mb.ca/research/community-health-assessment/community-area-profiles/.

World Population Review. (2022). *Northwest Territory population 2022.* https://worldpopulationreview.com/canadian-provinces/northwest-territory-population.

Yukon Hospital Corporation. (2021). *Our hospitals.* https://yukonhospitals.ca/yukon-hospital-corporation/our-hospitals.

# The Dollars and "Sense" of Health Care Funding

## LEARNING OUTCOMES

4.1 Explain the role of for-profit and not-for-profit organizations in the delivery of health care.
4.2 Outline the levels and mechanisms of health care funding in Canada.
4.3 Examine how hospitals are funded and identify their major expenses.
4.4 Discuss the funding challenges facing home, community, and continuing care in Canada.
4.5 Describe the reasons for, and the effect of, rising medication costs in Canada.
4.6 Discuss health expenditures related to human health resources.
4.7 Summarize the cost of advancing technology to the health care system.

## KEY TERMS

| | | |
|---|---|---|
| **Active ingredients** | **Nonprofit organization** | **Publicly funded health** |
| **Alternate level of care** | **(NPO)** | **care** |
| **(ALC)** | **Positron emission** | **Renal dialysis** |
| **Capitation-based funding** | **tomography (PET)** | **Residential care** |
| **Laparoscopic surgery** | **scanner** | |

Before you begin reading this chapter, write down—even if it is just a guess—what you think Canada spends on health care in one year and how much you think a visit to your family doctor for an intermediate assessment (e.g., for an earache, a sore throat, or a cold) might cost. Next, write down how much you think a knee replacement, a hip replacement, and an appendectomy might cost, or being hospitalized with COVID-19, acute anxiety, or depression. Keep these numbers handy to compare with the figures you will see later in the chapter for the true costs of these services.

Can you imagine going to the doctor for an ear infection and having the administrative assistant ask for cash or a credit card to pay for the visit? Or a parent, aunt, or uncle having cardiac bypass surgery or critically required heart surgery and being sent an invoice? Remember that, in addition to these procedures, the patient would need a preoperative physical examination, blood work, and perhaps an X-ray, magnetic resonance imaging (MRI), an arteriogram, or a computed tomography (CT) scan. They would have to pay for the hospital stay, tests, nursing care, and supportive care (e.g., physiotherapy, respiratory therapy)—and would even be charged for the use of the equipment to remove the sutures and the bandages covering the wound. What would you do if you needed such a procedure and knew it would cost you thousands of dollars? Even worse, can you imagine needing the heart surgery and being denied because you did not have the money to pay for it?

Many Canadians feel fortunate to have insured health care services. When they are sick, they seek care, present their health card, and ultimately receive the medical attention they need. If their case proves urgent, the appropriate care is almost always provided within a reasonable time frame. Most of the time, they do not pay for their care. Many Canadians believe that health care is free, perceived because they do not have to pay at the point of service, at the end of the month, or when discharged from a hospital. The reality is that Canadians do pay for their publicly funded health care services. The money comes from the taxes they pay to all levels of government. Only residents of Ontario pay health care premiums (see Chapter 3).

It is also true that today our health care system is facing extraordinary challenges resulting in long waits for surgery and diagnostic procedures, long waits to be seen in the emergency department, and a shortage of health professionals. Many describe the Canadian health care system as being on the verge of collapse and without the capacity to care for the number of people requiring health care services. Also up for debate is how to meet these challenges. Is more funding the answer? Better use of the funds already in the system? Restructuring of the entire system? Perhaps it is a combination of all of these factors.

This chapter examines the actual costs of health care and how health care is funded. The numerous statistics and dollar values presented are approximate, because costs change yearly, monthly, and sometimes even daily.

## THE ROLE OF PROFIT AND NONPROFIT FUNDING FOR HEALTH CARE SERVICES

The funding and delivery of Canada's health care are accomplished through a mix of public and private—both for-profit and nonprofit—businesses and organizations. *Funding* refers to how health care is paid for, and *delivery* refers to how health care services are managed, structured, and distributed.

In Canada, all medically necessary services are publicly funded but, for the most part, are delivered by either private for-profit or private not-for-profit businesses or organizations. For example, physicians (unless salaried) operate as private for-profit businesses. They deliver health care services and are paid, using varying payment formulas or plans by the government, or both (see Chapter 5). The services they deliver however, are very much controlled by the government.

*Physicians* in private practice pay for their own business expenses, including office space, supplies, and addition to staff salaries and medical software systems (although sometimes these are subsidized by external funding). Physicians who work in and are employed by hospitals are paid by the facility in which they work. The cost of their services comes out of the hospital's budget.

*Hospitals* and other facilities (which include those providing acute care, extended and chronic care, rehabilitation and convalescent care, as well as psychiatric care, and nursing stations or outpost hospitals) are licensed or approved as such either by a provincial/territorial government or are operated by the federal government. Other institutions that are publicly funded include group homes and **residential care** facilities, which also must be approved by provincial or territorial governments. In these facilities, there is a mix of health care and social services provided; most direct patient care is provided by registered nurses, registered practical nurses, and personal support workers (or the equivalent).

Although hospitals are primarily private, not-for-profit organizations, the majority of services in a hospital—food and meal preparation, maintenance, cleaning, security (including cybersecurity), and sometimes IT support, and laundry—are delivered by private, for-profit businesses. The hospital negotiates for cost-effective services and pays for them out of the funds allotted them by the government. The majority of laboratory and diagnostic services are other examples of private, for-profit services. Some nonessential services within a hospital—for example, a semiprivate or private room, television, or telephone—must be paid for directly by the patient or by a third party, such as through private insurance. That said, most patients have cell phones, tablets, or laptops which they are permitted to use in the hospital. Most facilities offer free Wi-Fi access to the internet, but usually with some limitations.

Patients also have choices with respect to some treatment options. For example, if Paul fractures his leg, he can have a plaster cast applied, or opt for a lighter fibreglass cast. If he is having cataract surgery he can opt for a superior-grade lens to be inserted rather than the standard lens. Because the fibreglass cast and the superior lens are considered enhanced products, legally, he can be charged for them. An analogy would be buying a car with standard features and wanting an upgrade (e.g., leather instead of cloth seats), which the customer would have to pay for. A patient must also pay for any diagnostic services or treatment not deemed medically necessary, such as an ultrasound to determine the gender of an unborn baby. Any cosmetic surgery not deemed medically necessary is not covered by insurance (either public or private). Patients are also charged for some laboratory tests that are not included in the province or territory schedule of benefits (e.g., prostate-specific antigen [PSA], vitamin D levels).

## LEVELS OF HEALTH CARE FUNDING

Canada's public health insurance is funded, for the most part, by the federal, provincial, territorial, and municipal governments through a blend of personal and corporate taxes and by Workers' Compensation Boards. Some provinces also use revenue from sales taxes and lotteries for health care. At the community level, many volunteer organizations (e.g., hospital auxiliaries, service clubs) also raise money for local hospitals to support such initiatives as expansion, updating the facilities, and purchasing new equipment or building a hospice. Often the provincial, territorial, or municipal governments will match funds raised or a portion thereof. A significant portion of health care that is not deemed medically necessary is funded privately, through private insurance, particularly services such as massage therapy, physiotherapy, eye examinations, physical assessments requested by a third party, and some eye examinations. Chapter 8 discusses private health care in Canada that is provided in conjunction with the law.

### Federal to Provincial Funding Transfers

The exact dollar figure that the federal government transfers to the provinces and territories is almost impossible to calculate, and the amounts given are continually debated among the jurisdictions. This has become even more challenging given the complexities of the 2016 health accord negotiated between provinces, territories, and the federal government (see Chapter 1).

The exact amount of money spent on health care at the provincial and territorial level is also difficult to determine, in part because of the complexity of the various formulas used to calculate the federal government's transfer payments to each jurisdiction, which are made in the form of both cash and tax points (see Chapter 1). Federal funding mechanisms are calculated using a complex formula and are distributed through four main transfer models, discussed below.

### Canada Health Transfer

The Canada Health Transfer (CHT) is the largest annual cash transfer of funds from the federal government to the provinces and territories and is based on the funding formula discussed in Chapter 1, wherein the amount paid to provinces and territories is tied to the gross domestic product (GDP) and guaranteed not to fall below 3% of the GDP (Department of Finance Canada, 2017). The CHT is estimated to increase from $43.1 billion in 2021–2022 to $55.2 billion by 2029 (Department of Finance Canada, 2021). The CHT payment grew by

**TABLE 4.1    Total Federal to Provincial/Territorial Funding Through Four Major Programs (in millions of dollars)**

| Year of Payment | 2019–2020 | 2020–2021 | 2021–2022 | 2022–2023 |
|---|---|---|---|---|
| Canada Health Transfer | 40,373 | 41,870 | 43,126 | 45,208 |
| Canada Social Transfer | 14,586 | 15,023 | 15,474 | 15,938 |
| Territorial Formula Funding | 3948 | 4180 | 4380 | 4553 |
| **Total Equalization Payments** | **19,837** | **20,573** | **20,911** | **21,920** |

Note that the 2019–2020 and the 2020–2021 payout excludes a one-time top-up to the CHT of $500 million in 2019–20 and $4 billion in 2020–2021 to support the response to COVID-19. Another $1 billion was provided to support vaccine rollout campaigns across the country.
**Source:** Based on Department of Finance Canada. (2019, August 29). *Federal transfers to provinces and territories.* https://www.canada.ca/en/department-finance/programs/federal-transfers.html

4.8% in 2020–2021 (Department of Finance Canada, 2021). See Table 4.1 for year-over-year payouts from 2019 to 2023 by jurisdiction.

### Canada Social Transfer

The Canada Social Transfer (CST) provides funding to the provinces and territories through a two-part payment formula, cash and tax points. The dollar value of the CST transferred is calculated on an equal per capita cash basis to ensure that the funds are equally distributed. Table 4.2 shows the amount of money by jurisdiction for 2022–2023. The CST is supposed to continue to increase at 3% per year until 2024, although there is no current plan to change this beyond that date.

The CST funding targets social programs, including post-secondary education, social assistance, and services programs for children (e.g., child care, early childhood education, and early child development and learning programs). Although provinces and territories can allocate the money as they see fit, it must be assigned to the programs outlined by the federal government. In 2022 and 2023, continued requests by provinces for increased funding (primarily through the CST) were met with resistance as the federal government wanted the jurisdictions to be accountable for how the money was spent, something the provinces opposed. See Table 4.1 for year-over-year increases between 2019 and 2023.

### Territorial Formula Financing

The federal government uses the Territorial Formula Financing (TFF) to calculate money given to the territorial governments for public services. This money is allotted to these jurisdictions because of their unique geography, population distribution, and related high cost of delivering health care and other public services. Funding is provided by the federal government through taxes paid by Canadians across the country.

In 2022–2023, TFF projected payments to the territories are $4.553 billion: $2.037 billion for Yukon, $1.579 billion for Nunavut, and $1.256 billion for the Northwest Territories. The TFF payments are in place of the equalization payments (discussed below) and are calculated by a different formula.

### Equalization Payments

*Equalization payments* refer to the federal-to-provincial transfer of funds to address fiscal inequities among the provinces (note that equalization payments are not made to the territories). Some provinces have more money than others and thus can provide more public

| TABLE 4.2 | Estimated CHT and CST Payments from the Federal Government (in millions of dollars) and Per Capita Allocations for 2022–2023 (in dollars) | | |
|---|---|---|---|
| **Jurisdiction** | **CHT** | **CST** | **Per Capita Allocation** |
| Alberta | $5250 | $1851 | $1592 |
| British Columbia | $6185 | $2181 | $1592 |
| Manitoba | $1633 | $576 | $3706 |
| New Brunswick | $934 | $329 | $4565 |
| Newfoundland and Labrador | $610 | $215 | $1592 |
| Northwest Territories | $54 | $19 | $34,716 |
| Nova Scotia | $1175 | $414 | $4101 |
| Nunavut | $47 | $17 | $48,353 |
| Ontario | $17,532 | $6181 | $1592 |
| Prince Edward Island | $196 | $69 | $4607 |
| Québec | $10,149 | $3578 | $3177 |
| Saskatchewan | $1390 | $490 | $1592 |
| Yukon | $51 | $18 | $28,497 |

*CHT,* Canada Health Transfer; *CST,* Canada Social Transfer.
**Source:** Department of Finance Canada. (2017, February 2). *Major federal transfers.* https://www.canada.ca/en/department-finance/programs/federal-transfers/major-federal-transfers.html

services to their residents. Provinces with less money cannot provide equivalent services and therefore receive equalization payments to ensure that they have sufficient revenues to provide reasonably comparable levels of public services at reasonably comparable levels of taxation. Money for equalization payments, for the most part, comes from federal taxes. Provinces do not contribute money to this program. Moreover, there are no restrictions on how this money is spent. Provinces with more money are sometimes referred to as the "have" provinces and those that have less money, the "have not" provinces.

A province receiving equalization payments will receive the difference between *its fiscal capacity* (i.e., its ability to generate income) and *the 10-province standard* (i.e., the national average). Without equalization payments, these provinces would have to raise their taxes significantly to generate revenue. Table 4.3 shows the amount of money received by eligible provinces from 2022 to 2023.

The concept of equalization payments was established in the Constitution in 1982. The related legislation is reviewed by the government on a periodic basis. The next review is due in March 2024. All provinces are consulted before the program is renewed.

### Controversy Over Equalization Payments

There is controversy among some provinces as to how fair the process is of determining what jurisdictions should receive equalization payments. For example, the Alberta government is dissatisfied with how the federal government determines what provinces receive equalization payments. The government added a referendum question to the ballot during the municipal elections in October 2021 asking Albertans if they wanted the equalization program reviewed (Box 4.1). A majority "yes" vote would mean that Albertans are calling on the federal government and other provinces to enter into discussions on a potential amendment to the Canadian Constitution regarding equalization payments (e.g., how they are calculated and the formula determining what provinces receive them). The ballot results were that 61.7% voted "yes," so the Government of Alberta is pursuing the issue with the Government of Canada.

**TABLE 4.3    Estimated Equalization Payments for Provinces and TFF for Territories 2022–2023 (in millions of dollars)**

| Province/Territory | Amount | Province/Territory | Amount |
|---|---|---|---|
| Alberta | None | Nova Scotia | $2458 |
| British Columbia | None | Nunavut (TFF) | $1859 |
| Manitoba | $2933 | Ontario | None* |
| New Brunswick | None | Prince Edward Island | $503 |
| Newfound and Labrador | None | Québec | $13,666 |
| Northwest Territories (TFF) | $1519 | Saskatchewan | None |
| Yukon (TFF) | $1174 | | |

*Ontario received has not received equalization payments since 2018–2019.
Note: The territories receive Territorial Formulae Financing (TFF) instead of equalization payments.
**Source:** Department of Finance Canada. (2017, February 2). *Major federal transfers.* https://www.canada.ca/en/department-finance/programs/federal-transfers/major-federal-transfers.html

**BOX 4.1    Alberta's Referendum Question**

On October 19, 2021, those voting in municipal elections were presented with a referendum regarding equalization payments: "Should Section 36(2) of the *Constitution Act,* 1982—Parliament and the government of Canada's commitment to the principle of making equalization payments—be removed from the Constitution?"

See the following video for a brief explanation of equalization payments:

CBC News: *The National. How equalization payments work.* https://youtu.be/ys80Xc-esrU?t=72

Sources: Based on Rusnell, C. (2021, October 26). *Elections Alberta posted incorrect information on equalization referendum, law experts say.* CBC News. https://www.cbc.ca/news/canada/edmonton/elections-alberta-referendum-vote-misinformation-1.6225333

### Financing for the COVID-19 Pandemic

In addition to these major transfers, the federal government continues to provide provinces and territories with financial assistance to support initiatives related to the COVID-19 pandemic. Amounts transferred are fluid and respond to changing trends related to variants of the coronavirus and the needs of provincial/territorial health care systems. This makes it difficult to predict, even in general terms, what spending in this category will be in the future.

Provinces and territories collaboratively estimated spending on COVID-19 health-related initiatives was $3.6 billion in 2020 and 22.9 billion in 2021 (Canadian Institute for Health Information [CIHI], 2022a). In March 2022, the federal government authorized the transfer of $2.2 billion as a one-time transfer to address the backlog of surgeries and other procedures resulting from the pandemic. The money has been distributed equally per capita to provinces and territories.

In addition, a new spending category called the *COVID-19 Response Fund* takes up about 7% of the total health budget. This has included federal, provincial, and territorial spending for such activities as treatment, testing, contact tracing (as required), and vaccines. The cost of antiviral medications has been an added expense. By April 2022, Health Canada had authorized the use of the antiviral drugs nirmatrelvir and ritonavir (Paxlovid) to treat symptomatic adults who are at risk of serious illness. These were the first (oral) medications authorized to be taken at home.

There is no doubt that health care in Canada, by federal, provincial, and territorial governments, has changed significantly as a result of the COVID-19 pandemic and will continue to do so over the next few years. There will likely be continued shifts in health care spending as well as spending categories, such as in long-term care. This will include investigating ways to minimize the spread of the coronavirus and its variants and the corresponding mortality and morbidity rates within the facilities. Funding primary care initiatives will also change, as evidenced by the move to virtual and telephone visits between patients and physicians and the increasing roles of non-physician primary care providers. The role of public health is likely to remain more prominent, which will involve continued investments to maintain and advance population health initiatives.

## Trends in Health Care Spending

Canada's total health care spending in 2019 was an estimated $265.5 billion, representing 11.5% of Canada's GDP. This expenditure rose to about $308 billion in 2021, following an upswing in spending in response to the COVID-19 pandemic in 2020. This represents a 12.8% increase in expenditures (three times the growth rate experienced between 2015 and 2018, which was 4.4% per year). The estimated growth rate for 2021 was a comparably modest 2.2%, more in line with prepandemic growth rates.

Over the past few years, spending on health has consumed approximately 40% of both provincial and territorial health care budgets. As a result of the pandemic, health care resources have been strained to almost unthinkable limits, with spending on the health sector reaching heights not seen in recent memory.

The economic decline and the unprecedented spending on health care resulting from the pandemic will undoubtedly result in future financial constraints and have a significant impact on health care spending and system growth.

## Per Capita Spending

A number of factors influence the per capita spending among the provinces and territories, including the services paid for by the public plan (i.e., what is considered medically necessary), the type and extent of social programs, the mix of health care providers delivering health care, the relative age of the population (e.g., community and home care programs), the number of individuals in publicly funded health care facilities (e.g., long-term care), and the population density versus geographic profile of the jurisdiction. Note in Fig. 4.1 that per capita health spending in the Northwest Territories, Yukon, and especially Nunavut is considerably higher than in other jurisdictions. These regions have a lower population base, but their large geographic area and distance between communities make the delivery of health care more complicated and more expensive. For example, population health initiatives, such as doing routine screening for colon and breast cancer and educating people on disease prevention and health promotion, are more difficult to achieve, as is managing diagnosed chronic health problems.

Health-related expenditures of the federal, provincial, territorial as well as municipal governments have increased exponentially over the past two and a half years because of the pandemic. This includes both direct and indirect health spending. The average estimated per capita spending on health care in Canada was $7,932 in 2019 and an estimated $8,019 in 2021 (CIHI, 2022b). Compared to this average, Ontario's per capita spending was lowest, at $7,773, and excluding the territories, Newfoundland and Labrador's spending was the highest, at $9,585 (CIHI, 2021a). Of the territories, Nunavut had the highest per capita spending, at $23,023.

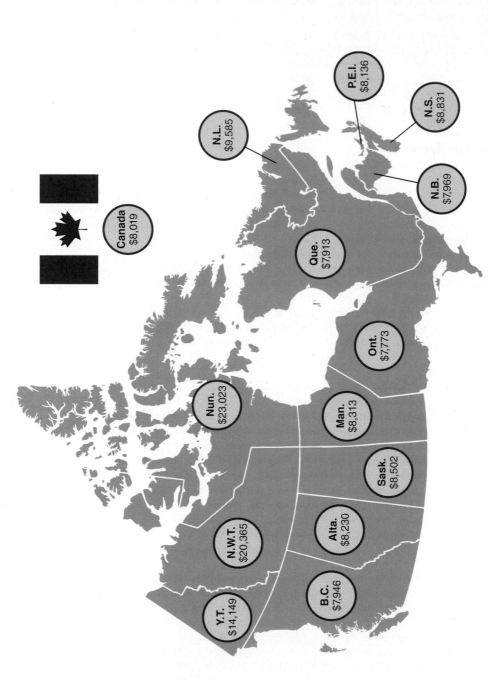

**Fig. 4.1** Estimated provincial and territorial health care spending per capita 2020–2021 (in dollars). (Sources: Department of Finance Canada. (2017, February 2). *Major federal transfers.* https://www.canada.ca/en/department-finance/programs/federal-transfers/major-federal-transfers.html; and Canadian Institute for Health Information. (2021). *National health expenditure trends, 2021—Snapshot.* https://www.cihi.ca/en/national-health-expenditure-trends-2021-snapshot#:~:text=National%20Health%20Expenditure%20Database%2C%20Canadian,2020%2C%20due%20to%20the%20pandemic)

**DID YOU KNOW?**

***How Per Capita Calculations Are Made***

To determine federal and provincial per capita spending, analysts use the most recently revised population estimates, as reported by Statistics Canada. These statistics (found in the Appendices of the NHEX database) are applied to the reported spending data for the respective year and jurisdiction. This is done at a national level as well as for each jurisdiction.

## The Cost of Poor Health

We often think that the cost of poor health relates only to the expenditures associated with direct health care services and treatments required to provide care for individuals who are unwell. Direct health care services include nurses' salaries, the cost of hospitalization, doctor visits, surgery, diagnostic services, rehabilitation, and long-term care. However, loss of productivity and earnings while workers are incapacitated because of a disability or illness is staggering for the general Canadian economy, as well as for individuals. Indirect costs of health care are greatly affected by the socioeconomic determinants of health, almost always negatively.

It is not a surprise that governments at all levels want to find ways to reduce health care costs while still providing high-quality health care. Disease prevention and health promotion, early diagnosis, and prompt intervention are deemed some of the most effective approaches to achieve this goal. Financial investments in such initiatives (e.g., focusing on primary care models that educate individuals about a healthy lifestyle to reduce the incidence of such conditions as diabetes, and heart disease) are believed to be effective upstream strategies with long-term cost-saving benefits.

The social determinants of health directly and indirectly affect the physical and mental health of Canadians, the economy, and the health care system, both in terms of resource utilization and expenditures. As discussed in Chapters 6 and 7, these determinants include a person's socioeconomic status, their level of education (which impacts the type of employment they have), where they live and living conditions, employment circumstances (income level, job satisfaction, including work—life balance), and their social support networks (particularly in times of high stress and adversity). Absenteeism costs Canadian employers approximately $1.6 billion annually. This loss in productivity amounted to an estimated $20 billion in 2020. A large portion of absenteeism from work is due to mental health issues, affecting roughly 72% of all employees (Mercer, 2018). Stress and other mental health issues are the leading cause of disability and absenteeism in Canada.

Addressing the social determinants of health is important for improving health and reducing longstanding disparities in health and health care. Inequities and disparities associated with the social determinants of health affect the physical, mental, and emotional wellness of a person. Increased funding for social programs (what some refer to as Canada's "social safety net") is as necessary as providing adequate funding across the health care spectrum. Canada's social safety net refers to any programs that provide benefits to individuals, their families, or both. Examples include social security and employment insurance (EI), as well as medicare. To truly address inequities related to the social determinants of health, all levels of government must work together, collaborating with numerous organizations. Providing affordable housing is just one (albeit a significant) example.

Ensuring that the minimum wage across Canada is congruent with a living wage (which differs with regions and jurisdictions) would also help individuals to pay for the necessaries of live (lifting many out of low-wage poverty) and promote improved physical and mental health. A *living wage* refers to an income level that allows an individual or a family to afford to pay for a place to live and adequate food and maintain a reasonable standard of living, one that,

| TABLE 4.4   Minimum Wages Across Canada, 2022 | |
| --- | --- |
| **Province** | **Minimum Wage** |
| British Columbia | $15.65 |
| Alberta | $15.00 |
| Saskatchewan | $13.00 |
| Manitoba | $12.35 |
| Ontario | $15.50 |
| Québec | $14.25 |
| New Brunswick | $13.75 |
| Nova Scotia | $13.35 |
| Prince Edward Island | $13.70 |
| Newfoundland and Labrador | $13.20 |
| Nunavut* | $15.20 |
| Yukon | $15.70 |
| Northwest Territories | $16.00 |

*Reviewed every 2 years.
Most jurisdictions review their minimum wage amount annually.
**Source:** Retail Council of Canada. (2022, June 1). *Minimum wage by province.*
https://www.retailcouncil.org/resources/quick-facts/minimum-wage-by-province/

at least in the best case scenario, prevents them from living in poverty. Although all jurisdictions have a minimum wage, what would be considered a living wage in any region is frequently higher. Table 4.4 illustrates current minimum wage by jurisdiction. Note that minimum wage in some jurisdictions are reviewed annually, while others have a phased-in plan for increasing minimum wage over a designated time frame. For example, Nova Scotia is in the midst of a five-step plan to bring the wage to $15/hour by April 1, 2024. Beginning April 1, 2025, the minimum wage rate will be adjusted with inflation plus an additional 1% each year. Saskatchewan is also moving to link minimum wage rates to inflation.

## THINKING IT THROUGH

### Minimum Wage versus Living Wage

Are you in favour of communities providing a living wage in place of a minimum wage?
1. What is the minimum wage in your jurisdiction and how often is it reviewed?
2. How does the minimum wage compare with the recommended living wage where you live?
3. What do you see as the risks and benefits for an employer who pays employees a minimum wage?
4. During the pandemic, some organizations paid essential workers a higher wage. Some made this change permanent, others removed it. Has this happened in your region, and do you think it is fair to remove these increases? Why or why not?

A study published by the Canadian Medical Association supports a strategy of spending less on direct health care and more on social programs that address inequities related to the social determinants of health. The study concluded that this strategy would, in essence, equate to treating the root causes of disease and illness but would be far more effective both in terms of the health of Canadians and the cost to both the economy and the health care system. (Dutton et al., 2018).

## HOSPITAL FUNDING AND EXPENDITURES

As mentioned previously, most Canadian hospitals are not-for-profit facilities. Community-based not-for-profit corporations, religious organizations, and sometimes universities or municipal governments "own" and run these facilities. The province or territory is the main source of revenue for most hospitals. Hospitals are, by far, the leading health care expenditure in Canada, as is evident in Fig. 4.2.

Many different types of health care facilities exist, including general and acute care facilities, long-term care facilities, chronic care facilities, rehabilitation centres, and psychiatric hospitals. All are publicly funded, in part or in whole.

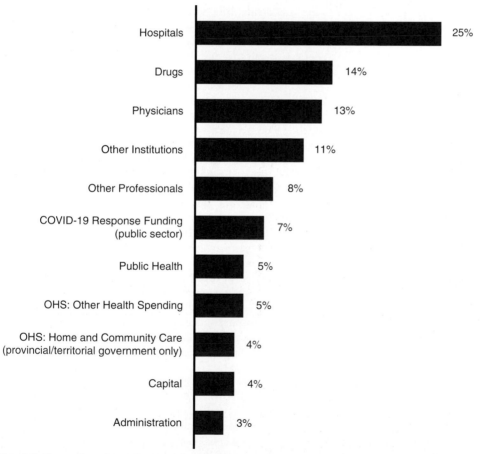

**Fig. 4.2** Share of total health expenditure by health spending category,* Canada, 2021 (forecast). Notes: *Administration expenditures in the National Health Expenditure Database (NHEX) are related to the cost of providing health insurance programs by the government and private health insurance companies and all costs for the infrastructure to operate health departments. This category includes, for example, expenditures for the human resources and finance departments within ministries of health. *OHS,* Other health spending. Numbers do not add up to 100 due to rounding. (Source: Canadian Institute for Health Information. (2022). *National health expenditure trends, 2021—Snapshot.* https://www.cihi.ca/en/national-health-expenditure-trends-2021-snapshot)

Other facilities may be covered only in part by provincial or territorial health plans, in which case patients pay a portion of the services they use. This varies with jurisdictions. Psychiatric hospitals and also the services of psychiatrists are fully covered in all provinces.

National problems that have faced hospitals, communities, and individuals over the past few years include cuts to health care services, reductions in acute care and alternative level of care hospital beds, closure or restricted hours of emergency departments (EDs), centralization of some specialized services, reductions in staff members amidst a shortage of human health resources, and outright closure of smaller hospitals. The following sections will examine how hospitals are funded, how they operate, why operational costs are high, and what is being done to lower costs.

## Hospital Funding Mechanisms

The provincial or territorial ministry, or department of health, provides the majority of funds to hospitals to deliver services to the community. The hospital is then expected to operate as a business, ending the fiscal year with a balanced budget. In all jurisdictions, hospitals are accountable for their operational plan and how they manage their funding allotment. To whom they are accountable may vary, but it is usually to a ministry of health or a central or local health authority. Much like any business arrangement, most hospitals sign agreements outlining target goals, as well as financial and performance outcomes. The specific terms and conditions under which this money is allotted depend on the funding model that guides a hospital's function. As previously mentioned, in all jurisdictions the government is the largest source of funding, with monies flowing from the provincial/territorial ministry of health (or federally in the territories), either through a provincial/territorial health authority or through local regional authorities as approved by provincial/territorial budgets. On average, this funding covers anywhere from 85 to 100% of the costs of operating hospitals, with additional revenue obtained from such sources as parking, cafeterias, and additional federal revenue, including services rendered to veterans (covered by the federal government). Funds are also raised by community organizations (especially for specific expenditures such as a new wing or diagnostic equipment), grants, donations, and charitable giving, through hospital foundations, for example. Many hospitals also operate on a 3P platform—a public/private partnership/government—where required services are provided by a third party based on a revenue-sharing agreement.

There are numerous funding models used to determine the amount of money the government provides to a hospital. Almost without exception, the bottom line is how efficiently a facility operates both in terms of cost-effectiveness and the provision of quality care using best practices guidelines. The more efficiently a hospital operates, the more funds it usually receives. For example, a given hospital may be allotted a certain amount of money for 100 hip replacements within a certain time frame. If the hospital achieves the set goal (under budget), the government, seeing that the hospital is performing efficiently, may provide the hospital with additional funds to do more joint surgeries. Governments will also compare hospitals offering similar services and address concerns if one ED, for example, is spending less than another, which may identify both efficiencies and inefficiencies relative to patient volume in how the ED is managed. There are several funding modes used for hospitals across Canada. Two that are widely used are activity-based funding and global or block funding.

### Activity-Based Funding

The activity-based funding model is popular and used in several jurisdictions (Esmail, n.d.; Wittevrongel & St. Onge, 2020). This model pays hospitals in accordance with the number and types of (selected) services the facility provides to each patient based on the condition that needs to be treated, including any complications that may arise. The goal of this model is to make the facility more efficient and reduce wait times. Implemented first in Ontario, the model was used to reduce wait times for services such as cataract surgery, cardiac bypass surgery, and joint replacement. Under activity-based funding, patients are deemed a source of revenue, where fewer patients result in reduced revenue. Alberta has recently moved to activity-based-funding from the global funding model.

### Block or Global Funding

A hospital's funding amount is determined by its previous year's expenditures and an annual lump sum of money is provided on the basis of that analysis. The block funding model can be problematic, as there is no consideration of the population the hospital serves, or their specific health care needs. In addition, there is no incentive for a hospital to provide high-quality care using a best practices approach. Global funding is also thought to disconnect funding from the provision of services to patients. This model does, however, encourage administrators to implement protocols to discharge patients early to either home care or other facilities in an effort to control costs. Saskatchewan is one example of a jurisdiction using a global funding model, overseen by the Saskatchewan Health Authority (Health Canada, 2022). Additional funds may be provided to hospitals for specialized services and for unforeseen emergency services, such as the pandemic program response.

### Requirements for Funding

Every hospital must be accountable for the funds it requests. After completing its budget, the hospital assesses its financial needs, prepares documentation, and negotiates with the minister of health for appropriate funding. To facilitate these activities, the hospital must track the expenses of all departments and services.

At the end of the fiscal year, a hospital must report on its financial status—whether it is in the black (i.e., posting a surplus) or in the red (i.e., posting a deficit). A hospital in the red must look for ways either to reduce costs or to be approved for extra funding—not an easy task. It must critically examine the services it offers and the cost of each and determine where cuts can be made. A hospital may have to reduce services and staff, close beds, or decrease operating time to keep within its budget. Under certain circumstances, the ministry or department of health may grant extra money to hospitals with budget shortfalls. This is the case with most hospitals as a result of the COVID-19 pandemic.

---

### THINKING IT THROUGH

#### *Are Hospital Services Free?*

Many Canadians think that being admitted to hospital and all the treatments and services they receive have no financial consequence. In addition, there is usually little thought given to the cost of items ranging from sundries such as facial tissues, toothpaste, meals and snacks to cleaning and laundry services. These items come out of the hospital's budget (which is reliant on government funding generated through tax dollars). In attempts to save money, some hospitals actually require patients to bring many items formerly given to patients "for free" (such as facial tissue, soap, toothpaste, even diapers for newborns).

1. If people were given a receipt showing an itemized list of all costs incurred during their hospital stay, do you think they might use health care services more prudently?
2. How would you feel or respond if you were given a list of things to bring in for personal use because the hospital would not pay for them? Or if you were charged for every nonmedically necessary item you used?
3. Can you suggest some reasonable cost-saving measures a hospital in your jurisdiction could employ?

## The Cost of Hospital Care

Hospitals offer diagnostic tests, treatment, and both inpatient and outpatient (also referred to as *ambulatory*) care. Patients admitted to hospital usually have serious illnesses and diseases in an acute phase, which cannot be managed outside of the hospital setting. In outpatient or ambulatory care, or day surgery, patients are admitted to hospital, but not for an overnight stay, sometimes also referred to as *same-day discharge*. These visits can include diagnostic services, clinic visits, outpatient surgery, and ED visits. Many services will include a physician's assessment and treatment or a consultation (usually with a specialist), but these costs are, in many cases, billed separately and do not come out of the hospital budget.

In 2021, the total amount of money (public) spent on the hospital sector was 25% of the total health care expenditure (for the calendar year 2020–2021) of $308 billion (see Fig. 4.2). This represents the largest financial output of any other health care spending category (CIHI, 2021b). As a result, hospitals are under significant pressure to operate as efficiently and cost effectively as possible—not an easy task. It can also generate concern among Canadians, especially when they experience long wait times, and in many cases, actual or perceived deficiencies in care, but are unaware of the financial parameters that a hospital must function within.

### Factors That Affect Hospital Costs

The types and mix and location of hospitals in any jurisdiction affect hospital expenditures, as do the mix of inpatient and outpatient admissions and related procedures. Larger hospitals with more inpatient beds, such as teaching hospitals and those that conduct research, typically have higher expenditures. For example, larger hospitals typically carry out more complex surgeries and have higher admission rates of acutely ill patients; both groups of patients have longer hospital stays (see Fig. 4.3 for the average length of stay [LOS] for various conditions). A major factor increasing a hospital's expenditures are employee wages and collective bargaining goals achieved by hospital unions.

### Costing Details

The average cost of a *standard hospital stay* in Canada in 2020 was $6,349. The costs vary across the country, as illustrated in Fig. 4.3. The highest costs were in British Columbia, Alberta, Saskatchewan, Manitoba, Nova Scotia, Prince Edward Island, Yukon, and the Northwest Territories. Ontario, Québec, New Brunswick, and Newfoundland and Labrador were in the mid-range.

The largest cost driver for hospitals is staff compensation (salaries), consuming about 71% of the total budget. Hospital supplies consumed 11.2%; sundry, 6.4%; equipment, 5.3%; in-hospital drugs, 4.9%; building and grounds, 4.8%; and lastly, services that were contracted out, 4.6%.

Physicians' services are excluded from hospital-based salaries because they are typically paid directly by provincial/territorial medical plans (CIHI, 2021c). There are some exceptions, for example, physicians hired by a hospital and who are paid a salary (either full-time or on contract) for specific services. This may include hospitalists and emergentologists (Fig. 4.4).

In terms of services within hospitals (referred to as *functional areas*), nursing services were the most expensive, responsible for 19% of expenditures, followed by support services at 17%. Administrative support takes up 4.9% of the expenditures (more than the operating room or the ED). Surprisingly, operating rooms consumed just under 7% of expenditures; medical imaging, 4.6%; and the EDs, 4.5%. In an attempt to reduce expenditures, many hospitals limit the amount of time an operating room can be used (Fig. 4.5).

In 2020–2021, across Canada approximately 3 million people were admitted to acute care hospitals. When grouped by category, the top five reasons for admissions to an acute care hospital were (in order of the numbers of admissions per category) patients giving birth, chronic obstructive pulmonary disease (COPD and bronchitis), heart attacks, heart failure (HF), and osteoarthritis (CIHI, 2022c). Osteoarthritis often results in surgery for joint replacements.

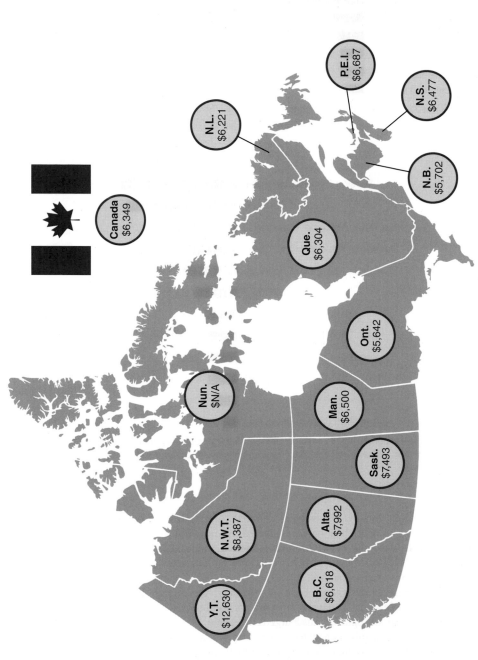

**Fig. 4.3** Average cost of a standard hospital stay by jurisdiction in Canada in 2020. *N/A,* Not available. (Source: Canadian Institute for Health Information. (n.d.). *Your health system: Cost of a standard hospital stay.* https://yourhealthsystem.cihi.ca/hsp/inbrief?lang=en#!/indicators/015/cost-of-a-standard-hospital-stay/;mapC1;mapLevel2;l)

### Patient Care Costs

Health care professionals providing patient care at various levels include registered nurses, licensed/registered practical nurses, nurses' aides, orderlies, and personal support workers. In analyzing their costs, most hospitals calculate the cost of nursing services for inpatient care separately, although these expenditures must be included in the facility's overall costing allowance. Expenditures for other nursing staff may be accounted for in the costs of specialized departments (e.g., outpatient clinic, renal dialysis, and chemotherapy units).

Using the funds allotted to a hospital, various departments are expected to function within given parameters—even an individual nursing unit must be mindful of how much it spends on all costs, from communication tools to paper. Each unit also calculates the number of hours nurses spend delivering direct care to patients. This is calculated using a workload or time-based costing formula and dictates the number and mix of nurses required by a patient care unit for a given time frame (discussed below). Other hospital departments, such as the operating room, for example, have specific expenses, including costs for its use, supplies, instruments, and other equipment (e.g., devices implanted into a patient, such as an artificial hip) and staff with specialized skills. Likewise, those managing an ED must do so with their budget in mind. Some EDs employ nurse practitioners to see patients with less serious conditions to offset the costs of an employed emergentologist as well as to increase efficiencies.

### COVID-19 Admissions

According to the Public Health Agency of Canada (PHAC), between September and October 2022, an average of 4,700 individuals were admitted to Canadian hospitals with COVID-19. Québec was among the provinces showing the largest number of admissions. The average cost of a hospital stay for a patient admitted with COVID-19 is often in excess of $23,000 per patient per hospital stay. This is roughly three times more than the cost of a hospital stay for a patient admitted because of a major heart attack, and almost as much as a person admitted for a kidney transplant, which costs approximately $27,000. Moreover, a patient admitted with COVID-19 typically has a much longer hospital stay than other patients (an average of 11.9 days). A COVID-19 patient is also more likely to require treatment in a Critical Care Unit (CCU), sometimes also referred to as an ICU or Intensive Care Unit. For patients requiring care in a CCU the average cost is $50,000, more than three times the cost of a patient admitted to the unit with a heart attack ($8400). The estimated total cost of caring for patients with COVID-19 in Canada (excluding Québec) in 2020–2021 was a staggering $1 billion.

### Cost-Reduction Strategies

Reducing both the number and length of hospital admissions are two of the most successful strategies to reduce overall hospital costs. This is punctuated by the move from hospital-based to home and community care. There are concurrent advantages to patients, who tend to recover more quickly at home, along with the reduced risk of developing a hospital-acquired infection (nosocomial infection). The following strategies have helped to reduce the length of stays in hospitals across Canada.

### Length of Stay and Bed Capacity

The longer a patient stays in the hospital, the higher the cost, detracting from the hospital's operational budget. Therefore, decreasing the length of hospital stays is an important way to reduce costs and make beds available for new admissions. The province or territory determines the cost of an insured bed in a hospital (paid for out of the allotted budget) by estimating the services required by the person occupying the bed. For example, a patient in an acute care bed recovering from cardiac bypass surgery would be deemed more expensive than one recovering from an appendectomy. It is worth noting that a hospital "bed" does not refer simply to a bed in a hospital room. A "bed" includes all of the services, care, interventions, and treatments the person occupying that bed requires. The person recovering from cardiac surgery will require more care (perhaps specialized care) than the patient recovering from an appendectomy. Likewise, the cost of a "bed" occupied by a patient recovering from an organ transplant would cost the hospital more than the person who had the bypass surgery.

During the COVID-19 pandemic it was not uncommon for hospitals to have physical beds available for patients but lack the other elements required to care for the patient, from nurses trained to care for critically ill patients and physicians to respiratory therapists and sometimes medical equipment such as ventilators. To cope with such situations, hospitals deferred elective procedures in addition to adding more CCU beds and redeploying qualified staff. Some hospitals transitioned recovery rooms and operating rooms to temporary CCUs. When a hospital had no more capacity to provide the care patients required, they were transferred to other hospitals, many out of their province or territory of origin. All of these albeit necessary but expensive interventions related to bed capacity placed added strain on the hospital's budget as well as taking an immeasurable toll on the hospital staff and paramedics.

### Type of Accommodation

The type of room (referred to as the *type of accommodation*) the hospital bed is in is also part of the cost of that bed. In some cases, the type of accommodation the patient has can generate income for the hospital. Public health insurance covers the cost of a "standard" room or ward. If the patient wants a private or a semi-private room, they must pay for the difference. Most often, this is covered by private insurance (Case Example 4.1). There are exceptions to this. If a patient is very ill, or palliative, the attending physician might order that the patient be placed in a private room. The hospital would absorb the cost. The same holds true if a patient must be placed in isolation (e.g., patients admitted who are COVID-positive).

### Same-Day Admissions

In the past, patients scheduled for major surgery were admitted a day or two before the operation for preoperative preparation (tests) and patient education (about what to expect from their hospital experience and recovery). Now, in most cases, required diagnostic tests and patient education are completed prior to admission, shortening the patient's hospital stay and reducing costs.

### Day Surgery

Because of technological advances in many fields, particularly in laparoscopic surgery, an increasing number are now done on an outpatient basis. These procedures range from routine removal of the gallbladder (called a *cholecystectomy*), hernia repairs, and some surgeries for cancer to knee and hip arthroplasties (for selected patients).

---

### CASE EXAMPLE 4.1   The Cost of a Semiprivate or Private Room

M.G. is scheduled to be admitted to a hospital in Vancouver for a knee replacement next week and would like to have semi-private or private accommodation. Provincial health insurance will only pay the basic rate for a standard room (also referred to as a *ward*, which may be a three- or four-bed room). Assume a semi-private room (i.e., a room containing two beds) would cost approximately $165 more per person per day than a ward or standard bed, and a private room would cost $195 more per person per day. Based on a 3-day stay, M.G. would pay the hospital $585 for a private room, or $495 for a semi-private room.

No matter what the procedure, a patient seldom remains in hospital longer than 2 or 3 days unless there are complications. However, some patients having designated day surgical procedure may encounter difficulties, which prolong their hospital stay, each hospital day adding to the cost.

### Bed Management

Efficient bed management is a priority for health care facilities across Canada because of chronic bed shortages, costs associated with prolonged hospital stays, and inappropriate assignment of beds to patients. Bed management is sometimes called *bed allocation management, patient access and flow, electronic bed management*, or *patient navigation*. All terms refer to a system of policies and procedures used by hospitals to coordinate efforts that will facilitate patient access to *the right care* in the *right place* at the *right time*. These systems address the need for timely admission and discharge from an acute care hospital to the appropriate discharge destination. Bed management systems collaborate with home and community care and long-term care facilities to optimize efficiency.

### Timely Discharge

Even in the presence of effective bed management strategies, hospitals endeavor to discharge inpatients before noon, setting routine discharge times as 10 or 11 o'clock. Hospitals will be charged for an additional 24-hour period if a patient is not discharged in a timely manner (usually noon). If a discharged patient cannot arrange to leave before the discharge time, the nurses will, if possible, have the patient vacate the bed and wait in a lounge so that the room can be cleaned and readied for an admission, as well as to avoid incurring the cost of an extra day for the patient going home.

### Outpatient and Community Support

Many patients can be managed on an outpatient basis, including those taking chemotherapy for various types of cancer and those on renal dialysis. Outpatient cancer treatments are made possible, in part, because of improved chemotherapy drugs and related management regimens, which result in fewer adverse effects, especially severe nausea and vomiting.

Patients needing intravenous antibiotics used to be hospitalized; now they are also managed as outpatients. A patient can either return to the hospital or to a designated clinic when their antibiotic is scheduled to be given, or a nurse can come to their home to administer the medication if the patient is not ambulatory. A device called a *saline lock/PRN adaptor* (or similar) is inserted into a vein in the patient's arm, keeping a vein patent. Patients receiving chemotherapy have a more complicated device inserted that can remain in place for long periods of time and through which chemotherapeutic agents are administered (called a *PICC line*, or a peripherally inserted central catheter). Home care services provide nursing assessments and care, managing many of the medical needs of patients that were previously done in hospital and, on occasion, teach family members to do some procedures.

### Tax Credits for Caregivers

Financial relief is available for individuals who care for infirmed family members, in the form of nonrefundable tax credits. Prior to 2017, there were three categories under which individuals could apply for a nonrefundable tax credit when caring for family members at home: the infirm dependent credit, caregiver credit, and family caregiver credit. From 2017 onward, these credit options were consolidated into the Canada Caregiver Credit (CCC), which was revised in January 2022. This remains a nonrefundable tax credit that an individual can claim if they support a spouse, common-law partner, or a dependent with a physical or a mental impairment. Dependents include parents, grandparents, siblings, aunts, uncles, nieces, and nephews. These individuals are eligible if they reside in Canada at any time during the year in which the claims submission is made. The amount a person can claim depends on such variables as the claimant's relationship to the person they are claiming the tax credit for and the person's net income (Government of Canada, 2022).

### Centralizing and Integration of Services

The concepts of merging and integrating services were introduced in Chapter 3. Here we expand on these concepts, looking at how they affect the cost of health care services.

A *merger* may involve two to several facilities and include acute care hospitals, specialty hospitals, or long-term care facilities. Mergers typically involve hospitals that are located in one geographic area and are headed by a single administrative body or corporation.

Hospital mergers occur in two main ways:
1. The *horizontal model* merges several hospitals under one administration—one board, one CEO, one budget—but maintains several sites.
2. The *vertical model* merges specific programs within a single organization; however, the administration of various programs may remain independent of one another, thus not be under the direction of one board.

The advantages of merging are broad: reduced duplication of services, higher levels of efficiency, lower administration and management costs, and the ability to offer more services with better results for patient care and recovery. Larger institutions are also believed to attract more staff. However, studies have shown some negative outcomes when larger hospitals merge, particularly the adverse effects on staff. Mergers often result in disruption of a hospital's culture, lost seniority, and displacement of staff members, either through a reorganization of positions or layoffs. Mergers of smaller hospitals appear to be more successful because the resulting facility broadens its service base while retaining staff and improving care. Whether or not successful mergers reduce costs remains controversial.

The aim of *integrating services* is to prevent the duplication of services, provide care at the necessary level within a community, and use resources more effectively. For example, in Kitchener, Ontario, cardiac and cancer services are centralized—St. Mary's Hospital has become the cardiac centre, and Grand River Hospital, the cancer centre. Government funds are invested in both hospitals to continually update, upgrade, and expand services in these specialty areas. Obstetrical services are offered only at Grand River Hospital, although both hospitals maintain a viable ED. Eliminating the duplication of services saves money and improves the level of care. In addition, more sophisticated and technologically advanced equipment can be purchased and operated by highly skilled health care providers.

Many smaller, rural hospitals have been closed over the past few years, whereas others have remained operational through relocation of services. For example, in one mid-sized community, cataract surgery and rehabilitation services were moved from a larger hospital to a smaller one several kilometers away. Although more cost-effective, this is a disadvantage to patients who have to travel out of their community to receive care.

## HOME, CONTINUING, AND LONG-TERM CARE IN CANADA

As of July 2022 there were about 7,329,910 Canadians 65 years of age and older. This accounts for approximately 18.8% of the total population, who, collectively, use 45% of the total health care expenditures. The average spending on someone over the age of 60 is seven times more than that for those under the age of 60 (CIHI, 2022b). By 2030, those in the over-75 population group is expected to double. The Canadian population over the age of 65 is expected to increase by 68% over the same time frame (by 10.4 million people) (CIHI, 2017). The population in Nunavut (of those over the age of 65) is expected to increase by 5.7 times its current population (the largest increase in Canada) and by 1.9 times in Saskatchewan (the smallest increase). Statistics Canada estimates that the number of Canadians over the age of 65 will account for one-fifth of the total population by 2025. This significantly outnumbers the population growth involving children between birth and the age of 14 years, which is expected to remain stable at about 15% over the same time frame (Statistics Canada, 2020).

People in the older age category are more apt to have complex medical conditions, often combined with mobility limitations and dementia, and therefore require more intensive support, both medically and in terms of general care (Fig. 4.6).

---

### DID YOU KNOW?

#### *The Impact of COVID-19 on Canadian Population Statistics*

In Canada there were over 300,000 deaths in 2020, with just over 16,000 of those related to COVID-19 (5.3% of the total deaths in the country in that year). According to Statistics Canada, the average life expectancy for Canadians dropped by 7 months the same year. Mortality rates linked to the COVID-19 pandemic are thought to have contributed significantly to this decline. COVID-19 was the leading cause of death in 2020, followed by cancer and heart disease, respectively.

Sources: Dion, P. (2021). *Reductions in life expectancy directly associated with COVID-19 in 2020.* Statistics Canada. https://www150.statcan.gc.ca/n1/pub/91f0015m/91f0015m2021002-eng.htm; Statistics Canada. (2020). *Canada's population estimates; age and sex, July 1, 2020.* https://www150.statcan.gc.ca/n1/daily-quotidien/200929/dq200929b-eng.htm; CBC News. (2022, January 24). *COVID-19 blamed for greatest drop in life expectancy in Canada since 1921.* https://www.cbc.ca/news/canada/life-expectancy-covid-decrease-1.6326089#:~:text=Pandemic%20was%203rd%20leading%20cause%20of%20death%20in%202020%20in%20Canada&text=Statistic

---

### Financing and Continuing Care

*Continuing care* refers to measures necessary to support and care for individuals who cannot manage independently; these services can be provided in their private homes, in a seniors' residence, or in long-term care facilities. Under the *Canada Health Act*, continuing care is described in vague terms as "extended" services that are not subject to the terms and conditions of the Act. As a result, individuals can be charged for continuing care services. Moreover, services do not have to be publicly owned or operated, offered on a universal basis, or accessible to everyone.

The provinces and territories select which continuing care services are publicly funded, by whom and by how much. All jurisdictions publicly fund a huge portion of home care, community care, and long-term care services, although configuration and delivery of these services vary. Despite these variables, provinces and territories are collectively examining frameworks to improve the sustainability of continuing care in a cost-effective manner. This involves examining existing models of delivering care within the community and in residential and long-term care facilities. The challenges are greater in jurisdictions with older populations. The 2022 figures show that Newfoundland and Labrador have the oldest population with a median age of 47.8 (Table. 4.6). New Brunswick is next, where the median is 45.7 years, and then Nova Scotia, with a median age of 44.2. The jurisdictions with the youngest median age are Nunavut, Northwest Territories, and Manitoba. British Columbia is the only Western province whose population is older than the Canadian average of 41.4 years. It is also the only jurisdiction with a higher-than-average population of individuals over the age of 65 (Dimmell, 2021).

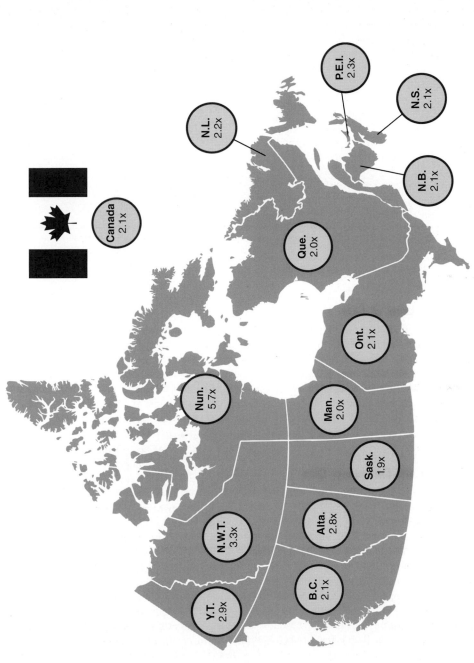

**Fig. 4.6** The population growth of older persons (age 75+) in each province and territory by 2037 (× its current size). (Source: Canadian Institute for Health Information. (2017). *Canada's seniors population outlook: Uncharted territory.* https://www.cihi.ca/en/infographic-canadas-seniors-population-outlook-uncharted-territory)

| TABLE 4.6 Median Age of Resident Population of Canada in 2022, by Province | |
|---|---|
| **Province/Territory** | **Median Age (years)** |
| New Brunswick | 45.7 |
| Nova Scotia | 44.2 |
| Prince Edward Island | 41.7 |
| Québec | 43.1 |
| Ontario | 40.4 |
| Manitoba | 31.7 |
| Saskatchewan | 38.2 |
| Alberta | 38.1 |
| British Columbia | 42 |
| Yukon | 39.5 |
| Newfoundland and Labrador | 47.8 |
| Nunavut | 25.1 |
| Northwest Territories | 34.9 |

**Source**s: Provinces: https://www.statista.com/statistics/444816/canada-median-age-of-resident-population-by-province/; Northwest Territories: https://www.populationu.com/ca/northwest-territories-population, Nunavut: https://www.populationu.com/ca/nunavut-population#:~:text=Total%20Nunavut%20private%20dwellings%20are,of%20the%20population%20is%2025.1

### Alternative Level of Care

The rising need for continuing care services across the country is, in part, demonstrated by the large numbers of individuals in hospitals who cannot return to independent living and are waiting for home care services or placement in a long-term care facility. These individuals are referred to as alternate level of care (ALC) patients, those who occupy more expensive acute care beds that should be used by those requiring an intensive level of care. This creates a backlog of acute care patients who languish in the hallways of EDs and nursing unit corridors. Some refer to this as *hallway medicine*, a costly scenario that imposes an emotional and physical burden on patients, their families, and health care providers, and a financial burden on hospitals.

### Home Care and Community Care

Home care and community care, although different, are closely connected, and the organizations collaborate with each other to provide seamless services for the individuals they support (see Chapter 3). In most communities, publicly funded home care is available through a central agency to which an individual must apply. In general, supporting individuals at home is more cost-effective than supporting them in long-term or residential care, and certainly more cost-effective than in an acute care bed in the hospital. The challenge is to find more efficient ways to use current resources and implement new strategies to contain the costs of home care and improve services to meet the growing demand (see Chapter 10).

Matching an individual with the proper community resources is an important step in deciding who can be managed at home instead of in long-term care. This decision making is highly dependent on the availability of community and health human resources.

### Residential Care

*Residential care* refers to living accommodations that offer a variety of support needs, usually for older persons. These accommodations include lodges (public or private), assisted living or supportive services in the community (e.g., supportive housing), and long-term care facilities. The cost of most residential facilities, or portions thereof, are covered by public health plans.

### Private residences

Older Canadians who can afford it and want to avoid long-term care facilities may choose to live in private residential facilities where they can select the type of accommodation and level of care required.

Private residential accommodation can be very expensive across Canada, with monthly fees ranging from $1453 to $4500 and higher (Comfort Life, 2020). Monthly costs vary with location and the "luxury" components of the facility. Choice of accommodation ranges from a single room to larger, more spacious suites. The more services required, the higher the cost. Maximum care would be similar to that provided in a long-term care facility. Federal, provincial, and territorial governments are not responsible for any costs incurred, and the resident pays the facility directly. A person living in a private residence can still have the services of publicly funded home and community care.

### Long-Term Care Facilities (Nursing Homes)

Most jurisdictions use the term *long-term care facilities*, or *nursing homes*, although *personal care homes* is used in Manitoba, *special care homes* in Saskatchewan, *continuing care homes* in Alberta, and *residential care homes* in British Columbia. These facilities provide varying levels of care to individuals—from those who require less support but are unable to live on their own, to those who require total care and supervision for physical or cognitive reasons—24 hours a day, 7 days a week. Levels of care are classified as independent, semi-independent, and dependent (Case Example 4.2).

Provincial or territorial governments oversee long-term care for all Canadians, with the exception of those individuals eligible for federal care through Veterans Affairs Canada, Workers' Compensation Boards, federal government acts, and medical health insurance. Licensed by the provincial and territorial ministries of health, long-term care facilities (often privately owned) must meet standards regarding staffing levels, training, food preparation, pricing, and medical care, including the administration of medications. Unsubsidized and unlicensed residences also exist, but they offer limited or no nursing care and are usually regulated by municipal bylaws, which do not control the quality of care.

Provincial and territorial governments control the number of publicly funded long-term beds in their jurisdiction. Public funding provides revenue to subsidize these nursing home beds; however, in addition to the fact that beds in public (or government-funded) nursing homes in most jurisdictions are subsidized, the patient must pay a flat rate for basic accommodation (called a *copayment*). The exception is Nunavut. The portion of costs that residents must pay may depend on their financial circumstances (Case Example 4.3) and whether they

---

**CASE EXAMPLE 4.2   A Long-Term Care Facility or a Secure Unit?**

Seventy-two-year-old O.P. has had a stroke. She is fully cognizant and can manage some activities of daily living but needs assistance with dressing, eating, and moving about. Because she was unable to manage at home despite home care support, she is now in a long-term care facility, semi-dependent, and receiving a moderate level of nursing supervision and supportive care.

However, if O.P. had advanced Alzheimer's disease (i.e., had little or no memory, wandered, and could not feed herself) and fell and broke her hip, she would be placed in a secure unit with maximum nursing supervision and be almost completely dependent.

---

**CASE EXAMPLE 4.3   The Cost of Moving to a Long-Term Care Facility**

After falling and breaking her hip, 80-year-old I.B. can no longer live independently at home. Arrangements have been made for her to move to Happy Meadows, a long-term care facility close by. I.B. has concerns about being able to afford long-term care and is even more worried about what will happen to her life's savings and her house. "They will take all of my money," she laments. "What will happen to my house? I heard they take everything to pay for staying there!" What might happen to I.B.?

The answer depends on what province or territory I.B. lives in and the type of long-term care facility she is moving to. In most jurisdictions, the patient's monthly income must be used toward payment for the accommodation. I.B. need not worry about her house and savings, however. These assets would be protected (although the amount of protection varies across jurisdictions) and would not be accounted for in the assessment of her ability to pay. If I.B.'s monthly income from her pensions is $2000 and the copayment is $3000/month, I.B. would have to surrender the bulk of her income for her accommodation, but would not be required to make the full copayment. The government would cover the balance, leaving her with enough money for personal expenses. I.B. would be eligible only for basic accommodation.

If I.B.'s monthly income were $3000 and the cost of her standard accommodation were $2,500 monthly, I.B. would be required to pay the full amount, leaving her with $500 left over to spend as she pleases.

---

have a spouse living in the community. If they have a spouse, payment would be adjusted so that the spouse can retain enough money to remain in their home. All jurisdictions have alternative funding options for those unable to pay, and no one can be denied accommodation or care.

During the first 2 years of the pandemic, the highest mortality rates were among residents in long-term care facilities (both private and publicly owned and operated). As a result, the quality and sustainability of long-term care facilities (under current circumstances) across Canada have been brought into question. Numerous problems have been exposed, ranging from the (until recently) absence of a national long-term care strategy, inadequate funding, lack of human health resources, and the built environment, to infection prevention and control policies and related resources (see Chapter 10).

Rates for a standard long-term care bed, copayments residents are required to pay (usually based on after-tax income), and the breakdown of how those copayments are used (e.g., for meals, accommodation) vary across Canada. Regardless of an individual's financial situation, all jurisdictions leave a percentage of the resident's income for their personal use (on average, 15%). This means that if the resident is unable to pay even the minimum amount for standard accommodation, the person's stay (as with I.B.) will be subsidized and they will be left with a stipulated percentage of their income for personal expenses. Table 4.7 shows the cost of long-term care across Canada.

Some facilities offer standard accommodation (up to three or four people in a room), although that level of accommodation is becoming increasingly rare. Depending on what type of accommodation is "basic" in a facility, if a person wants to change that accommodation, they must pay the difference between whatever is considered basic and the preferred accommodation.

Beyond the costs of long-term care are concerns around quality—for example, substandard resident and patient care, abuse of residents by staff members, abuse of staff members by residents, and abuse among residents themselves, racism being one of the factors. Other causes include

| TABLE 4.7    The Cost of Long-Term Care Accommodation Across Canada | |
|---|---|
| **Province** | **Monthly Cost of Long-Term Care for Basic/ Standard Accommodation** |
| British Columbia | $1700 |
| Alberta | $1753 |
| Saskatchewan | $1634–$4719 |
| Manitoba | $1743 |
| Québec | $1256 |
| Newfoundland and Labrador | $2990 (maximum) |
| Nova Scotia | $3315* |
| New Brunswick | $3437 |
| Prince Edward Island | $2765.70* |
| Northwest Territories | $844 |
| Yukon | $1217 |

*Calculated based on a 30-day month.
**Sources**: Government of Alberta. (2021). *Continuing care—Accommodation charges.* https://www.alberta.ca/continuing-care-accommodation-charges.aspx; Government of Nova Scotia. (2021). *Long-term care rates schedule.* https://novascotia.ca/dhw/ccs/FactSheets/Long_Term_Care_Rate_Schedule.pdf; Government of Yukon. (n.d.). *Find information on long-term care in Yukon.* https://yukon.ca/en/health-and-wellness/care-services/find-information-long-term-care-yukon

inadequate staffing levels and poor training of staff members. Underlying it all is chronic underfunding, with the result that nurses and other staff are underpaid, and insufficient numbers of care providers are hired for the number of residents, who increasingly have more complex needs. These problems have been exacerbated during the pandemic, prompting all jurisdictions to review the whole concept of long-term care facilities and how care is delivered.

### Public, for-profit private and not-for-profit long-term care facilities in Canada

Currently there are 2,076 long-term care homes in Canada. Of these, 46% are publicly owned, and 54% are privately owned. Of the privately owned facilities, 29% are for profit, and 23% are not-for-profit (CIHI, 2021d) (Table 4.8). In Yukon, Nunavut, and the Northwest Territories, long-term care facilities are all funded publicly. Of the long-term care facilities in Newfoundland and Labrador, 98% are publicly funded, and in Québec, 88%. In contrast, New Brunswick has no publicly funded long-term care facilities, and in Ontario only 16% of the 627 long-term care facilities are publicly funded. See Fig. 4.7, which illustrates the number of long-term facilities in Canada.

## THE RISING COST OF MEDICATIONS

According to the Canadian Institute for Health Information (CIHI, 2022d), spending on medications increased by 4.6% in 2020, compared with a slightly lower increase in 2019. What public programs spent on prescription medications varies with jurisdictions, which in 2020 ranged from just under 32% in New Brunswick, 34% in Newfoundland and Labrador, to about 47% in Manitoba. Private insurance spent $12.7 billion on prescription medications, and Canadian households spent approximately $6.9 billion (out-of-pocket) (CIHI, 2020).

Note that public drug spending estimates do not include medications used in hospitals or those dispensed through specialized public programs such as cancer agencies. Calculated

TABLE 4.8 **Total Number of Long-Term Care Facilities in Each Jurisdiction, Number Publicly Funded, Number of Private-for-Profit Facilities, and Number of Private Not-for-Profit Facilities**

| | BC | AB | SK | MN | ON | QC | NB | NS | PEI | NL | NWT |
|---|---|---|---|---|---|---|---|---|---|---|---|
| Number of facilities | 308 | 186 | 161 | 125 | 627 | 440 | 70 | 84 | 19 | 19 | 3 |
| Public | 35% | 46% | 74% | 57% | 16% | 88% | 0 | 14% | 47% | 98% | 100% |
| **Private** | | | | | | | | | | | |
| For-profit | 37% | 27%** | 5% | 14% | 57% | 12%* | 14% | 44% | 47% | 2% | — |
| Not-for-profit | 28% | 27% | 21% | 29% | 27% | | 86% | 42% | 6% | 47% | — |

*Breakdown of private for-profit and not-for-profit status is unknown.

**Information for one facility in Alberta related to private for-profit and private not-for-profit status was unavailable.

**Source:** Based on Canadian Institute for Health Information. (2021, June 10). *Long-term care homes in Canada: How many and who owns them?* https://www.cihi.ca/en/long-term-care-homes-in-canada-how-many-and-who-owns-them

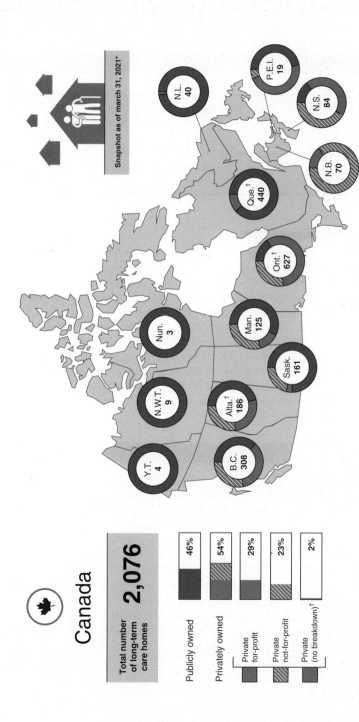

Canada

Total number of long-term care homes

**2,076**

Snapshot as of march 31, 2021*

| | |
|---|---|
| N.L. 40 | |
| P.E.I. 19 | |
| N.S. 84 | |
| N.B. 70 | |
| Que.† 440 | |
| Ont.† 627 | |
| Man. 125 | |
| Sask. 161 | |
| Nun. 3 | |
| N.W.T. 9 | |
| Alta.† 186 | |
| Y.T. 4 | |
| B.C. 308 | |

Publicly owned — 46%
Privately owned — 54%

Private for-profit — 29%
Private not-for-profit — 23%
Private (no breakdown)† — 2%

CIHI

**Notes**
* Data for all jurisdictions is as of March 31, 2021, except Québec (as of April 1, 2021) and Alberta (as of February 28, 2021).
† Private for-profit and not-for-profit ownership breakdown information for some long-term care homes in Québec, Ontario, and Alberta was not available at the time of publication.

**Fig. 4.7 Long-term care facilities in Canada.** (Source: Canadian Institute of Health Information. (2021, March 31). *Long-term care homes in Canada: How many and who owns them?* https://www.cihi.ca/en/long-term-care-homes-in-canada-how-many-and-who-owns-them)

separately, the Canadian Agency for Drugs and Technologies and Health (CADTH, 2021) reported that spending on medications administered to patients in Canadian hospitals in 2020 cost $4.9 billion.

## THINKING IT THROUGH

### Percentage of Drug Spending

In 2020, 2.7% of the population in Canada accounted for a staggering 42.9% of total drug spending. That means that the rest of the Canadian population accounted for about 58% of drug expenditures.

1. With the costs of newer medications rising, do you think that the money spent on medications for a small percentage of the population is sustainable? Why or why not?
2. Do you think it is equitable? Support your answer.

## Major Cost Drivers for Drug Expenditures

Increased drug expenditures can be attributed to several factors, including the rising cost of some newer medications and the fact that more people are taking more medications. Medications used for high blood pressure, high cholesterol, and gastrointestinal disorders are among those most commonly prescribed. Older Canadians have a significantly higher per capita spending related to medications, compared to other cost drivers.

Pharmaceutical companies are researching and producing more specialized—and more expensive—medications. These include a class of drugs called *biologics* (e.g., immunosuppressants, anti-inflammatory, and cancer drugs). Biologics are derived from living material and are growing in popularity, along with "targeted drugs" that require biomarker testing to ensure they are right for the patient. In 2021, the top four spending categories were used to treat rheumatoid arthritis and Crohn's disease, age-related macular degeneration, autoimmune diseases, and antirejection drugs (for organ transplant recipients) (CIHI, 2022d).

## DID YOU KNOW?

### Biologic versus Biosimilar Drugs

Biologic drugs are among the most expensive medications used in Canada. They are used for such conditions as rheumatoid arthritis and other autoimmune and inflammatory diseases. They are made from living cells, human or animal protein. The annual cost of some biologics can be overwhelming, between $10,000 and more than $50,000/month.

A biosimilar drug is one that is similar to a biologic drug, but not identical. A biosimilar drug enters the market only after the patent of the biologic drug it mimics has expired, and after the drug has been authorized for use; in this case, approval must be given by Health Canada. There were only 18 biosimilar drugs approved by Health Canada as of January 2022. Biosimilar drugs are not the same as generic drugs, which are chemically sourced and more or less identical to their brand-name counterparts. Biosimilar drugs are, on average, 30% cheaper than biologics.

Sources: Health Canada (2019, August 27) *Biosimilar biologic drugs in Canada: Fact sheet.* https://www.canada.ca/en/health-canada/services/drugs-health-products/biologics-radiopharmaceuticals-genetic-therapies/applications-submissions/guidance-documents/fact-sheet-biosimilars.html; Canadian Society of Intestinal Research. (n.d.) *Biologics and biosimilars available in Canada.* GI Society. https://badgut.org/information-centre/a-z-digestive-topics/biologics-in-canada/

## Drug Coverage

All provinces and territories provide some kind of drug insurance to certain groups, such as older Canadians, people with disabilities, and individuals who earn low incomes or are on social assistance. A copayment or deductible may apply (see Chapter 9), but some pharmacies will waive deductibles and copayments in certain circumstances.

Canada is one of only a few developed countries without a national drug plan. However, most provinces and territories have some form of catastrophic drug coverage, meaning they will assume the cost of very expensive medications for specific health conditions when the family is unable to cover the expense. Québec has had a provincial drug plan since 1997 for those who do not have private drug insurance. However, as discussed in Chapter 3, there are plans under consideration to implement a national pharmacare plan, which, when implemented, should result in lower overall costs for medications (collectively) for provinces and territories (Canadian Health Coalition, 2021).

A drug's accessibility and coverage through an insurance plan are determined by its category; over-the-counter (OTC) medications can be purchased without a prescription and are rarely covered by public or private health plans; prescription medications can be purchased only with a prescription from a health care provider (e.g., family doctor or specialist, nurse practitioner, midwives, or, in some jurisdictions, a pharmacist or a holistic doctor [allowed to write prescriptions in Ontario and British Columbia]). There are limitations on medications that providers (other than physicians) can prescribe.

Occasionally, a province or territory will remove a drug from the list of drugs that may be obtained only with a prescription. Once removed, however, insurance will no longer cover the drug, and the drug is considered to be OTC.

## Brand-Name and Generic Drugs

Brand-name drugs—those that are owned and sold by the company that developed them—cost more than generic drugs. They are protected under a piece of legislation called the *Patent Act*. Currently, patents last 20 years from the time the pharmaceutical company applies to the board for approval to sell the drug in Canada. Once a patent expires, any p company can produce the drug (called a *generic drug*) and sell it at a lower cost (a quarter to a half of the brand-name counterpart). Brand-name drug names are always capitalized; generic drug names are not (e.g., *ibuprofen* is a generic drug; *Advil* is the brand-name for the same drug).

Because they do not have to spend money on research and development, companies producing generic drugs can do so at a greatly reduced cost. Generic drugs contain the same active ingredients, although the other ingredients (called *nonmedicinal ingredients*) vary. All generic drugs go through an approval process and analysis similar to those of brand-name drugs. Some claim that brand-name drugs are of a higher quality and that different non-medicinal ingredients can alter the action and efficacy of the medication. Unless a doctor specifically indicates on a prescription "no substitution," pharmacists may substitute a generic drug for a brand-name one.

Over the next few years, patents on a large number of brand-name drugs will expire; generic equivalents will become available, reducing the cost of prescription medications for patients. Most provincial and territorial formularies use generic drugs, although brand-name drugs are allowed by special permission if there is not a generic equivalent to effectively treat a specific condition.

## Controlling the Cost of Patented Drugs

An independent government agency, the Patented Medicine Prices Review Board (PMPRB), regulates the price at which patentees—pharmaceutical companies—sell their patented medicines in Canada to wholesalers, hospitals, pharmacies, and others (e.g., clinics), called the *factory-gate price.* Although the PMPRB can ensure that drug companies themselves do not charge excessive prices, the board does not have jurisdiction over the prices retailers charge customers or pharmacists' dispensing fees. For the duration of the patent, the PMPRB regulates the prices of all *patented* products, including medication available only through prescription, sold over the counter, and available through Health Canada's Special Access Program. This program provides physicians with access to existing medications not currently on the market that might prove effective for treating serious or life-threatening conditions when mainstream medications have proven ineffective, are not readily available, or cannot be tolerated by a specific patient. The PMPRB has no authority to regulate the prices of non-patented drug products (i.e., drug products that were never patented or for which the patent has expired).

## HEALTH HUMAN RESOURCES

The term *health human resources* (HHR) refers to almost all people who work in the health care field, from primary care providers and nurses, to technologists and administrative management. See the video on Evolve for a complete explanation. Nurses, followed by physicians, are the largest group of regulated health professionals in Canada. Physicians and nurses are also the two largest cost drivers of health human resources.

How a health care organization best manages the skills and expertise of its employees greatly affects its financial bottom line. For example, it is essential to find the proper balance of nursing staff in hospitals to deliver high-quality care within budgetary guidelines. Achieving this balance without patient care suffering, or negatively impacting nursing staff, is a difficult task. Organizations assess the level of care that their patients or residents require and decide who can best competently deliver that care. Acute care hospitals employ registered nurses, licensed or registered practical nurses, and personal support workers. Typically, CCUs employ only registered nurses, most of whom have had additional training specific to the specialized unit they work in, where patient care is both complex and acute. On patient care units, there is likely to be a mix of registered nurses, licensed or registered practical nurses, and personal support workers working as a team depending on the nurses' level of skill and scope of practice. Long-term care facilities usually employ more licensed or registered practical nurses and personal support workers than registered nurses.

Money to pay employees in hospitals and other facilities comes out of the funding envelope assigned to the facility by the government. The mix of health professionals employed to fit within the budget is determined by the facility. It is important, for example, to ensure that the mix of professional nurses employed fits within budgetary guidelines. Hospitals frequently exceed their financial limits, ending up in the red. This is often because of the cost of human health resources. When hospitals and other facilities have to make up a deficit, it is often nursing staff that is reduced. Nurses in primary health clinics are paid through the clinic or by the physicians for whom they work. Nurse practitioners are paid by the government or by physicians directly.

### The Cost of Nurses

Nurses working in hospitals usually are paid a higher wage than those working in other facilities such as long-term care, doctor's offices, or a primary care setting. Other considerations related to how much a nurse makes include additional education and how long they have been in the workforce (this is for all categories of nurses).

In 2022, the average remuneration for a registered nurse was $71,103, with a low of $57,336 for an entry-level position to a high of $81,628 for a nurse with more experience.

The average annual remuneration for a registered/licensed practical nurse is $55,044. An entry-level position starts at approximately $50,479 annually, with more experienced nurses making approximately $64,327 per year (Talent.com, 2022).

A personal support worker in an entry-level position makes between $30,000 and $35,100 yearly, with a more experienced personal support worker making up to $44,312 annually. These numbers vary and differ with jurisdictions as well as within jurisdictions.

## The Cost of Physicians

In 2020, there were 92,173 physicians licensed to practice in Canada. Total gross clinical payments to physicians that year were $29.4 billion, which is an increase of 4.3% over 2019. The average payment made to physicians (before taxes) was $354,000, representing a 20% increase over the previous year (CIHI, 2021c). Of these physicians, 62% were paid fee-for-service (FFS), and 28% via alternate payment formulas. The payments were paid by provinces and territories for insured medical services—the majority for consultations and physician visits, including virtual and telephone visits (which have increased dramatically since 2020 because of the pandemic). Physicians and other providers saw selected patients in their offices or clinics but managed a large portion of their patients' appointments virtually. In terms of specialties, 52% of the total number of physicians were working in family medicine, the rest in either medical or surgical specialties.

## Physician Funding Mechanisms

As mentioned above, FFS is the oldest and, for the moment, most widely accepted method of physician payment in Canada. Using this method, doctors charge the provincial or territorial plan for every service they perform (see Chapter 1). Doctors (or more likely, their medical office assistant) must submit a claim to the ministry in their province or territory for each insurable assessment made and service provided. Each province or territory has slightly different parameters for FFS billing. Invariably, though, the amount the doctor bills relates to the complexity and length of the patient visit as well as the location of that visit. Most jurisdictions have three or four main categories for "visit fees" that a physician can charge for a minor assessment, an intermediate assessment, and a full assessment (e.g., a physical examination). In Ontario, a physician would bill about $36.85 for an intermediate visit and assessment, such as P.K.'s visit described in Case Example 4.4.

Within the FFS model, doctors can also bill for things other than the actual office visit. For example, doctors who make house calls can charge more to ensure they are compensated for travel, for seeing a patient away from the office, for the time of day or night the house call is made, and for the office patient visits cancelled if making a house call during office hours (although that is rare these days). Doctors may also bill for procedures, such as giving an injection or suturing a wound, or for visiting a patient in hospital.

In general, family doctors across Canada are claiming that they are underfunded for the amount of work they do, which, more recently, includes enormous amounts of administrative work. This situation is, at least in part, discouraging new graduates from choosing family medicine as a career and contributing to doctors leaving the profession. In late 2022, British

---

### CASE EXAMPLE 4.4 A Quick Visit for Gallstones

P.K. went to see his family doctor, complaining of pain just under the rib cage (substernal). The family doctor did a brief physical examination, took a medical history, and ordered several tests, one of which revealed that P.K. had gallstones. The visit took about 15 minutes.

Columbia introduced a new funding formula for family doctors which includes remuneration for the administrative work that doctors do.

### Capitation- or Population-Based Funding

Capitation-based funding (also called *population-based funding*) pays the doctor an annual fee for each patient in their practice. Some primary care groups have the option of rostering patients. How much the physician receives for each patient depends on the patient's age, general health status, and sometimes gender. Under this model, the amount the doctor is paid remains the same regardless of how many times they see the patient. Capitation-based funding is also applied to primary care groups that roster patients. Rostering requires a patient to sign an agreement with the physician stating they will only seek nonemergent care from that physician. If they go elsewhere, the doctor that the person is rostered to loses the amount of money charged for that other visit. Assume a patient who is rostered to one doctor goes to see a different doctor for a health problem. The second doctor submits a claim to the ministry for $25. The ministry, knowing that the patient is rostered to the first doctor, will pay that claim, but will also deduct $25 from the first doctor's next payout from the ministry.

The fundamental components of capitation-based funding are summarized as follows:

- The physician receives a guaranteed income based on the defined population base of their practice.
- The physician may enter into other compensation schemes; for example, a portion of their practice may still be FFS.
- Incentives provided to the physician incorporate a strong element of disease prevention and health promotion to result in better health outcomes for patients of the practice.

### Global Budget

Doctors practising in underserviced areas are paid a certain fee for maintaining these practices. The global budget plan also usually includes ample vacation time and educational leave.

### Salary and Contract

Doctors on salary receive a negotiated amount of money per time frame (usually a month). Larger hospitals, medical centres, clinics, and some nonprofit clinics often employ this model. A physician would be paid on a contract if hired for a specific period of time by either a hospital or a clinic. Specialists employed by hospitals, emergentologists, and hospitalists are salaried positions. Specialists usually have private practices as well and bill fee-for-services for patients they see.

### Blended Funding

Most physicians in Canada who engage in a form of funding other than FFS also partake in another method of payment. For example, a physician in a primary health care network group can have a certain portion of their practice non-rostered and on an FFS funding scheme, and another portion calculated on capitation-based funding.

### Telephone and Virtual Visits

During the COVID-19 pandemic, most primary care physicians began to conduct patient "visits" virtually or over the telephone in order to reduce viral transmission. Provincial and territorial governments issued physicians with special billing codes so that they could submit a claim for each visit. This was welcomed by many patients, but viewed with some skepticism by others who would rather see their provider in person. Not all health complaints can be adequately assessed unless the patient sees the provider in person, while others can be managed quite adequately without an in-person visit.

## INFORMATION TECHNOLOGY

Funding for IT services in public facilities such as hospitals and long-term care facilities ultimately are provided by the provincial and territorial governments. For the most part, physicians are responsible for any expenses related to medical software systems used in their offices, primary health groups, or clinics, although in some jurisdictions the provincial/territorial government will offer grants to selected recipients (see Chapter 10).

The information systems in hospitals are both complex and varied. There are currently several major platforms used in hospitals across Canada, including Cerner, Meditec, and Epic. All hospitals are digitalized, but to varying degrees. Hospitals assume the financial responsibility for both changing and upgrading their systems, although under some circumstances, the ministry will allot extra funds for this purpose. Hospitals tailor the system they use to suit their own needs. Systems are managed by a busy IT department and numerous IT experts who both initiate and implement changes as well as troubleshoot for hospital staff as required—all of these activities are expensive. IT departments also manage IT security.

### The Canada Health Infoway

Canada Health Infoway is an independent **nonprofit organization (NPO)** that was established by the Canadian government in 2001 to provide digital solutions for Canada's health care system. The Infoway invests in projects that contribute to a national digital framework that expands and improves information technology and connectivity across the health care spectrum and provides prompt access to digital charts. Canada Health Infoway's most recent projects include PrescribeIT and ACCESS Health. The PrescribeIT project, in collaboration with Health Canada, provinces, territories, and health care organizations, began expansion in 2018. The goal is to replace the current patchwork of pharmacy-related connectivity among prescribers and organizations with a national system offering enhanced security management, connectivity to Canada-wide electronic health record systems, and seamless integration with current facility and clinic operating systems (Canada Health Infoway, 2022a).

ACCESS Health is a digital solution enhancing patient accessibility to their own health information, facilitating the concept of patient-centred care. Canada Health Infoway also supports e-mental health solutions, including online help and crisis support (phone line assist, text support, access to online chat and support groups, and hot-spot notifications). The organization supports a national initiative called the *Circle of Care Project* (overseen by Indigenous organizations) to improve health care services through the integration of community electronic medical records and a citizen health portal (Canada Health Infoway, 2022a).

Over the past several years, funding from the federal government for the Infoway totalled over $2.5 billion for over 370 e-health projects Canada-wide. This includes a $50 million commitment for virtual care made in 2020 (Canadian Health Infoway, 2022b).

---

### DID YOU KNOW?

#### Security Breach in Newfoundland

In early November 2021, the health care system in Newfoundland and Labrador experienced a cyberattack that some called the worst in Canadian history. The attack all but paralyzed the Newfoundland and Labrador health network for several days, necessitating the cancellation of thousands of procedures and appointments. Information regarding such cyberattacks is often kept secure for a number of reasons. In this case, the provincial government felt that revealing too much information would jeopardize investigations and impede efforts to restore the system.

### Diagnostic and Imaging Devices

Although offering improved diagnostic outcomes, imaging options such as CT scanners, MRI scanners, and positron emission tomography (PET) and PET/CT scanners are expensive to purchase, maintain, and operate. Added to that is the cost to our publicly funded system each time a diagnostic imaging is ordered for a patient. The least expensive devices are CT and MRI scanners, with the most expensive being PET scanners and PET/CT scanners. PET/CT scanners produce specialized views fusing images from two platforms, giving the physician views of the targeted body part or organ on two different planes with one examination.

CT scans and MRI scans are publicly funded services when considered medically necessary. Both services can also be purchased privately in some regions. The cost of having a CT scan ranges from just over $200 to approximately $650; an MRI examination costs between $900 and $2500. Prices fluctuate with jurisdictions and the specific imaging ordered.

For hospitals or diagnostic facilities to purchase these devices, a CT scanner can cost as little as $65,000 for a basic refurbished device. A larger and brand-new CT scanner can cost as much as $2.5 million. An MRI device costs on average about $3 million.

The average cost of an installed PET/CT scanner is $7 million. This would include the construction of the nuclear and molecular facility required to accommodate the scanner, and the price of other necessary equipment needed to run it, such as a cyclotron, which generates the nuclear power to run the scanner. The PET/CT scanner itself costs between $2.5 and $4 million.

In terms of diagnostic imaging ordered for patients, the cost of a single PET scan varies from $956 in Québec (possibly because of the large number of scans done there) to $1500 in Ontario and $1800 in Manitoba (Statista, 2022).

The manner in which equipment is funded varies with provinces and territories. In 2020, Québec had 23 PET/CT scanners, the most in Canada. Ontario has 20 such scanners, Alberta has 4, and British Columbia has 4, with 3 in Alberta, 2 in New Brunswick, 1 in each of the remaining provinces, and none in Yukon, Nunavut or the Northwest Territories (Tolinsky, 2020). In Ontario, such scanners are usually funded by local organizations along with money from the local hospital's operational costs. Most jurisdictions cover the cost of PET scans only for specific conditions, such as selected cancer and cardiac conditions. Scans are also covered for people who are part of a Health Canada clinical trial.

In 2020, Québec's Ministère de la Santé et des Service Sociaux funded a $7 million project (including another $3.8 million to construct a facility to accommodate the PET scan). The device was installed in the hospital in the mining town of Val d'Or, 525 kilometres north of Montreal, The PET/CT scanner serves 135,000 people in the town and surrounding community. The project was part of a strategy initiated on the part of the Québec government to ensure that advanced medical imaging was available to individuals outside of major centres. Kelowna, British Columbia, and Sudbury, Ontario also acquired PET/CT scanners in 2020 (Tollinsky, 2020). Information from the Canadian Agency for Drugs and Technology in Health (CADTH) indicates that in 2019 there were 67,849 PET/CT scans done in Québec and only 23,554 in Ontario. This equates to 1.6 scans per 1000 individuals for Ontario and 8 per 1000 individuals in Québec (CADTH, 2021).

In most jurisdictions, selected diagnostic imaging services are contracted out to private facilities. The provincial/territorial plan covers the cost of the scans, paying the facility for their services. The financial arrangements made with private companies vary among jurisdictions.

## CONCLUSION

Have you found the answers to the questions you were asked at the beginning of the chapter? How close were your estimates? Review the prices noted in the chapter. Were your estimates close? Did you expect the cost of the services to be less, or more? How would paying out-of-pocket for some of these services impact you or your family?

What does the future of health care in Canada hold? It is nearly impossible to know, although change is certain. Resources are limited, and services may need to be rationed—an alien concept to Canadians. Excluding people from the treatment they need (or want) based on factors such as age, health status, or type of disease seems unthinkable, but it may become a reality. We must use health care resources wisely and continue to promote healthy lifestyles and disease prevention. During the pandemic, several hospitals came close to having to ration services, particularly for those requiring a CCU bed and ventilators. Larger centres across Canada had to develop triage protocols. Risk assessments were based on the patient's chances of survival beyond a certain time frame, considering risk factors such as age, comorbidities, and acuity of their current illness. Can you imagine how difficult a decision that would be for some physicians to make? How would you feel if your loved one had COVID-19 and required a ventilator but was triaged with a decision made that the ventilator went to someone else who had a higher chance of survival? Simply preserving the level of care in hospitals across the country as it is today will require enormous increases in funding by all levels of government. To improve this care and be prepared for the next pandemic will require even more funding, as well as a coordinated and critical look at how and where current funds are spent in addition to improving system-wide inefficiencies.

## SUMMARY

4.1  In Canada, all medically necessary services are publicly funded but, for the most part, are delivered by either private for-profit or private not-for-profit businesses or organizations. For example, most hospitals are private nonprofit facilities, and although funded by the government, many of the services they deliver are done so by private businesses. Often publicly funded health services contract businesses to deliver those services, including some home care organizations. Doctors, although paid for with public funds, can be considered small business owners. They are responsible for all of their expenses and either bill the province/territory for services rendered or are remunerated with alternative payment plans. Although medically necessary services are covered by public health insurance, Canadians either pay directly or through insurance or employee benefits plans, or both, for supplementary health services.

4.2  Public funding for health care in Canada is provided by the federal, provincial and territorial, and municipal governments through a blend of taxes and tax points as well as by Workers' Compensation Boards. Some jurisdictions also use revenue from sales taxes and lotteries for health care. Only Ontario residents pay health care premiums. At present, the federal government makes transfer payments to the provinces and territories through the Canada Health Transfer, the Canada Social Transfer, the Territorial Funding Formula, and equalization payments (which remain controversial, especially in Alberta). In addition to these major transfers, the federal government continues to provide provinces and territories with financial assistance to support initiatives related to the COVID-19 pandemic. The indirect costs of health care, including illness, injury, and premature mortality, have a negative effect on the Canadian economy.

4.3  Hospitals, medications, and human health resources represent the three top health care expenditures in Canada. The provincial or territorial ministry or department of health provides the majority of funds to hospitals to deliver services to the community. Most hospitals are nonprofit facilities and in addition to government funding use an array of private businesses and organizations to deliver their services. Human health resources account for the bulk of hospital spending. The major funding models for hospitals are global funding and activity-based funding. Many Canadians are unaware of the high cost of hospitalizations. The *average* cost of a hospital stay for a patient admitted with COVID-19 is often in excess of $23,000. This is roughly three times more than the cost of a hospital stay for a patient admitted because of a major heart attack.

4.4   Canada has an aging population, which is proving costly when it comes to providing for the health care system. Currently, older persons (over the age of 65) account for about 18% of the total population, who, collectively, use 45% of the total health care budget. The average spending on someone over the age of 60 is seven times more than for those under that age. Care provided for older Canadians (and others) is provided by home and community care services, residential accommodation, and long-term care facilities. It is more cost-effective to care for individuals at home with the support of home and community care services. Long-term care facilities in Canada are primarily publicly funded and are regulated by the provincial and territorial governments. The copayment that residents make is largely dependent on their annual income. Private facilities are popular but can be expensive, offering varying levels of care and accommodation.

4.5   After hospital services, medications represent the next largest health care expenditure. Spending on medications increased by 4.6% in 2020, slightly more than the previous year. Contributing factors include increased use of prescription medications, particularly by older persons with multiple health problems. A major contributor is the high cost of newer medications, in particular biologics, although biosimilar drugs, which are slowly being approved by Health Canada, are less expensive. Generic drugs are less expensive than brand-name drugs. Most physicians order generic drugs for that reason, although there are occasions when a brand-name drug takes priority. A pharmacist can fill a prescription with a generic drug unless the physician notes that there is to be no substitution. Canada does not have a national drug-funding program, but all jurisdictions cover the cost of most medications for certain groups, including older person, disabled persons, and those on assisted income.

4.6   Human health resources (HHR), collectively, are a significant expense to the health care system, with physicians and nurses being the two largest cost drivers. Physicians and nurses are the largest of the regulated professions and account for the largest financial output for the HHR sector. How a health care organization best manages the skills and expertise of its employees greatly affects its financial bottom line. For example, it is essential to find the proper balance of nursing staff in hospitals to deliver high-quality care within budgetary guidelines. Achieving this balance without patient care suffering or negatively impacting nursing staff is a challenge. Registered nurses (the most costly nurses) are almost exclusively employed in specialty settings such as critical care and cardiac units. However, a mix of levels of nursing skills delivers high-quality, cost-effective care. Registered nurses, registered practical nurses, and personal support workers each work within their own scope of practice. Physician remuneration is primarily fee-for-service in many jurisdictions, although blended funding is popular in family health groups and teams.

4.7   Technological advances have been seen in all facets of health care, including surgical procedures, diagnostic equipment, and health and medical records. Medical software systems are used in physicians' offices, primary care groups, and hospitals. At times the acquisition of software systems may be subsidized by the provincial/territorial government but remain a significant expense. It is safe to say that most hospitals are using electronic software operating systems, but many are still using a blend of electronic and manual environments. The Canada Health Infoway is an organization that provides digital solutions for Canada's health care system, investing in projects that contribute to a nationwide digital framework that improves patient care and enables prompt access to a patient's digital or electronic chart. New technologies related to medical imaging promote early diagnosis, prompt treatment, and improved treatment outcomes, but they come at a price.

## REVIEW QUESTIONS

1. Why do some Canadians regard health care as "free"? Do you feel that way? Why or why not?
2. Why don't the territories receive the Canada Health Transfer?
3. Explain the concept of equalization payments, including why they are given and how they are calculated.
4. What types of services are covered by provincial and territorial insurance both in and out of hospitals?
5. What is the difference between direct and indirect health care?
6. What are the three largest expenditures for provincial and territorial health plans?
7. Explain the principle behind equalization payments.
8. How does the average cost of a hospital stay for a person with COVID-19 compare to a hospital admission for someone without COVID-19? Give two examples.
9. List five strategies for reducing the length of hospital stays and thus hospital expenses.
10. What assistance does the government provide for family members who care for family members who are cared for at home? What is the criterion for this assistance?
11. What are the key differences between prescription medications and over-the-counter medications?
12. Are biosimilar drugs the same as generic drugs? Explain.
13. How has advanced technology contributed to rising health care costs?

### Activity

a. Investigate what type of hospital funding is used in two hospitals within your region. Explain how the funding mechanism is managed and if it is deemed efficient for the population base it serves.
b. How are hospital services delivered in your community? Have services been centralized? Explain.

## REFERENCES

Canada Health Infoway. (2022a). *About us*. https://www.infoway-inforoute.ca/en/about-us.

Canada Health Infoway. (2022b). *Our history: Working towards a more connected and collaborative health system*. https://www.infoway-inforoute.ca/en/about-us/our-history.

Canadian Agency for Drugs and Technologies and Health (CADTH). (2021). *New in the canadian journal of health technologies — canadian trends and projections in prescription drug purchases: 2001—2023*. www.cadth.ca/news/new-canadian-journal-health-technologies-canadian-trends-and-projections-prescription-drug#:~:text=The%20researchers%20found%20that%20total,%2C%20an%20increase%20of%20165%25.

Canadian Health Coalition. (2021). *Pharmacare*. www.healthcoalition.ca/project/pharmacare/#:~:text=Public%2C%20universal%20pharmacare%20could%20save,health%20and%20good%20for%20business.

Canadian Institute for Health Information (CIHI). (2017). *Canada's seniors population outlook: Unchartered territory*. https://www.cihi.ca/en/infographic-canadas-seniors-population-outlook-uncharted-territory.

Canadian Institute for Health Information (CIHI). (2020). *Prescribed drug spending in Canada, 2020: A focus on public drug programs*. https://secure.cihi.ca/free_products/prescribed-drug-spending-in-canada-2020-report-en.pdf.

Canadian Institute for Health Information (CIHI). (2021a). *Health expenditure data in brief*. https://www.cihi.ca/sites/default/files/document/health-expenditure-data-in-brief-en.pdf.

Canadian Institute for Health Information (CIHI). (2021b). *What are hospitals spending on?*. https://www.cihi.ca/en/what-are-hospitals-spending-on.

Canadian Institute of Health Information (CIHI). (2021c). *Physicians in canada*. https://www.cihi.ca/en/physicians-in-canada.

Canadian Institute for Health Information (CIHI). (2021d). Long-term care homes in Canada: How many and who owns them?. https://www.cihi.ca/en/long-term-care-homes-in-canada-how-many-and-who-owns-them.

Canadian Institute for Health Information (CIHI). (2022a). *National health expenditure trends, 2021—Snapshot.* https://www.cihi.ca/en/national-health-expenditure-trends-2021-snapshot.

Canadian Institute for Health Information (CIHI). (2022b). *Age-adjusted public spending per person.* https://yourhealthsystem.cihi.ca/hsp/inbrief?lang=en#!/indicators/014/age-adjusted-publ/;mapC1;mapLevel2;/.

Canadian Institute for Health Information (CIHI). (2022c). *Hospital stays in Canada.* www.cihi.ca/en/hospital-stays-in-canada#:~:text=Key%20findings,-In%202019%E2%80%932020&text=The%20most%20common%20reason%20for,myocardial%20infarction%20(4.9%20days.

Canadian Institute for Health Information (CIHI). (2022d). *Prescribed drug spending in Canada.* https://www.cihi.ca/en/prescribed-drug-spending-in-canada.

Comfort Life. (2020). *Costs of senior care. What type of retirement care can you afford?*. https://www.comfortlife.ca/retirement-community-resources/retirement-cost.

Department of Finance Canada. (2017). *Major federal transfers.* https://www.canada.ca/en/department-finance/programs/federal-transfers/major-federal-transfers.html.

Department of Finance Canada. (2021). *Federal government announces major transfer amounts for 2022—23.* https://www.canada.ca/en/department-finance/news/2021/12/federal-government-announces-major-transfer-amounts-for-2022-23.html.

Dimmell, M. (2021). *Canada's younger, western population.* Canada West Foundation. https://cwf.ca/research/publications/canadas-younger-western-population/#:~:text=Canada's%20population%20is%20getting%20older,to%20the%20rest%20of%20Canada.

Dutton, D. J., Forest, P., Kneebone, R. D., et al. (2018). Effect of provincial spending on social services and health care on health outcomes in Canada: An observational longitudinal study. *Canadian Medical Association Journal, 190*(3), E66—E71. https://doi.org/10.1503/cmaj.170132.

Esmail, N. (n.d.). *Activity-based funding is good for alberta.* The Fraser Institute. https://www.fraserinstitute.org/article/activity-based-funding-good-alberta.

Government of Canada. (2022). *Canada caregiver credit.* https://www.canada.ca/en/revenue-agency/services/tax/individuals/topics/about-your-tax-return/tax-return/completing-a-tax-return/deductions-credits-expenses/canada-caregiver-amount.html.

Health Canada. (2022). *2020—2021 Canada health act annual report.* https://www.canada.ca/content/dam/hc-sc/documents/services/publications/health-system-services/canada-health-act-annual-report-2020-2021/canada-health-act-annual-report-2020-2021-eng.pdf.

Mercer. (2018). *Our thinking: How much are you losing to absenteeism?*. https://www.mercer.ca/en/our-thinking/how-much-are-you-losing-to-absenteeism.html#:~:text=Costs%20employers%20%2416.6%20billion%20annually.

Statista. (2022). *Number of positron emission tomography CT units in Canada in 2019/2020, by province.* https://www.statista.com/statistics/821438/number-of-pet-ct-units-in-canada-by-province/.

Statistics Canada. (2020). *Canada's population estimates: Age and sex*, 2020. https://www150.statcan.gc.ca/n1/daily-quotidien/200929/dq200929b-eng.htm.

Talent.com. (2022). *Registered nurse average salary in Canada*, 2022. https://ca.talent.com/salary?job=registered+nurse.

Tollinsky, N. (2020). *Québec continues leadership in PET/CT.* Canadian healthcare technology. www.canhealth.com/2020/10/29/quebec-continues-leadership-in-pet-ct/#:~:text=The%20%247%20million%20project%20%E2%80%93%20%243.2,outside%20the%20province%E2%80%99s%20major%20urba.

Wittevrongel, K., & St Onge, P. (2020). *Entrepreneurship and universality: The way forward for health care in alberta.* https://www.iedm.org/entrepreneurship-and-universality-the-way-forward-for-health-care-in-alberta/.

# Practitioners and Workplace Settings

5.1 Describe three categories of health care providers.
5.2 Explain the purpose and benefits of regulated health professions.
5.3 Discuss the role and educational requirements of selected health care professionals.
5.4 Describe practice settings in which health care is delivered.
5.5 Summarize the current state of primary care in Canada.

## KEY TERMS

Accredited program
Alternative practitioner
Community-based care
Complementary health
    professional
Controlled act
Delegated act
Evidence-informed
Geriatrics

Health care provider
Hospice
Interprofessional
    collaboration
Intubate
Practice setting
Primary care
    organization

Refraction
Rostering
Scope of practice
Specialist
Telehealth
Title protection

The provision and delivery of health care depend entirely on human health resources: numerous, broad categories of individuals each with unique educational backgrounds, skill sets, and **scope of practice**. Most, in one way or another, are interdependent at some level. Responsibilities of those providing health care services differ, but collectively, their contributions contribute to the viability of the health care system and, importantly, to the well-being of the patient.

This chapter will look at some of the different health care workers in Canada—who they arc, what they do, and where they work. It will briefly examine some of the professional organizations that support these people, and the regulations, policies, and procedures in place to ensure that care is given by individuals qualified in their field. This chapter focuses mainly on the evolving team-based models of delivering primary care in Canada. The list of health care professionals discussed in this chapter represents a cross-section of these providers. Please note that the order of the health professionals described does not reflect any hierarchy (that any one profession is deemed more valuable or important than another) and is as such purely for organizational purposes.

Health care in Canada is provided by a wide variety of health care professionals —from conventional (or mainstream) medical practitioners to those who practise complementary and alternative medicine. Also integral in delivering care are informal workers: volunteers of community organizations as well as friends and family members who care for loved ones at home.

**Practice settings** include hospitals, residential care facilities, rehabilitation centres, community care facilities, **hospices**, a variety of clinics, **primary care organizations**, and the home. Who delivers health care, when, where, and how, is continually changing. This is largely an attempt to provide Canadians with timely, cost-effective access to community-based primary, secondary, and tertiary care to accommodate the health needs of a diverse population in an unbiased, culturally safe manner. The COVID-19 pandemic has impacted all aspects of health care, affecting how services must be adapted to meet the physical, spiritual, psychological, and mental health needs of both **health care providers** and those seeking health care.

Strategies to improve patient access to primary care providers have been underway for a number of years, initially referred to as *primary care reform*. One of the most successful approaches has been the implementation of centralizing primary care services administered by interprofessional teams. This approach is called **interprofessional collaboration**. Primary care organizations are introduced in Chapter 3. This concept facilitates improved access to primary care in that patients can capitalize on the expertise of other health care providers according to their individual needs.

There are glaring gaps in the provision of health care despite the increasing popularity and efficiencies of primary care groups. Providers other than physicians have gone a long way to close these gaps while maintaining continuity of patient care. Nurse practitioners, for example, provide much of the primary care in rural and northern regions, in addition to being an integral part of the health care team in urban settings as well as in hospitals. Midwives assume primary care for mothers and initial care for newborn babies. Moreover, physician assistants, nurses and nurse **specialists**, physiotherapists, respiratory therapists, dietitians, social workers, mental health specialists, pharmacists, and podiatrists are only a few health professions that also render primary care services, working collaboratively within the interprofessional team environment.

The move away from hospital-based care has become the norm across Canada, utilizing home and community-based services (see Chapter 3) and keeping individuals as independent for as long as possible in their own homes. See Box 5.1 for a summary of **community-based**

---

**BOX 5.1    Community-Based Care: A Summary**

- An approach to health care that integrates the elements of primary and community care as well as home care
- Care and services that are delivered in a variety of community settings: providers' offices or clinics, hospices, patients' homes, public health units, workplace settings, and schools (e.g., immunizations, educational programs)
- Care and services that are responsive to economic, social, language, cultural, and gender differences within a community
- Care and services that respond to the needs of each community (e.g., within an urban or rural setting or in remote communities in northern regions of the country, where community needs vary greatly)
- Community-based primary care provides community members with a full spectrum of services, including patient education, disease prevention and health promotion strategies, counselling, curative and rehabilitative services
- Addresses the social determinants of health as required in each region or community; primary care providers collaborate with community agencies and other stakeholders to promote a healthy environment. This may include food security, safe water, proper sanitation, maternal-child health, mental health support (e.g., drug and alcohol use and addiction), and immunization protocols.

---

**BOX 5.2   Shift to Patient-Centred Care**

Typical of Western medicine, physicians assess a patient's needs, form a health care plan, and advise the patient what to do. Patient-centred care involves the skills of a variety of health care practitioners (as seen in primary care organizations) to maximize health outcomes for the patient. In addition, over the past several years, patients have played an active part in their own health and health care, assuming responsibility for healthy lifestyles and managing their own risk behaviours. Treatment options are discussed with the patient, who is an active participant in the decisions made regarding their treatment plans.

---

**care**, and Box 5.2 for patient-centred care. The long-term care system across Canada is currently being assessed, and strategies are being developed to avoid the problems that came to light during the pandemic (see Chapter 10).

## CONVENTIONAL, COMPLEMENTARY, AND ALTERNATIVE PRACTITIONERS

**Health care providers** have traditionally been divided into three categories: conventional, core, or mainstream (e.g., physicians, nurse practitioners, midwives, nurses, dentists); **complementary health professionals** (e.g., dental hygienist, dietitians, optometrists, psychologists, social workers); and complementary and **alternative practitioners** (e.g., Indigenous healers, naturopathic doctors, homeopathic practitioners, massage therapists). Some sources simply refer to health professionals as either regulated or nonregulated, others refer to health professionals as physician and non-physician practitioners, dispensing with the previously discussed categories. See Table 5.1 for one categorization of some of Canada's many health care providers.

How health care providers are grouped remains controversial, especially since managing the care of patients has taken on a team approach, with numerous health professionals participating in and contributing to the patient's diagnosis, treatment, and ongoing care. Interdisciplinary team members are regarded as partners with respect to rendering patient care, contributing differently but equally, relative to their professional expertise and scope of practice.

### Conventional Medicine

Conventional medicine is frequently referred to as *orthodox, mainstream, traditional, allopathic* medicine, *biomedicine,* or *Western* medicine. Conventional medicine typically encompasses all those modalities not performed by alternative practitioners. "Conventional" practitioners typically diagnose and treat prediagnosed health problems and render technical, therapeutic, or supportive care with scientifically proven therapies, medication, surgery, or a combination of these modalities.

### Complementary and Alternative Care

Complementary and alternative medicine (CAM) is practised by all health care providers not generally considered mainstream. The terms are sometimes used interchangeably but, strictly speaking, there is a difference. As the names suggests, *complementary medicine*, meaning "in

| TABLE 5.1    Some of Canada's Health Care Providers | |
|---|---|
| **Conventional Health Care Providers** | **Complementary and Alternative Health Care Providers** |
| Chiropodists (Podiatrists) | Acupuncture practitioners |
| Dental assistants | Aromatherapists |
| Dental hygienists | Chiropractors |
| Dentists | Homeopathic doctors |
| Licensed/Registered practical nurses | Indigenous healers |
| Medical laboratory technologists | Naturopathic doctors |
| Medical radiation technologists | Registered massage |
| Midwives | therapists |
| Nurse practitioners | Reflexologists |
| Occupational therapists | Reiki practitioners |
| Opticians | Therapeutic touch |
| Optometrists | practitioners |
| Osteopaths | Traditional Chinese medi- |
| Paramedics | cine practitioners |
| Personal support workers (health care aides) | Yoga practitioners |
| Pharmacists | |
| Physician assistants | |
| Physicians | |
| Physiotherapists | |
| Psychologists | |
| Registered dietitians/Nutritionists | |
| Registered nurses | |
| (Registered) clinical nurse specialists | |
| Registered psychiatric nurses | |
| Registered respiratory therapists | |
| Social workers | |
| Speech-language pathologists audiologists | |

Note: This list is neither exclusive nor definitive. Titles, roles, and categorization vary by region. For example, chiropractors and acupuncture practitioners may well be considered conventional health care providers by some people.

addition to" supports, or complements, conventional medical treatments and services. *Alternative medicine* usually involves an option, an alternative treatment modality that can be used in conjunction with or in place of conventional treatments. These treatments may or may not be to the exclusion of conventional medicine.

What is considered alternative and what is considered complementary is somewhat fluid and very subjective. There is often no one "right" category to place a particular modality in. Is chiropractic mainstream, complimentary, or alternative? What about holistic medicine? Are doctors of holistic medicine considered complimentary or alternative because they focus more on natural treatments? What category would you put therapeutic touch or ear candling in? Ask 10 different people and you are likely to get a variety of answers.

**THINKING IT THROUGH**

*Treating a Sore Back*

A doctor sees a patient in their office. The patient is complaining of a sore back resulting from a fall. The doctor orders some diagnostic tests to rule out a physical injury, finding none. The doctor tells the patient to take ibuprofen as directed, and recommends that they make an appointment with a massage therapist to help relax the back muscles.

1. Would you consider a massage therapist a complimentary or alternative health practitioner? Explain your answer.
2. If the doctor sent the patient to a chiropractor, would you consider the chiropractor a complimentary or alternative practitioner? Why or why not?
3. Would you prefer to use the term *complimentary* instead of *alternative*? Explain why or why not.
4. Review Table. 5.1 Would you rearrange these categories? How?

The term *complimentary* has gained some prevalence over *alternative* as the latter can be interpreted as having negative connotations despite the fact that, for many people, modalities that traditionally come under that umbrella are both therapeutic and effective, with most founded deep in one's culture or traditions.

Moreover, what is considered standard treatment in one country, or even in one province or territory, may not be in another. Indigenous healers, for example, are well recognized in most jurisdictions and are free to treat individuals within their communities (with variable oversight).

*Acupuncture* is standard and mainstream medical care in China and considered by many in Canada to be either mainstream medical care or complementary. Acupuncture Canada offers a range of courses for regulated health professionals ranging from introductory to advanced courses, including some that teach traditional Chinese medicine assessment and treatment, resulting in certification to perform acupuncture. For example, physiotherapists often offer acupuncture as part of a treatment program. Traditional acupuncturists are regulated in British Columbia, Alberta, Québec, Ontario, and Newfoundland and Labrador.

Critics of alternative medicine believe that for treatments to be considered conventional, they should be scientifically proven before they can be claimed as effective treatments (also called an **evidence-informed** or evidence-based approach). Practitioners of therapeutic touch, for example, claim to use balance and energy, coupled with the healing force of the practitioner's hands, to facilitate a patient's recovery; however, no scientific evidence exists to prove it alters the course of a disease. That is not to say that therapeutic touch does not benefit the patient by reducing stress and promoting relaxation. For many, this in turn can certainly have an effect on the mind–body connection. For example, we know that stress reduction and feeling calm reduces a person's heart rate and blood pressure. Mindfulness is another modality that has gained popularity in recent years and has been shown to be very effective in reducing anxiety and stress and promoting a sense of well-being (see Chapter 7).

In Canada, the uptake in popularity of CAM is driven in part by Canadians themselves, as a significant number of people use CAM at some point in their lives. This may be due to several factors, including disillusionment with conventional treatment, difficulty getting appointments with their primary care provider, cultural influences and belief systems that contradict mainstream medicine, as well as information available on the Internet. In addition, many more people are actively participating in their own health care and treatment options. This includes, for most people, the desire to integrate all components of the care they seek and a move toward collaborative care by interprofessional health care teams. According to the most recent survey commissioned by the Fraser Institute, in 2016, Canadians spent $8.5 billion on providers on complementary and alternative health services, and an additional $2.3 billion on natural health products, including herbs, vitamins, and classes, between 2015 and 2016 (Esmail, 2017). In 2016, nearly 56% of Canadians used at least one CAM health care service (Esmail, 2017). Highest usage was in British Columbia and Alberta, followed by the Atlantic provinces and Québec (Table 5.2).

Almost all medical practitioners are aligned with complementary medical services, but some have reservations about modalities not supported by evidenced-informed criteria. That said, as long as an alternative therapy is safe and results in some benefits for the patient, many

**TABLE 5.2   Use of Complementary and Alternative Medicines or Therapies in Canada, by Region, in the 12 Months Preceding Interviews, 2016 (%)**

|  | B.C. | Alta. | Sask./ Man. | Ont. | Que. | Atlantic Provinces |
|---|---|---|---|---|---|---|
| Used at least one therapy in the past 12 months* | 65 | 65 | 55 | 58 | 46 | 52 |
| Massage | 46 | 71 | 51 | 53 | 53 | 62 |
| Relaxation techniques | 83 | 63 | 77 | 73 | 73 | 82 |
| Chiropractic care | 35 | 45 | 38 | 35 | 34 | 40 |
| Yoga | 53 | 59 | 65 | 59 | 50 | 63 |
| Prayer/spiritual practice | 80 | 74 | 84 | 74 | 78 | 93 |
| Herbal therapies | 72 | 71 | 80 | 67 | 60 | 48 |
| Aromatherapy | 76 | 74 | 67 | 70 | 91 | 100 |
| Acupuncture | 22 | 34 | 24 | 27 | 17 | 21 |
| Lifestyle diet | 74 | 53 | 80 | 50 | 68 | 56 |
| Naturopathy | 49 | 46 | 36 | 45 | 37 | 33 |
| Folk remedies | 60 | 46 | 56 | 59 | 6 | 22 |
| Homeopathy | 56 | 43 | 44 | 38 | 40 | 100 |
| Energy healing | 44 | 31 | 46 | 37 | 37 | 47 |
| Imagery techniques | 73 | 46 | 63 | 69 | 69 | 50 |
| Special diet programs | 30 | 39 | 56 | 32 | 13 | 41 |
| Spiritual or religious healing by others | 53 | 52 | 69 | 60 | — | 57 |
| Osteopathy | 50 | 38 | 33 | 26 | 56 | 38 |
| Self-help group | 26 | 39 | 40 | 27 | 28 | 50 |
| High dose/mega vitamins | 33 | 40 | 75 | 61 | — | 52 |
| Biofeedback | 44 | — | 20 | 35 | 75 | 50 |
| Hypnosis | 11 | — | 20 | 24 | 10 | 25 |
| Chelation | — | 50 | — | 50 | — | — |

*Total population.
Base: Those who have used therapies in their lifetimes.
**Source:** Esmail, N. (2017, April). *Complementary and alternative medicine: Use and public attitudes 1997, 2006, and 2016*. Fraser Institute. Table 5d, p. 26. https://www.fraserinstitute.org/sites/default/files/complementary-and-alternative-medicine-2017.pdf

medical practitioners have no objection to their use. Often individuals will seek alternative modalities when they feel conventional medicine is no longer effective, or if they do not want to endure the recommended treatment (such as chemotherapy for cancer), particularly when their prognosis is guarded at best.

---

**THINKING IT THROUGH**

*Seeking Alternative Treatment to Chemotherapy and Radiation*

J.D. was treated for breast cancer 2 years ago with an optimistic prognosis, although J.D. found the chemotherapy and radiation treatments difficult. Last month, she went to her physician complaining of shortness of breath. Magnetic resonance imaging (MRI) revealed metastasis to both lungs (the spread of cancerous cells from their original site). J.D.'s oncologist told her that her she could try another course of chemotherapy, but they were not optimistic it would make much difference to her prognosis and suggested that she try alternative or complimentary treatments that, although not likely curative, might be beneficial in other ways, and that she consider a hospice when the time was right. Based on her former unpleasant experience with the adverse effects of these treatments, J.D. decided to seek a homeopathic treatment. Her oncologist supported her decision completely.

1. Considering these alternatives, what would you do if you were in this position?
2. If you were a health provider and J.D. approached you for advice regarding her decision, considering your scope of practice, how would you respond?
3. What other courses of action might J.D. consider?

---

### Chiropractic: Conventional, Complementary, or Alternative?

Chiropractors (doctors of chiropractic medicine) form the largest group of CAM practitioners. To obtain a degree to qualify for clinical practice, chiropractors complete 4 to 5 years of postsecondary education. Working in individual or group practices, they diagnose and treat a wide range of conditions that deal primarily with disorders of the spine, pelvis, extremities, and joints, and the resulting effects on the central nervous system. Taking a holistic approach to patient care, chiropractors use various types of noninvasive therapies, such as exercise routines and spinal adjustments (treatments used by individual chiropractors may differ). Chiropractors are not licensed to prescribe medicine in the same manner as a medical doctor or to do surgery. Chiropractic care is not covered by most provincial or territorial plans, but most private insurance plans (extended health benefits) will pay for a specified number of visits and treatments.

Chiropractic medicine is still considered by many to be on the cusp of alternative and complementary medicine, but that is a subjective view. Increasingly, chiropractors are moving into the complementary and conventional stream, as primary care providers. The relationship between chiropractors and physicians is variable, some sharing a mutual respect, others preferring to keep their professional distance.

## REGULATION OF HEALTH CARE PROFESSIONS

The majority of health care professions are self-regulated, meaning that a professional body enters into an agreement with the government to exercise control over and set standards for its members. Some professions are entirely self-regulated while others are regulated under the umbrella of another professional organization. There are also professions regulated by the government, meaning that legislation controls the conduct and practice of the profession and its members.

Regulatory authority is granted through legislation, such as an act or statute that outlines the framework for behavior and values for a given profession. In Canada, provincial and territorial legislation (e.g., British Columbia's and Alberta's *Health Professions Act*, Ontario's *Regulated Health Professions Act*) provides the legal framework for regulating most health care professions.

Regulated professions have self-governing bodies called *colleges* (e.g., College of Registered Nurses of Nova Scotia, College of Massage Therapists of Newfoundland and Labrador), which regulate the conduct and practice of their members. Each province and territory has 20 to 30 regulated health care professions; professions regulated in some provinces and territories may not be regulated in all (Table 5.3). For example, registered psychiatric nurses in British Columbia are regulated by a college unique to their specialty—the College of Registered Psychiatric Nurses of British Columbia—while in Ontario, psychiatric nurses are under the umbrella of the College of Nurses of Ontario. Although regulated professions provide support for its members, the overriding objective of regulated professions is to protect the public, ensuring that safe care is rendered by health professionals who are properly educated and working within their scope of practice.

## Title Protection

Regulated professionals—those who belong to a professional body—are licensed to practise their profession and are legally entitled to use a specific designation, such as registered massage therapist (RMT). These professions receive **title protection**, meaning only properly trained persons registered and in good standing with their regulatory body can legally use that title. For example, people who have cared for loved ones at home but have no formal training cannot call themselves licensed or registered practical nurses. Likewise, someone who dropped out of college halfway through a respiratory therapy program cannot call themselves a respiratory therapist. Nor can health care aides call themselves nurses. Conversely, someone trained on the job can call themselves a health care aid or a personal support worker equivalent as there is no regulatory body legally protecting this title, although regulation of some type for health care aids (and the equivalent) is under review in some jurisdictions. Fully trained nurses registered in other countries cannot call themselves registered nurses here until they have met the standards set by and have been accredited by the college of nurses in the province or territory they want to practise in. Along with title protection, regulated professions share other collective elements (Box 5.3).

Any health care profession can apply to the government to become regulated, but it must meet strict criteria. The Minister of Health and some type of advisory body within the province or territory usually oversee the lengthy and often arduous application process.

Just as the possession of a legitimate driver's licence indicates that a person knows how to drive and has passed a driving test, regulation proves a person has undergone training and gained a predetermined level of knowledge, skill, or ability. Possession of a driver's licence, however, does not guarantee driving excellence; even in regulated professions, some individuals working in health care professions render substandard services.

All regulated professionals must practise within a framework of skills and services defined by their governing body (their **scope of practice**). Nurses have certain skills and acts they have been educated to carry out; physicians have a range of skills and services they have been educated to offer; and respiratory therapists, medical, and other health care practitioners, likewise, have a defined scope of practice. Even within a single profession, different levels of practice exist. For example, registered nurses with special education (e.g., advanced practice) may perform acts that those without this education cannot legally perform. Nurses usually

**TABLE 5.3  Regulated Health Care Professions in Each Province and Territory**

| Profession | PROVINCE/TERRITORY | | | | | | | | | | | | |
|---|---|---|---|---|---|---|---|---|---|---|---|---|---|
| | AB | BC | MB | NB | NL | NS | NT | NU | ON | PEI | QC | SK | YT |
| Cardiology technologists | ** | | | | | | | | | | ** | ** | ** |
| Chiropractors | ** | ** | ** | ** | • | ** | | | ** | ** | ** | ** | ** |
| Clinical assistants and physicians assistants | ** | ** | ** | | | | | | | | | | |
| Combined certified lab/X-ray technicians | ** | | • | • | | | | | | | | | |
| Dental assistants | • | ** | ** | ** | ** | • | • | | • | • | • | ** | ** |
| Dental hygienists | ** | ** | ** | ** | ** | ** | ** | | ** | ** | ** | • | ** |
| Dental technicians/Technologists | ** | ** | ** | ** | • | ** | • | | • | • | • | • | ** |
| Dental therapists | ** | ** | ** | ** | • | ** | ** | | • | | | ** | ** |
| Dentists | ** | ** | ** | ** | ** | ** | ** | • | ** | ** | ** | ** | ** |
| Denturists | ** | ** | ** | ** | ** | ** | ** | ** | ** | ** | ** | ** | ** |
| Dietitians/Nutritionists | ** | ** | ** | ** | | ** | ** | | ** | | ** | ** | |
| Hearing aid practitioners | ** | ** | ** | • | ** | | • | | •** | • | ** | •** | |
| Homeopaths | | | | • | | | | | ** | | | • | |
| Kinesiologists | | | | | | | | | •** | | | | |
| Licensed practical nurses/Registered practical nurses | ** | ** | ** | ** | ** | ** | ** | ** | •** | ** | ** | ** | ** |
| Massage therapists | | ** | | ** | • | | | | ** | | | | |
| Medical laboratory technologist | ** | | ** | ** | ** | * | ** | ** | ** | ** | ** | • | |
| Medical radiation technicians | ** | | ** | ** | | ** | ** | ** | ** | | ** | ** | |
| Medical radiation technologists | • | ** | • | • | • | • | • | •• | • | • | • | • | ** |
| Midwives | ** | ** | ** | ** | ** | • | ** | ** | • | | ** | ** | ** |
| Naturopathic physicians | ** | ** | | | ** | • | ** | | ** | | | | |
| Nurse practitioners (included as registered nurses in some provinces) | ** | ** | ** | ** | ** | ** | ** | ** | ** | ** | ** | •** | •** |
| LPNs/RPNs | ** | ** | ** | ** | ** | ** | ** | ** | ** | ** | ** | ** | |
| Occupational therapists | ** | ** | ** | ** | ** | ** | | | ** | ** | ** | ** | |
| Ophthalmic medical assistants | | | | | | | • | •• | | | | | |
| Ophthalmologists | • | • | • | • | • | • | • | • | • | • | • | • | |
| Opticians | ** | ** | ** | ** | ** | ** | ** | ** | ** | ** | ** | ** | ** |
| Optometrists | ** | ** | ** | ** | ** | • | ** | ** | ** | | ** | ** | ** |
| Paramedics, ambulance/emergency medical attendants | ** | ** | ** | ** | ** | ** | ** | ** | ** | | ** | ** | |
| Pharmacists | ** | ** | ** | ** | ** | ** | ** | ** | ** | ** | ** | ** | ** |
| Pharmacy technicians | ** | ** | ** | ** | ** | ** | ** | ** | ** | •** | ** | ** | ** |
| Physicians | ** | ** | ** | ** | ** | ** | ** | ** | ** | ** | ** | ** | ** |

*Continued*

## TABLE 5.3 Regulated Health Care Professions in Each Province and Territory—cont'd

| Profession | AB | BC | MB | NB | NL | NS | NT | NU | ON | PEI | QC | SK | YT |
|---|---|---|---|---|---|---|---|---|---|---|---|---|---|
| Physiotherapists | ** | • | ** | ** | • | ** | | ** | ** | ** | • | ** | ** |
| Physiotherapy assistants/Physical rehabilitation technicians | | | | | | | | | | | ** | | |
| Podiatrists/Chiropodists | ** | ** | ** | ** | | | ** | | ** | | ** | ** | ** |
| Psychiatric nurses | ** | ** | ** | | | | | | | | ** | ** | ** |
| Psychologists | ** | ** | ** | ** | • | ** | ** | ** | ** | ** | ** | ** | ** |
| Psychotherapists | | | | | | | | | ** | | ** | | |
| Registered nurses | ** | ** | ** | ** | ** | ** | ** | ** | ** | ** | ** | ** | ** |
| Respiratory therapists | ** | ** | ** | ** | ** | ** | ** | • | ** | • | ** | • ** | |
| Social workers | ** | * | ** | • | ** | • | ** | ** | • ** | • | ** | • ** | |
| Speech language pathologists and audiologists | | | | | | | | | ** | | ** | ** | |
| Traditional Chinese medicine and +acupuncture practitioners | +* | • ** | | | +* | | | | • ** | | +* | | |

Professions that are self-regulated and those regulated under the umbrella of another organization are not differentiated.

*+ Only acupuncture is regulated.

•Regulated health professions under the umbrella of another organization.

**Organizations that are self-regulated.

**Sources:** The Canadian Information Centre for International Credentials. (2021). *Find an occupation profile.* https://www.cicic.ca/934/search_the_directory_of_occupational_profiles.canada; Canadian Dental Association. (2022). *Laws, regulations and guidelines in health care.* https://www.cda-adc.ca/en/services/internationally-trained/laws/; Robinson, K. (2020). Chapter 8. The professional framework for midwifery practice in Canada. In E. K. Hutton, B. Murray-Davis, K. Kaufamn, et al. (Eds.), *Comprehensive midwifery: The role of the midwife in health care practice, education, and research.* https://ecampusontario.pressbooks.pub/cmroleofmidwifery/chapter/the-professional-framework-for-midwifery-practice-in-canada/#:~:text=In%20Canada%2C%20midwifery%20is%20a,midwifery%20legislation%20is%20enforced%2C%20effectively; Canadian Nurses Association. (2022). *Regulatory bodies.* https://www.cna-aiic.ca/en/nursing/regulated-nursing-in-canada/regulatory-bodies; Canadian Society of Cardiology Technologists: https://csct.ca/; Chiro-Med Rehab Centre. *Are chiropractors doctors in Canada?* (2014). https://www.chiro-med.ca/blog/are-chiropractors-doctors-in-canada/; Canadian Association of Physician Assistants. (2022). *Are physicians assistants regulated through a college?* https://capa-acam.ca/faqs/are-physician-assistants-regulated-through-a-college; Ontario Ministry of Health, Ministry of Long-Term Care. (2018). *Regulated health professions.* https://www.health.gov.on.ca/en/pro/programs/hhrsd/about/regulated_professions.aspx

> ## BOX 5.3  Regulated Professions: Common Elements
>
> - Educational standards
> - Provincial and territorial examinations
> - Practitioner's scope of practice, which outlines skills, acts, and services the practitioner is able to perform competently and safely
> - Curbing of individual's practice if standards are not met
> - Formal complaints process for the public
> - Complaints investigation and follow-up
> - Title protection
> - Competence and quality assurance

have to take specialized courses to acquire the skills to start an intravenous line or manage wound care. Similarly, a medical doctor in family practice is not qualified to remove a gallbladder or do a hip replacement; a licensed practical nurse is not qualified to do a complete physical, but a nurse practitioner is; and a massage therapist is not qualified to deliver a baby, but a midwife, nurse practitioner (depending on their education), or obstetrician is. In health care, many of these skilled procedures, some specific to certain professions, are called **controlled acts**.

## Performing Controlled Acts

Controlled acts (called *reserved acts* in British Columbia), if not performed by a qualified practitioner, may result in harm to a patient. Examples of controlled acts include giving an injection, setting or casting a fracture, passing a nasogastric tube, and prescribing a medication.

Controlled acts are identified by the *Regulated Health Professions Act* (RHA) or the equivalent in each jurisdiction. For example, the RHA in Ontario has identified 14 controlled acts that a registered nurse may perform; these are similar across the country. Acts related to each profession further define which controlled act(s) members of that profession can perform—for example, respiratory therapists and regulated radiation technologists can perform 5 of the 14 acts, physicians can perform 13, thus there is some overlap. Controlled acts may only be performed in response to an order (either direct or indirect) given by a physician or nurse practitioner, for example.

## Exceptions

Most provinces and territories allow controlled acts to be performed in certain situations by competent yet nonregulated individuals, including the following:
- A person with appropriate training providing first aid or assistance in an emergency
- Students learning to perform an act under the supervision of a qualified person, as long as that act is within the scope of practice of graduates of the student's professional program (e.g., a respiratory therapist student intubating a patient under the direct supervision of their clinical supervisor, who must be a registered respiratory therapist in good standing with their regulatory body).
- A person, such as a caregiver, trained to perform an act (e.g., giving injections to a person with diabetes)
- An appropriate person designated to perform an act in accordance with a religion—for example, a rabbi may circumcise a baby with a penis

Exclusions also apply in the case of body piercing for the purpose of jewellery, electrolysis, tattooing, and ear piercing.

## THINKING IT THROUGH

### *Performing Controlled Acts*

A personal support worker is looking after an older woman. The woman has been unable to urinate for several hours and is very uncomfortable because her bladder is full. The woman's visiting RN occasionally has to catheterize her; however, the nurse is unavailable for a few hours. The personal support worker, who is a fully qualified nurse from England, easily catheterizes the woman, making her comfortable. Clearly, the personal support worker is performing a controlled act that they are not qualified to do in Canada.

1. In your opinion, was making the patient comfortable more important than the legal implications of performing a skill not legally within the personal support worker's scope of practice? Explain your answer.
2. What might the legal implications be for the personal support worker for performing the procedure?
3. What other courses of action could the personal support worker have taken?

### Delegated Acts

As our health care system continues to evolve, health care providers' scopes of practice are also changing. Reforms in the health care system, in methods of delivery, and in health care providers' responsibilities, have affected the traditional roles of health care providers. The needs of patients also continue to change—more complex care is required more frequently. For patient needs to be met, occasionally the acts, procedures, and treatments rendered by health care providers must go beyond standard boundaries.

A **delegated act** by definition is the means by which a regulated health professional (authorized to perform the delegated act) transfers legal authority or permits another person to carry out a controlled act they are otherwise unauthorized to do (procedures that are not controlled acts do not require delegation). The person to whom the act is being delegated must be provided with education and observed performing the act to ensure understanding and competency to perform the act. A delegated act may include a specific procedure, treatment, or intervention that is not within the scope of practice of the person to whom the act is delegated. For instance, a registered nurse working in the community can delegate the act of giving an injection to a nonregulated provider (personal support worker), or to a daughter caring for her father at home. Physicians can delegate the act of obtaining a Pap smear to a qualified nurse.

Not all controlled acts can be delegated. Those that can, are defined by provincial and territorial regulations (under the jurisdictions of the *Regulated Health Professions Act*). For example, a nurse practitioner cannot delegate the act of prescribing a medication to a registered nurse or an occupational therapist. Acts in most jurisdictions cannot be subdelegated. This means that a person accepting the responsibility of performing a delegated act cannot assign someone else to carry out that act.

Guidelines and protocols for delegation of medical acts vary across Canada. In some jurisdictions, controlled acts can be delegated only to a person who is a member of a regulated profession, but in others, certain acts may be delegated by a regulated health professional to a nonregulated health care provider. Generally, the delegated act must be clearly defined and supervised accordingly. Supervision can be direct (i.e., the delegating health care provider is physically present) or indirect (i.e., the delegating provider is available for consultation).

In most health care organizations, authorities such as a board of directors or a medical advisory committee or their equivalents must agree to the rules and procedures for delegated acts. Delegated acts must also be approved by the health care agencies that specific people can take on the task. This may be agency specific, for example, identifying acts a registered nurse may delegate to a nonregulated care provider to perform. The health care provider with expert knowledge has a commitment to their patient to ensure that the person performing the act—called the *delegate*—is properly trained and demonstrates competence in completing the act.

The delegating health care professional, the delegate, and the facility or environment in which the act is performed share responsibility for the act. The health care professional who teaches or assesses the delegate's initial performance of the delegated act (and determines the delegate is competent) is accountable for ensuring the act is, in fact, carried out competently. The person carrying out the act is liable if they perform the act ineffectively.

Usually the patient or patient's power of attorney for personal care must give informed consent to allow someone other than the regulated health care professional (for whom the act is within their scope of practice) to perform a procedure. For acts typically performed by physicians, delegation will occur only with the patient's consent and only after the physician has assessed the patient, discussed the procedure, and answered any outstanding questions.

Details outlining regulations for delegated acts are available on provincial or territorial websites for related nursing and medical associations. It is worth noting that many colleges offer courses to nonregulated individuals on carrying out certain interventions.

## Complaint Process

Regulated professions have a system in place whereby the public can launch complaints against a health care provider. A designated committee investigates all complaints, protecting both the public, who can rest assured that legitimate complaints will be looked into and appropriate action taken, and health care providers, who will have illegitimate or unfounded complaints against them dismissed. Health care providers found to be at fault may face suspension, an order for additional training, the loss of their licence to practise, or even legal proceedings, such as a criminal investigation.

## Educational Standards

A regulator of a profession has the authority to set educational standards for the training of its professional members, including theoretical and practical components of their education as well as examinations for entry to practise. The educational process both prepares professional members and provides assurance to the public that the health care provider is competent to practise.

Professional bodies often use competency-based assessment programs to ensure the continued maintenance of practice standards, protecting both the health care provider and the public. The requirements may include the use of self-assessment tools, participating in continuing education programs, keeping a record of professional activities, or a combination of these. Often proof that these standards have been met is a requirement for renewal of a professional's license to practise.

## License to Practise

In each province and territory regulators of professions, in conjunction with educational facilities and in keeping with provincial and territorial requirements, oversee the licensing of their members. Regulated professions almost always require licence renewal annually. Many now have other criteria that must be met, such as peer reviews or other proof of ongoing education.

Moving from one province or territory to another can cause issues for some professionals since not all regulated professions have agreements and standards in place for members to practise in other jurisdictions (Case Example 5.1).

## Nonregulated Professions and Occupations

Table 5.2 illustrates the current professions that are regulated in the provinces and territories across Canada. All others work in the many professions and occupations that remain nonregulated, ranging from jobs that require university degrees and in-depth, specialized training, to those requiring less formal education.

People who work within nonregulated occupations do not have federal or provincial legislation governing their occupations. Like regulated professions, however, many nonregulated occupations have professional organizations or bodies that award certification when a person completes a set of written or practical examinations or both—for example, dental assistants are currently unregulated in Ontario, but dental assistants must complete a formal education and write certification examinations to practise.

When a profession is unregulated or a job applicant has not met the educational requirements of their regulatory body, the person or organization doing the hiring sets the requirements (Case Example 5.2). For example, to work as a medical secretary, an administrator in a doctor's office, or a clinical secretary (ward clerk) in a hospital, a person requires a

---

### CASE EXAMPLE 5.1    A Physician Moving Their Practice From One Jurisdiction to Another

Because physicians write a national examination, they are qualified to practise anywhere in Canada, but each jurisdiction must license physicians to practise. Dr. H., a licensed general surgeon in Newfoundland and Labrador, wants to practise medicine in British Columbia; therefore they must apply to the College of Physicians and Surgeons of British Columbia and follow provincial protocol before working in the province. Although the standards of practice for doctors are the same across the country, medical and legal issues are often different, and every physician practising in a particular jurisdiction must be aware of jurisdictional and legal guidelines that pertain to that region. Once licensed in British Columbia, Dr. H. will be assigned a billing number, which they must use to bill the provincial plan for services rendered.

---

### CASE EXAMPLE 5.2    Hiring and Educational Requirements

The CEO of a primary care organization in Alberta has decided that they want to hire a nurse to work with the health care team. The nurse must be a registered nurse (as opposed to a graduate nurse). An applicant, P.H., graduated 2 years previously from a university nursing program in the province but did not pass the national examinations. Therefore, P.H. is a graduate nurse and not a registered nurse. Another applicant, M.S., also a graduate from a university nursing program, successfully completed their national registration examinations (NCLEX-RN) a month earlier and met all requirements to become a member of the College and Association of Registered Nurses of Alberta. M.S. is a registered nurse, and because M.S. has this designation, they meet the criterion for the job.

specialized knowledge base; however, an employer may hire someone with or without a certificate or diploma. A doctor, for example, can choose to hire a person with related experience as a medical secretary and provide additional on-the-job training, or they can hire someone who has graduated from a 1-year certificate or 2-year diploma program in medical office administration. A hospital may require a clinical secretary to have a Grade 12 diploma with some administrative experience or, alternatively, a diploma from a 2-year health administration program (or the equivalent).

Many nonregulated disciplines have no specific standards to meet. For example, anyone can learn how to do ear candling or aromatherapy and put out a sign inviting the public to seek treatment.

## PRIMARY HEALTH CARE AND INTERPROFESSIONAL TEAM MEMBERS

Health care traditionally has been dominated by physicians—from family doctors to **specialists**. However, a shift toward a team approach to health care continues to evolve across Canada, maximizing the skills and expertise of a variety of health care providers, particularly in the primary care setting (see Chapter 3). The following descriptions of individuals working in health care is organized, for the most part, alphabetically and includes specialists, primary care practitioners, and collaborative health professionals who typically work as interprofessional teams.

### Dentists

Applicants usually complete a 4-year undergraduate degree (often in science) before applying to dental school at a recognized university where they must complete another 4 years to become a dentist. In Canada, a dental program must be accredited by the Commission on Dental Accreditation of Canada. The first 2 years are primarily spent in the classroom and laboratory while the second 2 years focus, in part, on applying theory to practice in the clinical setting. To become a licensed dentist, a graduate must pass an examination overseen by the National Dental Examination Board of Canada. Dentistry is a regulated profession in all jurisdictions.

### Dental Hygienists

There are both diploma and degree programs for dental hygienists in Canada. Diploma programs range from 2 to 3 years in length and can be completed at a community college. Universities offering degree programs include the University of British Columbia, University of Alberta, University of Manitoba, and Dalhousie University. Dental hygienists assess patients' oral health, carry out preventive and therapeutic dental hygiene treatments, as well as provide information about achieving and maintaining optimal oral health. Dental hygienists work collaboratively with other health care providers within the interprofessional health care team. Workplace settings include dental hygiene practices, dental offices, public health agencies, dental industries, and educational and research institutions.

### Dental Assistants

Most dental assisting programs are 1 year in length and obtained at a community college. Programs offer two levels of competence, each resulting in more responsibilities that the student can assume in the workplace setting. After completing the necessary educational requirements, a student can graduate and practise as a level 1 dental assistant or go on to achieve level 2 competencies. Responsibilities are diverse, from patient education, preparing and setting up dental instruments, processing X-rays and assisting with dental procedures, to chairside assisting.

Dental assistants in Canada are governed by different regulations in each jurisdiction, and the profession is either regulated by their own body or under the umbrella of an external organization (Canadian Dental Assistants Association, 2017). For example, in Saskatchewan dental assistants are self-regulated and licensed by the Saskatchewan Dental Assistants' Association, but in British Columbia the profession is regulated by the College of Dental Surgeons of British Columbia. The profession remains unregulated in Ontario and Québec. To become certified, dental assistants must pass the National Dental Assisting Examination Board examination(s).

## Family Physicians

Family doctors are also called *general practitioners* or *primary care physicians*. With a wide knowledge base not limited to any specific disease or system or to any particular gender or age group, the family doctor provides ongoing care to individuals of all ages and to families that includes the diagnosis and treatment of conditions and diseases not requiring the care of a specialist. That said, family physicians are considered "generalists"; although they do not come to mind with the term "specialist," they are now regarded as specialists in their field. Family physicians complete a residency in family medicine (Box 5.4).

Increasingly, family doctors are working in primary care groups with interprofessional teams, collaborating with other primary care providers to render seamless, comprehensive, patient-centered care. A few remain in solo practice, and some in various types of clinics or health centres, especially in more remote regions of the country. Many family doctors also oversee the medical care of patients in health care facilities such as long-term care facilities. Some still make house calls, most of which are covered by public health insurance if deemed medically necessary. More recently, many family doctors are choosing to give up their hospital

---

### BOX 5.4   Overview of Educational Requirements for Physicians

Entrance requirements for medical school vary across Canada, but most universities require the applicant to complete 2 to 4 years of undergraduate work, usually obtaining a bachelor's degree, and then write an entrance examination, called the Medical College Admission Test (MCAT), before applying for placement in one of Canada's medical schools. Medical school consists of 3 to 4 years of study, followed by a residency in the person's area of specialty (e.g., family medicine, internal medicine, pediatrics, or general surgery).

Many specialists work in solo practice; others work in private or public organizations or are employed by hospitals.

All physician specialists must first complete their undergraduate degree in medicine. Following undergraduate training, residency training in an accredited program must be undertaken. General surgeons will have 5 years of additional training before they can write the Royal College Exams to be certified as a specialist.

The Royal College of Physicians and Surgeons of Canada is the national professional association that oversees the medical education of specialists in Canada. They accredit the university programs that train resident physicians for their specialty practices and write and administer the demanding examinations that residents must pass to become certified as specialists.

The Royal College also oversees postgraduate medical education. A physician's credentials must be assessed by the Royal College before they are eligible to write an exam to be certified as a specialist.

---

**BOX 5.5   A Shortage of Family Physicians**

There is currently a shortage of family doctors across Canada for a number of reasons.

- Fewer physicians are choosing family medicine as a specialty, to avoid the increasing expectations placed on family doctors without the proper resources and what they feel are "stagnant" payment models.
- Many leave family medicine (e.g., to become hospitalists or emergentologists) for more appealing work hours, less overhead, and better remuneration.
- Many of those who stay in the profession tend to accept fewer patients and work fewer hours in pursuit of a reasonable work—life balance.
- Other family physicians diversify, practising part-time family medicine and part-time in another area, such as sports medicine or general practitioner (GP) anaesthesia.
- Since the COVID-19 pandemic, a significant number of family doctors are retiring early because of increased stress and exhaustion after working though the pandemic (not unlike what other care providers have experienced).

The result? Thousands of Canadians still do not have a primary care provider. Or, for those that do, even getting an appointment in a timely manner can be difficult, although that situation is improving. A shortage of family doctors is more acute in rural and northern regions across the country.

---

privileges, temporarily turning over the care of their hospitalized patients to a hospitalist or other specialist (Box 5.5).

## Medical Laboratory Technologist

Medical laboratory technologists work in both private and public facilities as well as in provincial laboratories. In order to become a laboratory technologist in Canada, a person must be certified by the Canadian Society for Medical Sciences (CSMLS). To prepare for this certification, a person must complete an **accredited program** such as the one offered at the Michener Institute in Ontario. Individuals who have received education outside of Canada and have successfully completed the CSMS Prior Learning Assessment process are eligible to write the certification examinations. CSMLS certification is accepted anywhere in Canada. This certification is the entry-level requirement for medical laboratory technologists in provinces where the profession is regulated. As well, most employers in jurisdictions where the profession is not regulated also require this certification.

## Midwives

Depending on the jurisdiction, pregnant persons experiencing normal pregnancies may choose to see a midwife. Midwives provide prenatal care (before the baby's birth) and intrapartum care, deliver the baby (either at the patient's home, in a birthing centre, or in the hospital), and provide postpartum (after the delivery) and newborn care for up to 6 weeks after the birth. Midwives, in accordance with jurisdictional guidelines, will refer a mother to a physician, usually an obstetrician, if their pregnancy becomes high risk or shows signs of other problems during any phase of the pregnancy, labour, or delivery. Pregnancy-induced hypertension, gestational diabetes, placenta previa (low-lying placenta), or a multiple pregnancy, for example, would be considered high risk. In most jurisdictions, a midwife can still provide prenatal care and work collaboratively with a physician (usually an obstetrician) until the time of and after delivery.

Midwifery, which has been practised by Indigenous people for years (Box 5.6), is now licensed in all jurisdictions in Canada. Prince Edward Island and Yukon territory are the last jurisdictions in Canada moving to regulate and fund this profession. New regulations regarding licensing midwifes in the Yukon territory came into effect in August 2021. Prior to the new legislation, a person could choose to have a home birth with a midwife, but they had to pay out-of-pocket for the service.

---

### THINKING IT THROUGH

#### Midwifery in Yukon

In August 2021, new regulations came into effect in Yukon that requires midwifes, upon completion their formal education, to practise elsewhere in Canada for 1 year prior to applying for registration with the Yukon government. The rationale, at least in part, is that new graduates would not get enough experience delivering babies during the first year after graduation in the territory because of its low birth rate. Yet, Christina Kaiser, a fully qualified midwife who has been practising in the territory for over 20 years had to leave her practice and her patients to work outside of the territory for a year as per regulation guidelines. Moreover, at the time the regulations came into effect, she was the only midwife in the territory. Her leaving has left a gap in care and numerous expectant parents scrambling for alternative plans for the upcoming birth of their babies (Desmarais, 2021).

1. Explain whether or not you think the Yukon government should have made an exception, based on the fact that Christina was a competent midwife as evidenced by her work experience?
2. Can you think of any other course of action the government could have taken rather than applying the regulations evenly with no exceptions?
3. What impact do you think this decision would have on Christina's current patients who suddenly found themselves without a midwife?

---

### Doula

A doula (sometimes referred to as a *labour coach*) assists a pregnant person and their family through the process of having a baby. A doula can be a "birth" doula, or a "postpartum" doula (or both), providing the birthing parent and their family with informational, emotional, and physical support throughout the antepartum, intrapartum, and postpartum phases of childbirth. Doulas work independently for the most part, but they may also provide collaborative care with a midwife. No formal education is required to be a doula, but there are certificate courses that can be taken. These range from 7 to 12 months in duration with a practical component at the end before certification is earned.

### Naturopathic Doctors

Naturopathic doctors are primary care practitioners who use a holistic approach to patient assessment, treatment, and care and are experts in natural medicine. Their focus of treatment is on health promotion and disease prevention considering the whole patient and is not symptom driven. British Columbia and Ontario have granted naturopathic doctors the authority to prescribe medications with the exception of controlled drugs under the *Controlled Drugs and Substances Act* (Canadian Association of Naturopathic Doctors, n.d.).

BOX 5.6  Indigenous Midwives in Canada

For generations, prior to colonization, Indigenous midwives provided their communities with safe, competent maternal—child health care services. In the nineteenth century, colonization and the medicalization of the birthing process led to a decrease in midwifery in Canada—almost to the point where there were no practising midwives among both the Indigenous and non-Indigenous population. The effect on the Indigenous population was striking, resulting in birthing parents having to leave their communities and support systems to give birth. Today, the number of Indigenous midwives (along with other Indigenous healers) is slowly increasing, which is congruent with Call to Action 23 of the Truth and Reconciliation Commission of Canada, which states: "We call upon those who can effect change within the Canadian health-care system to recognize the value of Aboriginal healing practices and use them in the treatment of Aboriginal patients in collaboration with Aboriginal healers and Elders where requested by Aboriginal patients" (Truth and Reconciliation Commission of Canada, 2015).

Currently, the National Aboriginal Council of Midwives is attempting to expand educational opportunities for those living in Indigenous communities wishing to pursue a career in midwifery and to improve access to midwifery programs. The Council's vision is to (1) outline core competencies specific to Indigenous midwifery as a major component necessary to broaden educational pathways—this will ensure the cultural and traditional practices of Indigenous people are addressed in the educational process; and (2) remove financial and funding barriers to midwifery programs.

Indigenous midwives offer their patients a unique set of competencies specific to the reproductive and sexual health of Indigenous people, respecting Indigenous culture, oral language, and traditions (Fig. 5.1). Their presence allows birthing parent to have uncomplicated deliveries within their own communities, surrounded and supported by loved ones. Birthing parents are encouraged to write their own birthing plan, which includes how they would like their birth experience managed and where they would like the birth to take place (e.g., home, birthing centre if available, or the hospital).

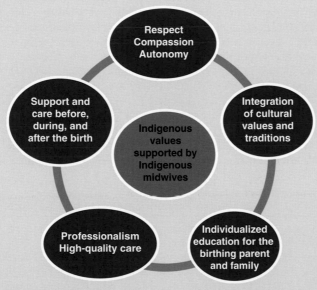

**Fig. 5.1** Indigenous values supported by Indigenous midwives.

Midwives also provide the birthing parent and the family with ongoing support in addition to facilitating parent—infant bonding, encouraging breastfeeding (promoting the related nutritional value to the infant), and infant care.

## Nurse Practitioners

Nurse practitioners (NPs) are registered nurses with advanced training and skills (RN Extended Class), authorizing them to practise in an expanded role with many of the skills and responsibilities formerly relegated to physicians. NPs can autonomously diagnose and treat health conditions, order and interpret some laboratory and diagnostic tests, and prescribe a wide range of medications, including certain controlled substances. As with other providers, NPs incorporate health education, disease prevention, and health promotion in their treatment plans. In addition, NPs can carry out specified controlled acts and activities that other nurses, by law, cannot. NPs can oversee medical aid in dying procedures in many jurisdictions.

There are numerous graduate and postgraduate nurse practitioner programs available in Canada, the majority at the master's and post-master's levels. Many of these programs are funded by their respective provincial/territorial governments. NPs need at least a master of science in nursing (MSN) degree, in addition to advanced clinical training, or completion of a nursing program with additional advanced or extended primary health care nursing education, and may require several years of practice as a registered nurse.

Licensure of NPs in Canada is dependent on the legislation and regulations established in each province and territory (personal correspondence with Dr. Stan Marchuk, DNP, MN, NP(F), CNeph(c), FAANP, President of the Nurse Practitioner Association of Canada). Each province and territory sets out the requirements for licensure, including what examination(s) an NP must successfully complete to become an NP. Some provinces utilize the Canadian Nurse Practitioner Family/All Ages exam for their Primary Care/Family Nurse Practitioner registrant, while others use the American Academy of Nurse Practitioners Exam or the American Nurses Credentialing Center Exam. There is currently no standardization of examination among provinces. All NPs must complete a written exam for licensure; however, British Columbia and Québec also require an oral exam. Registration examinations in most jurisdictions are overseen by the provincial/territorial College of Nurses.

NPs, like other regulated nurses, must renew their licence yearly. This usually involves completing a minimum number of practice hours and participation in designated quality-assurance programs, ongoing education, or both. Note that each province or territory endorses different streams of specialization (family, adult, pediatric, neonatal).

Practice settings include primary care and community settings, hospitals under specialty designations (e.g., pediatrics, cardiology), and emergency departments (Case Example 5.3).

## Optometrists

Most optometrists obtain an undergraduate degree, often in mathematics or science, before completing a 4-year university program in optometry at one of Canada's two schools of optometry (in Waterloo, Ontario, and Montreal, Québec). The minimum requirement for

---

### CASE EXAMPLE 5.3   Nurse Practitioners' Practice Settings

N.R. is applying for a nurse practitioner's licence in British Columbia. After completion of the nurse practitioner program, N.R. applies for, writes, and passes the College of Registered Nurses of British Columbia (CRNBC) examination, the province's clinical examination (OSCE) for adults, families, or pediatrics, and one of the written exams in their chosen specialty that is recognized by CRNBC. N.R. chose the family stream, or primary care stream. A person can choose from recognized examinations, including the Canadian Nurse Practitioner examination, the American Nurses Credentialing Center examination, or the American Academy of Nurse Practitioners in family examination.

entry to these programs is 3 years of undergraduate preparation, preferably in science. Graduates of a school of optometry are awarded a doctor of optometry degree. To practise, optometrists must be licensed by their province or territory. Skilled in assessing eye function and conditions, they may prescribe selected medications (topical and oral) to treat a variety of eye conditions (e.g., bacterial or viral eye infections, allergic conjunctivitis, glaucoma, and eye drops to dilate the eyes for examination). Optometrists also prescribe glasses and contact lenses to patients who need them. Most optometrists work in group or solo practices. Like all health care professionals in Canada, optometrists are regulated by their provincial regulatory authorities. The exceptions are Yukon, Northwest Territories, and Nunavut, where the *Optometry Act* is administered by the Government of Yukon, the Department of Health and Social Services, and the Department of Health, respectively (personal correspondence with Rhona Lahey, Director of Communications and Marketing, Canadian Association of Optometrists).

## Opticians

An optician completes a 2- or 3-year college program, sometimes followed by a practical component. Opticians can fill prescriptions for eyeglasses or contact lenses, fit glasses, help patients select frames, organize the grinding and polishing of lenses, and cut and edge lenses so they fit selected frames. They also do a considerable amount of health instruction related to contact lenses and glasses, including providing information about options such as lens coating and bifocal lenses. They may work independently or in a larger centre with other eye-care specialists. Opticians are regulated in nine jurisdictions across Canada.

## Pharmacists

To practise pharmacy, a person must earn a bachelor's degree or master's degree in pharmacy (or a doctorate), complete an internship, and successfully pass a national board examination through the Pharmacy Examining Board of Canada.

A licensed pharmacist, among other responsibilities, dispenses medications in response to prescriptions. Experts in their field, pharmacists provide other members of the health care team with valuable information about medications and medication interactions. The physician looks to the pharmacist for advice about current prescription medications and their interactions. The patient may look to the pharmacist for direction and advice about taking medications, their risks, and adverse effects. In most jurisdictions, the provincial or territorial plan will pay pharmacists to periodically review a person's medication profile, offer advice and counselling, or refer the person to their physician if needed.

Increasingly, pharmacists are assuming expanded roles, from giving vaccinations to prescribing certain medications. Their scope of practice differs among jurisdictions. In January 2023 pharmacists in Ontario were authorized to assess and prescribe medication for 13 more conditions ranging from urinary tract infections to skin irritations and fever. See Table 5.3 for a detailed account of the responsibilities pharmacists assumed across Canada in 2021. The goal of adding new responsibilities to the scope of practice for the pharmacist is to reduce the volume of work for doctors, clinics, and emergency departments, and to provide Canadians with more options and more convenient access to front-line services (Khaira et al., 2020).

Pharmacists are playing a significant role in providing vaccinations to Canadians. When vaccinations first became available, pharmacists were one of the most visible and accessible health care providers. Many felt safer visiting their pharmacy for their COVID-19 vaccination than they did going to larger vaccination centres, and the local pharmacy for many was closer to where they lived. Pharmacists have continued with this service, offering the third and fourth vaccinations for the COVID-19 series. The expanded responsibilities of pharmacists across Canada are summarized in Table. 5.4.

**TABLE 5.4   Pharmacists' Scope of Practice in Canada**

| | | BC | AB | SK | MB | ON | QC | NB | NS | PEI | NL | YT | NWT | NU |
|---|---|---|---|---|---|---|---|---|---|---|---|---|---|---|
| Prescriptive authority (Schedule 1 Drugs) Initiate[1,2] | Independently, for any Schedule 1 drug | X | Y[5] | X | X | X | X | X | X | X | X | X | X | X |
| | In a collaborative practice setting or agreement | X | Y[5] | Y[5] | Y[5] | X | Y | Y | Y | X | X | X | X | X |
| | For minor ailments and conditions | X | Y | Y | Y[5] | P | Y | Y | Y | Y[5] | Y | X | X | X |
| | For smoking and tobacco cessation | X | Y | Y | Y[5] | Y | Y | Y | Y | Y[5] | Y | X | X | X |
| | In an emergency | Y[7] | Y | Y[7] | Y[8] | Y | Y | Y | Y | Y | Y[7] | X | X | X |
| Adapt/ Manage[1,3] | Independently, for any Schedule 1 drug[4] | X | Y[7] | X | X | X | Y | X | Y | X | X | X | X | X |
| | Independently, in a collaborative practice[4] | X | Y[5] | Y[5] | Y[5] | X | Y | Y | Y | X | X | X | X | X |
| | Make therapeutic substitution | Y | Y | Y[9] | X | X | Y | Y | Y | Y | Y | X | X | X |
| | Change drug dosage, formulation, regimen, etc. | Y | Y | Y[9] | Y | Y | Y | Y | Y | Y | Y | X | X | X |

| | | | | | | | | | | | | |
|---|---|---|---|---|---|---|---|---|---|---|---|---|
| **Renew/extend prescription for continuity of care** | Y | Y | Y | Y | Y | Y | Y | Y | Y | Y | Y | X |
| **Injection authority (SC or IM)[1,5]** | | | | | | | | | | | | |
|   Any drug or vaccine | P | Y | Y | Y | X[10] | Y | Y | Y | Y | P | Y | X |
|   Vaccines[6] | Y | Y | Y | Y | Y | Y | Y | Y | Y | Y | Y | X |
|   Influenza vaccine | Y | Y | Y | Y | Y | Y | Y | Y | Y | Y | Y | X |
| **Labs**   Order and interpret laboratory tests | X | P[11] | X | Y[12] | X | Y | P | P[11] | Y[13] | X | X | X |
| **Techs**   Regulated pharmacy technicians | Y | Y | Y | Y[14] | Y | Y | X | Y | Y | Y | Y | X |

*IM*, intramuscular; *P*, pending legislation, regulation or policy for implementation; *SC*, subcutaneous; *X*, not implemented; *Y*, implemented in jurisdiction.

**(Source:** Canadian Pharmacists Association. (2022, February). *Pharmacists scope of practice in Canada.* https://www.pharmacists.ca/advocacy/scope-of-practice/)

[1]Scope of activities, regulations, training requirements, and limitations differ between jurisdictions. Please refer to the pharmacy regulatory authorities for details.
[2]Initiate new prescription medication therapy, not including medications covered under the *Controlled Drugs and Substances Act.*
[3]Alter another prescriber's original or existing or current prescription for medication therapy.
[4]Pharmacists independently manage Schedule 1 drug therapy under their own authority, unrestricted by existing or initial prescription(s), drug type, condition, etc.
[5]Applies only to pharmacists with additional training, certification, or authorization through their regulatory authority.
[6]Authority to inject may not be inclusive of all vaccines in this category. Please refer to the jurisdictional regulations.
[7]Applies only to existing prescriptions, i.e., to provide continuity of care.
[8]Pursuant to a Ministerial Order during a public health emergency.
[9]Applies only to pharmacists working under collaborative practice agreements.
[10]For education and demonstration purposes only.
[11]Pending health system regulations for pharmacist requisitions to labs.
[12]Authority is limited to ordering laboratory tests.
[13]Authority is limited to ordering blood tests. No authority to interpret tests.
[14]Pharmacy technician registration is available through the regulatory authority (no official licensing).

### Podiatrists (Chiropodists)

The term *podiatrist* is used internationally as the name for a foot specialist. In Canada, only Ontario uses the term *chiropodist*. Podiatrists specialize in the diagnosis, assessment, and treatment of foot disorders. They treat sports injuries, foot deformities (related to the aging process, as well as misalignments), infections, and general foot conditions, including calluses, corns, ingrown toenails, and warts. Included in their scope of practice is performing specified foot-related surgical procedures, administering injections to the feet, and prescribing medications (e.g., nonsteroidal anti-inflammatory medications and antibiotics, depending on the jurisdiction). Podiatrists refer patients to surgeons or other doctors when necessary.

In Canada, the chiropody/podiatry program is offered only at the Michener Institute in Toronto. Although Québec offers a podiatry program for residents of the province, students are required to do 1 year of training in New York. Chiropody/podiatry is not regulated in all Canadian jurisdictions.

Practice requirements and scope of practice vary from one jurisdiction to another. In jurisdictions with no regulatory body, there are no standards of practice; essentially anyone can call themselves a podiatrist and treat patients.

Practice settings include health care facilities, clinics, the community, primary care organizations, and private practice. Some podiatrists specialize in such areas as biomechanics, diabetic foot care, or foot care in long-term care facilities.

### Personal Support Workers

Most jurisdictions recognize this category of health care workers, who provide a wide variety of services to those in their care and that vary somewhat with the workplace setting. There are numerous titles for these health care workers: personal support worker (PSW), health care aide, health care assistant, continuing care assistant (used in Nova Scotia), health care support worker (commonly used in British Columbia), home care support worker, resident care aide, health care attendant, or patient service associate.

This category of health care worker provides invaluable support for patients across the health care spectrum. In most jurisdictions, individuals in this classification of caregivers must have a certificate from a community or private college in order to work for community agencies and in most health care facilities. Individuals can take a course that enables them to administer medications to stable residents in residential care (which is one step below care in a long-term care facility), usually under the supervision of a registered nurse or registered practical nurse/licensed practical nurse.

These health care providers work in long-term care facilities, home care organizations, adult day care programs, seniors' residences, and group homes under the direction of other members of the health care team. Other less common practice settings include hospitals, clinics, industry, interdisciplinary primary care practices, and private practice. This category of caregiver is currently not regulated in any jurisdiction in Canada.

### Disability Support Worker

Saskatchewan offers formal education and clinical application of skills for the designation of *disability support worker*. Workplace settings for disability support workers are residential and vocational settings where they provide personal care for residents.

### Psychiatric Nursing Assistant

In Manitoba, health care aids can further their education to become a psychiatric nursing assistant (PNA). PNAs are prepared at the college level, for they have not only the required college preparation for a health care aide but additional training specific to psychiatry.

## Psychologists

Psychologists graduate from university programs at the bachelor's, master's, or doctoral level. To practise psychology in Canada, psychologists must be licensed by the regulatory body in the province or territory where they work.

Psychologists work primarily as clinicians in hospitals, academic facilities, clinics, primary care facilities, correctional facilities, and private practice. Psychologists work with individuals and families to treat emotional and mental disorders, mainly through counselling. They administer noninvasive written and practical tests such as personality tests, intelligence tests, assessment tests for attention deficit disorder (ADD), and diagnostic tests for the early stages of Alzheimer's disease or dementia. Since psychologists are not medical doctors, they do not have the authority to prescribe medications, perform medical procedures, or order laboratory or diagnostic tests. Often, a psychiatrist and a psychologist will work as a team for more effective and ongoing patient treatment. Private insurance usually covers a specified number of visits to a psychologist, but usually only those with a PhD; for the most part, provincial and territorial plans do not cover these services.

## Physiotherapists

Physiotherapists (PTs) are regulated health care providers who graduate from university at the master's level and must pass a national exam to enter professional practice. An essential part of the primary care team, PTs work with individual patients to limit and improve upon physical impairments and disabilities, and to prevent and manage pain related to acute and chronic diseases and injury. They work in a variety of settings, such as health care facilities and clinics, as part of a primary care team, in the community (home care), and in private practice, often in groups. Some PTs specialize in such areas as **geriatrics**, sports medicine, or pediatrics. Most jurisdictions cover physiotherapy services under specific conditions and for limited time frames. Many private insurance plans also offer some coverage.

## Occupational Therapists

Occupational therapists (OTs) are members of a regulated profession who provide support, direction, and therapies to individuals in need of assistance in almost every aspect of everyday life, from recreation and work to the activities of daily living. For example, they help people learn or relearn to manage important everyday activities, including caring for themselves or others, maintaining their home, participating in paid and unpaid work, and engaging in leisure activities. OTs work with patients who have difficulties as the result of an accident, disability, disease, emotional or developmental problems, or aging. In most jurisdictions, individuals can visit OTs without a referral, although the decision to see an OT is usually made jointly with a primary care provider. OTs work in hospitals, private homes (usually through provincial or territorial home care programs), schools, long-term care facilities, mental health facilities, rehabilitation clinics, community agencies, public or private health care offices, and employment evaluation and training centres.

To practise as an OT in Canada, the minimal educational requirement is a baccalaureate degree in occupational therapy. All OTs must be registered with their provincial or territorial college. Upon passing the national certification exam, OTs can practise anywhere in Canada.

## Physiotherapy Assistants and Occupational Therapy Assistants

Physiotherapy assistant (PTA) and occupational therapy assistant (OTA) programs are offered at many community and private colleges in Canada. Most programs are 2 years in length and combine the two disciplines. A number of private colleges have single-discipline programs, usually for PTAs. Program names vary. For example, the Southern Alberta Institute of Technology offers a 2-year diploma program called Rehabilitation Therapy Assistant and graduates students with both OTA and PTA skills. All programs are in the process of becoming accredited through the Occupational Therapist Assistant and Physiotherapist Assistant Education Accreditation Program.

OTAs and PTAs work collaboratively with and under the direction of PTs or OTs to administer rehabilitation treatments to individuals who are experiencing physical, emotional, or developmental problems. Work settings include rehabilitation centres, long-term care facilities, the community (e.g., home care), physiotherapy clinics, and sports and medical clinics. Some jurisdictions, such as Alberta, have a professional therapy assistant association for PTAs, OTAs, speech-language pathologist therapy assistants, and recreation therapy assistants.

### Registered Respiratory Therapists

To become a registered respiratory therapist (RRT), one must successfully complete a respiratory therapy program from a college or university that has been accredited by Accreditation Canada. College programs are 3 years in length; university programs are 4 years long. The Canadian Society for Respiratory Therapists (CSRT) is the national professional association for respiratory therapists and the certifying body for RRTs who practise in nonregulated jurisdictions. In regulated provinces, provincial regulatory bodies provide the certification for RRTs. To obtain the RRT designation and be licensed to practise in Canada, graduates of accredited programs in respiratory therapy must write the national certification examination and meet designated registration criteria from CSRT and their respective regulatory bodies.

RRTs have expertise in caring for individuals with acute and chronic cardiorespiratory disorders and perform health-related functions—both in and out of hospital settings. In the hospital setting, they are available to evaluate, treat, and support inpatients and outpatients throughout the facility; however, they are especially vital within critical care areas such as the emergency department and in Critical Care or Intensive Care Units, where they manage advanced life support for patients with cardiopulmonary problems (e.g., persons on ventilators). With their advanced skills, respiratory therapists respond to emergencies (such as cardiac and respiratory arrests) and are able to **intubate** patients (a complex procedure of inserting a tube into the airway to facilitate breathing and initiate the use of a ventilator). Respiratory therapists are often required in the transfer of critically ill patients from one facility to another (e.g., transferring critically ill patients with COVID-19) or from an accident scene to a hospital. They are also required in the delivery room when doctors suspect the baby has or may develop respiratory problems. Respiratory therapists perform diagnostic testing, including arterial blood gases, and pulmonary function tests. In the hospital setting, the respiratory therapist is often responsible for setting up oxygen therapy or inhalation treatments. Respiratory therapists also work in medical centres, clinics, complex continuing care and rehabilitation facilities, and in the community.

### Registered Nurses

Many agree that the nurse, with skills across several disciplines, remains the backbone of the health care system, working in numerous settings, including hospitals, primary care settings, in the community, and in industry. Multiskilled and flexible, with a broad knowledge base, nurses frequently assume responsibilities typically assumed by other members of the health care team, particularly in the hospital setting. For example, when a respiratory therapist is not available, the nurse may do the inhalation treatments or set up oxygen for a patient; when a physiotherapist is unavailable, the nurse ambulates a patient and supervises their related exercises; when the chaplain is not available, the nurse counsels and comforts the patient and loved ones. When the clinical secretary is ill, the nurse may also assume administrative responsibilities for the patient care unit.

All Canadian jurisdictions except Québec require a bachelor's degree in nursing (BN or BScN) to enter the profession. In Québec, two pathways to becoming a nurse remain: one results in a college diploma (Diploma of College Studies) or a bachelor of science in nursing (Ordre des infirmieres et infirmiers du Québec, n.d.).

Degrees in nursing can be completed in 2, 3, or 4 years. Accelerated (2-year) programs are available across Canada. The related regulatory body in each province or territory must ensure that the individuals seeking to practise as nurses meet designated levels of competence. To that end, program graduates in all jurisdictions except Québec must write a national examination.

Introduced in 2015, the National Council Licensure Examination (NCLEX-RN) replaces the Canadian Registered Nurse Examination (CRNE) as Canada's national examination. Applicants for registration as a registered nurse (RN) are required to successfully complete the NCLEX-RN exam, administered by the National Council of State Boards of Nursing (NCSBN). Some jurisdictions require additional examinations. In Québec, in addition to a provincial examination, applicants must pass a Language Proficiency Licensure Examination administered by the Office Québécois de la Langue Française, in accordance with Article 35 of the Charter of the French Language. Those applying to practise in Ontario must also write a jurisprudence examination, which tests knowledge about provincial nursing and health care legislation.

Postgraduate and ongoing educational opportunities for RNs vary among provinces and territories. Some specialties include critical care, emergency nursing, community health nursing, hospice and palliative care, as well as perinatal and obstetric's health.

The RN usually assumes the most complex components of nursing care and also a variety of leadership roles both clinical and administrative. Many hospitals and other facilities employ RNs only in specific areas, such as Intensive or Critical Care Units, where their specific skill sets, particularly in assessment and decision making, are critical.

In 2021, there were approximately 459,005 *regulated* nurses eligible to practice in Canada. This figure includes 312,382 registered nurses (up 2.5% from 2020) and 7,400 nurse practitioners (an increase of 10.7% from 2020), representing the largest increase of all the nursing designations. There were 132,886 licensed or registered practical nurses (an increase of 1.6% from 2020) and 6,337 registered psychiatric nurses (an increase of 3.6% from 2020) (Canadian Nurses Association, 2022). Of interest, the Canadian Institute of Health Information (CIHI) reports that in provinces where the information was available, 4,186 RNs who either retired or left the profession for other reasons returned to the workforce to provide support that was badly needed during the pandemic. Most of the returning nurses were from Quebec and Ontario (CIHI, 2021a).

Most jurisdictions are offering various incentives to encourage individuals to apply to nursing programs in order to address the current national shortage of nurses. In addition, incentives are being offered to foreign-trained nurses. British Columbia, for example, in the fall of 2022, pledged $12 million to recruit foreign-trained nurses by simplifying the recertification process and making it more financially viable (Immigration Canada, 2022).

## Advance Practice Nurses

Advanced practice nurses are registered nurses with additional education. There are two categories of advanced practice nurses recognized in Canada: nurse practitioners (discussed earlier) and clinical nurse specialists.

### Clinical Nurse Specialists

Clinical nurse specialists (CNSs) are registered nurses who have a master's or doctoral degree in nursing in addition to wide-ranging nursing knowledge and skills and clinical experience in a specialty area (e.g., cardiology, oncology, mental health, geriatrics, neonatology). Usually in leadership positions, CNSs work in a variety of roles—as clinicians, consultants, educators, and researchers. In any setting, CNSs contribute to evidence-informed practices, continuity of care, improved patient experiences, and enhanced treatment and health care outcomes. CNS is not a protected title.

### Registered/Licensed Practical Nurses

To become a licensed practical nurse (LPN/RPN), called a registered practical nurse (RPN) in Ontario, a person must complete high school (or the equivalent) and a 2-year diploma program at a community or private college. All jurisdictions require graduates to write the Canadian Practical Nurse Registration Examination (CPNRE) for provincial or territorial registration and to use the professional designation (College of Licensed Practical Nurses of Manitoba, 2022). Some jurisdictions are replacing the CPNRE with the Regulatory Exam—Practical Nurses (REx-PN™) (College of Nurses of Ontario, 2022). This replacement took effect in Ontario and British Columbia in January 2022. There are no limits on how many times the writer takes this exam; it is computer based, and the system will automatically give the writer new questions each time they log in to rewrite it.

The skill set and scope of practice of LPN/RPNs have expanded dramatically over the past few years, with practical nurses now assuming many of the skills and responsibilities formerly limited to registered nurses. Their skill set includes doing dressings, dispensing medications, and, in some facilities, taking charge of units. The practical nurse collaborates with registered nurses and other members of the health care team to render patient care. Practical nurses can be found in almost all practice settings and in the community. The CIHI reports that there were 130,710 LPNs incensed to practise in Canada in 2020 with more of them practising part-time than other categories of nurses (CIHI, 2021b). LPNs also make up the largest number of regulated nurses working in long-term care facilities across the country. As with registered nurses, a number of LPN/RPNs who had retired or left the profession for other reasons returned to the workforce in 2020 to provide support where needed during the pandemic. Ontario and Québec accounted for the majority of those returning.

### Registered Psychiatric Nurses

Registered psychiatric nurses (RPNs)—not to be confused with registered practical nurses (RPNs) in Ontario—are recognized as a separate regulated health profession in Western Canada (Manitoba, Saskatchewan, Alberta, and British Columbia) and the Yukon. They form the largest body of mental health care professionals providing services in Western Canada. RPNs focus on the mental, developmental wellness (i.e., incorporating a holistic approach including mind, body, and spirit), mental illness, addictions and substance use, as well as the physical components of health of individuals within the context of their overall health and life situations. RPNs apply concepts from biopsychosocial and spiritual models of wellness, integrated with cultural norms, to maintain inclusion of a holistic approach to care and treatment.

RPNs work with a variety of other health care providers and mental health and community organizations. Practice settings are diverse and can include crisis stabilization and forensic assessment units, hospitals, the community, and academic facilities. Unique and separate from BN or BScN programs, education for RPNs (available only in western Canada) is offered at the degree level (bachelor's or master's degrees) and incorporates medical and surgical nursing skills with those specific to the area of mental health. RPNs are regulated to practice only in four Canadian provinces: British Columbia, Alberta, Saskatchewan, and Manitoba, and in the Yukon Territory.

The Registered Psychiatric Nurse Regulators of Canada (RPNRC) is the national umbrella organization for registered psychiatric nurses regulators in Canada. The provinces of British

Columbia, Alberta, Saskatchewan, Manitoba, and the Yukon territory regulate psychiatric nursing as a distinct profession.

## Specialists and Consultants

### Cardiologists

Cardiologists specialize in conditions and diseases of the heart, ranging from abnormal rhythms and heart attacks to related vascular problems. The cardiologist treats patients from a medical perspective, but does not do surgery. If surgery is required, the patient will be referred to a cardiac surgeon. Aside from seeing patients in the office setting, cardiologists with special training may carry out diagnostic procedures such as cardiac catheterizations in a hospital or private diagnostic facility.

### Emergentologists

Some physicians, called *emergentologists*, have chosen careers practising full-time emergency medicine. This specialty has developed because most emergency departments (EDs), also often referred to as emergency rooms, are choosing to hire full-time physicians, rather than staffing the ED with on-call physicians as in the past. Trauma surgeons also work in the ED.

### Geriatricians

Geriatrics focuses on the care of older people, typically those over 65. A geriatrician is usually an internist who has additional training in caring for older adults.

Geriatrics does not attract a large number of physicians. The assessment and treatment of an individual with complex medical conditions is time consuming. Additionally, geriatricians are typically paid less than other specialists. Most work in private practice, team-oriented practices, or health care facilities. There were just over 300 geriatricians working in Canada in 2019 (Glauser, 2019).

### Gynecologists and Obstetricians

Specializing in health of persons with a female reproductive system, gynecologists diagnose and treat disorders of the gynecological and reproductive systems. Obstetricians focus on the care of pregnant people and the delivery of their babies in both normal and high-risk situations. Closely related, these two specialties are usually undertaken together (resulting in the abbreviation OB/GYN). Midwives will refer a patient to an obstetrician if they determine that the patient is "high risk," meaning that the pregnant person needs specialized care and that there is a likelihood of a complicated delivery. The midwife will continue elements of care, collaborating with the obstetrician. Examples of a high-risk pregnancy include a history of a complicated delivery, diabetes, or pregnancy-induced hypertension (PIH).

### Internists and Hospitalists

An internist typically diagnoses and renders nonsurgical treatment for diseases of a person's internal organs (e.g., problems of the digestive tract, liver, or kidneys). An internist often refers patients to other specialists who deal with specific organs.

A hospitalist is a physician—usually an internist—who oversees the medical care of patients in the hospital, usually those who do not have a family doctor with admitting privileges to that hospital. Also, a hospitalist will collaborate with specialists as required. Usually employed by the hospital, a hospitalist may or may not have a private practice.

### Neurologists

A neurologist treats conditions of the nervous system, including chronic and potentially fatal conditions such as Parkinson disease and multiple sclerosis, sleep disorders, headaches, peripheral vascular disease, brain tumours, and spinal cord injuries. Neurologists do not perform surgery. Patients requiring surgery would be referred to a neurosurgeon.

### Ophthalmologists

Ophthalmologists, medical doctors who specialize in diseases of the eye, can carry out both medical and surgical procedures, such as cataract removal and ocular emergencies (e.g., glaucoma, eye trauma). Although ophthalmologists can perform **refractions** and prescribe glasses, these functions have largely been taken over by optometrists (who are doctors of optometry, different from medical doctors). Cataract surgery is done either in hospital or in free-standing medical facilities, such as Lasik MD clinics or the Canadian Centre for Advanced Eye Therapeutics Inc.

### Osteopathic Physicians

Osteopathy incorporates a holistic, manual approach to the diagnosis and treatment of disease. It considers, in particular, the musculoskeletal system and its relationship with the rest of the body in terms of self-healing, self-regulating capabilities.

In Canada there are osteopathic physicians and osteopathic manual practitioners or therapists. Osteopathic physicians are those individuals who have trained in the United States and who hold a medical degree from a university approved by the American Osteopathic Association. Their qualifications are the same as those for a medical doctor, and if they have completed the provincial/territorial requirements, may practise in Canada.

There are numerous schools of osteopathy across Canada graduating students who can practise as osteopathic manual practitioners or therapists. These programs are typically 4 years in length with a mandatory clinical component. Graduates from these programs are *not* medical doctors. Manual osteopathy and related educational facilities are currently not regulated in Canada.

### Oncologists

Oncology is the branch of medicine that deals with all forms and stages of cancer development, diagnosis, treatment, and prevention. Because cancer treatment has become so highly specialized, oncologists may specialize in only certain areas, such as radiation therapy, chemotherapy, gynecological oncology, or surgery. Oncologists usually practise in large hospitals or medical centres specializing in cancer treatment. They also provide ongoing treatment for patients in hospices and related facilities.

### Psychiatrists

Psychiatrists specialize in mental illness and emotional disorders, including depression, bipolar disorder, schizophrenia, obsessive-compulsive disorder (OCD), borderline personality disorder, bulimia, anorexia nervosa, and personal stress issues. As medical doctors, psychiatrists can order laboratory and diagnostic tests and prescribe medications, unlike psychologists who are not medical doctors. Psychiatrists do not perform surgical procedures. Geriatric psychiatry is an emerging field.

### Surgeons

General surgeons are qualified to perform a wide range of procedures, mostly involving the gastrointestinal tract. Many go on to further specialize in specific areas such as gynecology, neurosurgery, or cardiovascular surgery. A surgeon's scope of practice varies with experience, specialty training, and level of comfort with the type of surgery they are asked to perform (Case Example 5.4).

---

**CASE EXAMPLE 5.4   Surgeons' Scope of Practice**

A patient presents in the emergency department complaining of chest pain. Investigation reveals they have a blockage in a major artery serious enough to require surgery. A general surgeon is on call. The general surgeon is qualified to assess the patient's condition but has no special training in cardiovascular surgery. The patient is referred to a cardiovascular surgeon, who completes all required examinations and tests and performs the surgery.

---

## Speech-Language Pathologists and Audiologists

Speech-language pathologists are experts in disorders of human communication. They assess and manage persons with a wide variety of related conditions, including problems with swallowing and feeding, stuttering, and delays in speaking, and also social communication and literacy issues. Practice settings include hospitals, long-term care and mental health facilities, research and academic facilities (schools and universities), group homes, the community, and private practice.

Audiologists work with patients with problems related to sound, hearing, deafness, and balance. They provide ongoing education and diagnostic services, as well as create and manage treatment plans for all age groups. In most jurisdictions, audiologists can prescribe and fit hearing aids and other hearing devices. Practice settings are similar to those of the speech-language pathologist, with the addition of industrial settings.

In Canada, the minimal requirement to be a speech-language pathologist or an audiologist is a master's degree in the relevant course of study.

### Communications Disorders Assistant

Communications disorders assistants (CDAs) work with, or under the direction of, both speech-language pathologists and audiologists. They assist clients in communicating effectively or using alternative forms of communication, among other things. Their scope of practice includes initiating and carrying out diagnostic tests (e.g., audiology screening), assisting with treatments, and health teaching. CDAs require a graduate certificate along with an undergraduate degree or diploma in a related field such as linguistics, early childhood education, social work, or educational assistants.

## Administrative Roles

### Health Information Management

Health information management (HIM) professionals hold the designation of CHIM—Certified in Health Information Management. They provide leadership and expertise in the management of clinical, administrative, and financial health information in all formats and in a variety of settings (e.g., hospitals, community care, long-term care facilities, physician offices, clinics, research facilities, insurance companies, and pharmaceutical companies).

The Canadian College of Health Information Management (CCHIM) administers the National Certification Examination (NCE) on behalf of the Canadian Health Information Management Association (CHIMA), the national body representing approximately 5000 HIM professionals. To become a CHIM, one must graduate from a CHIMA-accredited diploma or degree program, offered at colleges and universities across the country, and successfully pass the National Certification Examination, which is offered at one level countrywide. This examination assesses the entry-level competencies of qualified applicants. Membership is classified as professional, student, retired, or affiliate.

Successful candidates receive a certificate of registration in the Canadian College of Health Information Management and are eligible to use the CHIM credential and the title Certified HIM Professional.

Certified members of CHIMA are required to participate in earning continuing professional education (CPE) credits to maintain their certification. Conestoga College in Ontario offers a bachelor of health information sciences (BAHIS) degree and will also consider graduates of CHIMA-accredited HIM diploma programs for advanced-standing opportunities. Detailed contact information on current CHIMA-accredited programs, including those offered through distance education, can be found on the CHIMA website.

The HIM profession has four domains of practice: *data quality* (the collection and analysis of health information, the coding of clinical information, and quality assurance); *e-HIM—electronic health information management* (the physical-to-digital conversion of health records, digital cloud storage and distribution of health information, and the management of complex communications systems); *privacy* (keeping health information confidential and secure, and enforcing privacy legislation as it pertains to the information for which they are responsible); and *HIM standards* (records management standards, documentation standards, terminology standards, etc.).

Health information managers are involved with almost every aspect of health information throughout its life cycle, from data and information collection, analysis, and retrieval, to the destruction of information once it is no longer needed. For example, when working with health records, health information managers facilitate the collection of health information and oversee proper access to and use of the information. They ensure that data are stored properly and safely, and when no longer needed, are disseminated and destroyed according to facility and legal guidelines. Health information managers also conduct quantitative analysis of health records, ensuring they are accurate and complete, and statistical analysis used for identifying trends, such as births, deaths, diseases, and health care costs.

In Canada, HIM professionals are trained in six core competency areas that include biomedical sciences; health care systems in Canada; health information, including the HIM life cycle; information systems and technology; management aspects; and ethics and professional practice. The HIM professional is playing a pivotal role as Canada continues to work toward the implementation of integrated electronic health information systems at local, provincial and territorial, and national levels. They will continue to be instrumental in directing and reshaping how health care is delivered.

## Health Office and Services Administration

Every aspect of health care requires some level of administrative support. The responsibility for the day-to-day administrative management of a hospital unit, a clinic, primary care organization, or a physician's office requires skill, knowledge, patience, commitment, and a high level of professionalism. The name for individuals working in these roles varies (depending on the workplace setting) from medical secretary or medical office/administrative assistant (in hospitals), to unit clerk, clinical secretary, or administrative coordinator. People in these roles must have a sound knowledge base in several areas, including pharmacology, diagnostic and laboratory testing, medical terminology, anatomy and physiology, disease pathophysiology, and the principles of triage. Those working in primary care settings must have both clinical and administrative capabilities to manage electronic health records, schedule and triage patients, and be able to do provincial or territorial billing. In the hospital setting, administrative staff have to navigate complex computer software systems for data-entry responsibilities and understand hospital policies and procedures. All must have the ability to multitask and to work efficiently under pressure, and they must be ethical, highly professional, flexible, friendly, empathetic, supportive, and comfortable around individuals experiencing any type of physical, emotional, or mental health problems.

Practice settings include doctors' offices and group practices, specialists' offices, all hospital units, and long-term care facilities. Health services or health office administrators are not regulated, so there are no provincial or territorial standards.. The International Association of Administrative Professionals (IAAP) welcomes members from any administrative discipline and has chapters across Canada.

## Other Non-physician Practitioners

Alternative practitioners are valuable contributors to the health and wellness of Canadians. Some disciplines have provincial or national organizations with varying levels of oversight by their associated bodies. Most are unregulated. Educational requirements vary greatly within the discipline, and across provinces and territories.

## Volunteer Caregivers

Friends, family, and volunteer caregivers (who work in partnership with professional caregivers) provide tremendous support to those who are ill, family members, and the general public when they interact with health care facilities. With current shortages in all categories of health care providers, many individuals depend on this group of people to fill in the gaps in their care that cannot otherwise be filled. The hours of care, direction, and support provided by these individuals are uncountable, the output unequalled, and the stress phenomenal. Many individuals interfacing with the health care system could not manage without this supportive network.

The importance of the role of volunteers during the COVID-19 pandemic cannot be underestimated. Volunteers, for example, were essential in organizing and staffing vaccination clinics, providing information for people, as well as support. Many agencies are staffed, at least in part, with the assistance of volunteer caregivers.

The exclusion of volunteers from long-term care facilities during the pandemic, justified with respect to infection prevention and control measures, was detrimental to residents in terms of their physical and mental well-being.

# WORKPLACE SETTINGS

Workplace (or practice) settings described here provide a cross-section of where health care is delivered. Included in some detail are practice settings that interprofessional teams work in. Several types of clinic settings are also described.

## Community and Home Care

You will recall from Chapter 3 that home and community care refers to the practice of effectively managing the health care needs of eligible Canadians in their homes or other community settings in which they reside. The objective is to reduce time in hospital or avoid hospital stays altogether, and delay or avoid admission to long-term care facilities. Strictly speaking, home and community care are different services, *community care* referring to the use of community resources and services to assist individuals being cared for at home; *home care* involving the services and support provided within the person's place of residence. More often than not, the services are interdependent.

The need for home and community care is increasing for several reasons, ranging from an aging population and the shift away from institutionalized care by our provincial/territorial health care system to the growing preference on the part of most Canadians to be cared for within their communities. *Home and community care* services are not covered under the *Canada Health Act.* Selected home care services (but not all) are identified, implemented, and paid for by provincial and territorial public health plans (see Chapter 4). If services provided for a person do not meet their needs, additional services must be paid for privately.

In January 2020, Statistics Canada released a report stating that approximately 3 million Canadians received some form of home care in 2018, with the majority of those being 65 years of age or older (Statistics Canada, 2020). In addition, one in six of those receiving home and community care services were between the ages of 15 and 24 (age is not a barrier to receiving home care). Collectively, the reasons for requiring home care services included individuals with acute or chronic illnesses; those recovering from surgery; those with physical disabilities, mental health issues, or complex health needs; those needing palliative care, respite, or rehabilitative care; and individuals with other matters related to aging.

Requests for home care can originate with several sources, including the person wanting home care, a family member, friend, or primary care physician; in the case of a hospitalized patient, the request may come from the health professionals within the patient's circle of care (e.g., physician, social worker, nurses, physiotherapist). In most jurisdictions, the initial point of contact for requesting home care services is made through a related community organization. After a referral has been received, the individual is assessed for the type and amount of care that would best meet their needs.

A hospitalized patient's needs may be short or long term in nature. If a patient's needs are considered to be long term, for example, if an older person with chronic medical conditions is assessed and home care services feel they cannot accommodate the patient's needs at home, other options must be considered, for example, long-term care. It can take days to weeks to find a long-term care bed, during which time the patient must remain in the hospital occupying either an acute care bed or be transferred to a bed considered an alternate level of care (ALC) bed, for example, in a step-down unit (Case Examples 5.5 and 5.6).

## CASE EXAMPLE 5.5  A Short-Term Need for Home Care Services

A 76-year-old patient who is paraplegic had an outpatient procedure done recently, and they require intravenous (IV) antibiotics and dressing changes. A referral for home care would result in a visiting nurse administering the IV antibiotics and changing the dressings. This would be considered a short-term need for home care services. If mobility was not an issue, an alternative would be for the patient to go to the hospital or other community facility for the required interventions.

## CASE EXAMPLE 5.6  A Long-Term Need for Home Care Services

An 84-year-old patient has heart disease and hypertension, chronic obstructive pulmonary disease (COPD), low vision, and some mobility issues related to arthritis. With family assistance they managed in their own home. The patient fell and broke their hip, requiring surgery and a period of rehabilitation. After the surgery, it became apparent that they could not manage at home without significant support. A home care assessment (part of the patient's discharge planning) determined they could go home with the proper home and community support, which involved several levels and types of interventions. An occupational therapist helped to make modifications to their home, addressing the patient's mobility issues. Meals on Wheels were engaged to provide them with seven meals a week. A community nursing agency was contacted to provide the patient with a personal support worker for 3 hours daily, helping with bathing, dressing, and some home management. An LPN was also made available to attend to the patient's medical needs. The support the patient requires is considered long term.

In Canada there is a shortage of long-term care beds. It is estimated that the number of long-term care beds in Canada will need to double to accommodate the demographic needs by the year 2035. Shortfalls in this type of accommodation are due to increasing need, system organization (or lack thereof), a lack of health human resources, and insufficient funding.

Home care services that are typically funded for a designated number of service hours per week are determined at the intake assessment (see Chapter 4). If a patient feels they need additional hours of care (e.g., housekeeping, general maintenance, and more supportive care), those services must be hired and paid for privately. In some regions it is difficult to find additional care, especially from nurses or personal support/care workers, because of the shortage of health human resources.

### Home Care Management in Saskatchewan

Some jurisdictions have alternative funding models, such as individualized funding provided by the Saskatchewan Health Authority. This option is offered through the province's home care program and allows the patient or their family/guardian to accept the responsibility of managing and directing supportive services (e.g., personal care or home management services such as meal preparation, house cleaning, or grocery shopping). The level of funding provided for these services is based on the assessed need. Professional services (e.g., those provided by registered nurses or therapies) are excluded from individualized funding and are provided instead through the Saskatchewan Health Authority. People who choose individualized funding are responsible for hiring, training, and terminating workers, managing payroll under the *Employment Act*, and reporting to the Saskatchewan Health Authority at designated intervals.

## Clinics

### Urgent Care and Walk-in Clinics

Canadian residents who do not have a family doctor, are away from home, or cannot get an appointment with their primary care physician can seek medical care from an urgent care or walk-in clinic. These clinics reduce the burden on emergency departments by providing nonemergency care to patients who would otherwise clog up the ED. Typically, clinic visits are less costly to the health care system than visits to the ED. Some urgent care clinics offer more immediate access to diagnostic testing, such as ultrasound, and to minor procedures, such as suturing, whereas walk-in clinics often refer the patient elsewhere for these procedures.

### Ambulatory Care Clinics

In the most literal interpretation, ambulatory care clinics have traditionally encompassed any clinic—for example, a walk-in, urgent care, or private clinic—that offers services and discharges the patient when their health care issue has been addressed. Ambulatory care, therefore, may include day surgeries, cast changes, postsurgical assessments (perhaps after hip or knee surgery), and cancer treatment. Within the past 5 years, the term has referred more specifically to facilities that offer groups of services in one location—often, a hospital.

### Outpatient Clinics

Outpatient clinics offer services that vary from hospital to hospital and community to community in an effort to meet the unique needs of a particular area. An outpatient clinic can operate under the umbrella of an ambulatory care clinic—a clinic within a clinic. Services may include family doctor care, minor surgery, screening procedures (e.g., vascular screening), laboratory and diagnostic procedures, and foot care. Outpatient clinics in large hospitals offer an even wider range of services. Some hospitals divide clinics into areas of specialty and related services; others offer many disciplines within one clinic.

### Mental Health Clinics

Most jurisdictions have clinics that respond to the specific needs of individuals with mental health disorders, although services provided are rarely adequate. Some services focus on youth and young adults and include addiction support. For the most part, these clinics collaborate with other organizations and hospital outpatient services to provide short-term, problem-focused therapy, peer support, and system navigation to help individuals find the services they need. For example, a mental health counsellor can fast track a person to a psychiatrist.

Almost all jurisdictions have adult mental health clinics (for individuals age 18 years and older). Some accept walk-in patients, others require referral from a primary care provider or have a self-referral option. For example, clinics in Saskatchewan offer a variety of services, from individualized to group sessions, which may or may not be problem specific. These clinics also provide access to wellness programs, support groups, counselling for victims of sexual violence and abuse, addiction services, and treatment for common conditions such as depression, acute anxiety, and eating disorders. Clinics in most regions also provide access to a mobile crisis team (also called a *crisis response team*) staffed by health care professionals with crisis response training (e.g., registered psychiatric nurses and counsellors) who will respond to mental health emergencies within a given geographic area.

### Nurse Practitioner—Led Clinics

Nurse practitioners in some jurisdictions have taken the lead role in seeing patients in a clinic setting. The purpose of these nurse practitioner—led clinics is to provide care for individuals who do not have access to a primary care physician or primary health care team. Individuals register with a clinic (not with a specific provider) and are offered routine health and preventive educational services (e.g., prenatal or well-baby care, managing a chronic condition) similar to those received in any other primary care delivery model, theoretically over the course of a lifetime. Basic primary health care services are provided by the nurse practitioner, not a physician. Other team members are similar to any primary health care team model: registered nurses, registered psychiatric nurses (in the western provinces), social workers, pharmacists, dietitians, psychologists, occupational therapists, physiotherapists, and others. Teams can be designed to meet the needs of the community they serve. The nurse practitioner can refer patients to specialists and other community resources as required.

### Why Clinics Make Sense

Clinics have gained prominence for a number of reasons, including the following:
- *Cost effectiveness.* New technologies have shortened surgeries and made them less invasive, allowing for earlier discharges and follow-up in clinics. It costs less to care for patients at home than to maintain them as inpatients. Many tests and procedures formerly done in a hospital are now done in a clinic on an outpatient basis. Having patients see a specialist or other health care provider in the clinic setting on a first-come, first-served basis usually costs less than having them make an appointment with a specialist or other health care provider. Organizations can staff clinics more efficiently according to perceived need. In addition, equipment booking, if handled centrally, can result in available equipment being maximized.
- *Timely access, fewer patient visits, and convenience.* With proper organization, patients can access more services faster, possibly in one clinic visit. The move toward interprofessional health care teams in clinics, similar to those found in primary care groups, has enabled clinics to readily provide the patient with a variety of services (Case Example 5.7). With centralized resources, the patient should have to make fewer visits, which is especially beneficial to patients with multiple health problems and those with mobility or transportation

---

**CASE EXAMPLE 5.7   Interprofessional Health Care Teams in Clinics**

J.L. fell, which resulted in a complex fracture of their leg, requiring a cast. They were able to have their cast checked 5 days later. Instead of having to make an appointment with the orthopedic surgeon, J.L. went to a "cast" clinic at the local hospital. A nurse specialist working in the clinic checked their cast, the circulation in their foot, and answered any questions they had. J.L. then saw the orthopedic surgeon working in the clinic, who briefly reviewed their progress, and told J.L. to return to the clinic in 2 weeks, unless complications arose.

   This clinic not only reduces the cost to the health care system (avoiding a visit to the orthopedic surgeon), but is also more convenient for the patient.

---

issues. Walk-in and similar clinics also provide patients without a primary care provider with access to one, reducing the number of visits to the ED.

- *Patient focus.* Specialized clinics are usually better prepared to work with patients, to consider their individual needs, and to offer streamlined and patient-friendly health education. Clinic staff members typically have experience dealing with a specific condition and take the opportunity to learn from their patients, which increases the professionals' overall effectiveness in meeting patients' health care needs.

## ABOUT PRIMARY CARE SETTINGS

### Strategies for Improvement

According to the Canadian Medical Association, access to prompt or same-day appointments (also known as *advanced access*) has been identified by many Canadians as being one of the most important elements of primary care. To facilitate same-day access, the College of Family Physicians of Canada introduced a number of guidelines and strategies, most of which have been implemented, in whole or in part, by Canadian physicians and with growing success. These include the use of interprofessional teams, extended office hours or after—office hours clinics (shared among providers), the use of email, and other communication technologies to manage patients' needs. For example, in chronic disease management, patients can take their own blood pressure and enter the results electronically to be tracked and assessed remotely by a health care provider. Blood glucose profiles can be managed in this manner, as can monitoring blood test results for patients on first-generation anticoagulant therapy (newer anticoagulant medications do not require such close monitoring). Some primary care teams have portals through which patients can address questions to the appropriate team member and access their chart and laboratory information.

### Forming a Primary Care Organization

In Chapter 3, we introduced various types of primary care organizations and explained which models were used in each province and territory to deliver primary care. This section explores how some primary care organizations are formed and provides additional detail regarding their structure, function, and remuneration mechanisms.

   A number of family physicians can unite to create a primary health care organization. They first need to choose what particular model or framework they want to use (it must be an acceptable model within their province or territory). In most jurisdictions, the physicians must apply to the provincial or territorial government or the appropriate body for permission to form the organization. Once approved, they enter into a formal contract with their provincial or territorial government, which details the organizational structure, funding mechanisms, and their professional obligations to the organization and patients. The obligations and funding for other members of the group (depending on the mix of health care providers) is also determined by the type and nature of the model. Organizations can also be modified to reflect the contextual, cultural, and geographic needs of the communities they serve.

### Basic Structure and Function

In some organizations most of the team members will be located in one facility; others will network with their team members who are in various locations. For the most part, physicians (or nurse practitioners in some regions more than others), are at the hub of each organization. The physicians or nurse practitioners are responsible for certain aspects of the patient's treatment, refer the patient to other resources within and outside of the organization as required, and provide oversight for the patient's overall treatment plan and well-being.

The responsibilities of most health care team members are fairly straightforward; those of physicians and nurse practitioners may be more complex (e.g., on-call hours, clinic availability, **telehealth** access, expectations related to other services offered, and patient care).

### Community Health Centres (CHCs)

CHCs, as you will recall, are located in many jurisdictions. These CHCs are community-based, nonprofit health care organizations, whose boards are comprised of members from within the communities they serve. The clinic's physicians and other health care providers are most often salaried and paid by the provincial, territorial, or federal government. Nurse practitioners (more than in other primary care organizations) often lead clinics and provide a wide range of care. In many regions, physicians, nurse practitioners, nurses, and mental health and addiction counsellors, using a mobile van, go out into the community to deliver care and address the needs of vulnerable population groups, providing support and counselling and health education.

CHCs stress an intersectoral and interdisciplinary approach to care. They partner with numerous organizations within the community to address concerns related to social and environmental determinants of health which impact the health and well-being of individuals within their geographic area.

CHCs found in rural and urban areas are especially important to those with limited access to health care (known as *hard-to-serve communities and populations*). In addition to disease prevention and related health teaching, CHC professional staff also examine the underlying social, built, and environmental conditions that may affect a community (e.g., chronic disease, seniors' needs, poor diet, housing issues, and drug and alcohol use). These centres provide a central location for the community, offering a place to gather and address health and related concerns.

A person does not have to have a health care provider to access a CHC. New Canadians are welcome with or without provincial or territorial coverage.

Table 5.5 compares primary care organizations and CHCs.

### Patient Enrollment and Primary Care Models (Rostering)

Many primary health care groups (including all groups in Ontario) require that a certain percentage of patients formalize their relationships with the group by signing a form agreeing to become part of the doctor's practice, a process called **rostering**, *patient attachment*, or *formal registration*. The idea is that the physician and patient establish a mutual commitment for care.

**TABLE 5.5 Comparison Between Primary Care Organizations (PCOs) and Community Health Centres (CHCs)**

| PCOs | CHCs |
|---|---|
| • Community based | • Community-based not-for-profit |
| • Interprofessional teams | • Interprofessional teams |
| • Not usually overseen by a board | • Overseen by boards composed of |
| • Physician led (usually, but not always) | members within the community |
| • Deliver care in a central location. Do not usually venture into the community to render care | • More likely to have nurse practitioner; may be more in lead clinics |
| • Patients must present their provincial/territorial health card | • Centrally located, but practitioners are more likely to deliver care within the community, often using a mobile approach attending to vulnerable populations, including addiction and mental health counselling, |
| • Offer full range of primary care services | |
| • Offer extended hours, enhancing patient care | • Patients can be seen without a provincial/territorial health card |
| • Usually found in urban settings | • Provide comprehensive primary care; articulate with community partners for mental health and addiction services; support community initiatives to improve health of community members |
| • Mix of funding mechanisms, usually fee-for-service, capitation-based funding, or both | |
| | • Offer extended hours |
| | • More likely to serve rural populations and those with limited access to health care |
| | • Practitioners more likely to be on a salary paid for by the province or territory |

Signing the form is purely voluntary and not binding; a patient may leave the agreement at any time or become de-rostered. Being rostered, however, entitles the patient to all of the services and benefits offered by that particular primary health care organization, such as access to after-hours clinics and a telephone helpline (see Chapter 4). If a rostered patient visits another medical doctor for a routine health problem (i.e., not an emergency), the government may deduct from the family doctor's monthly stipend the fee for that visit (Case Example 5.8).

**CASE EXAMPLE 5.8 When a Rostered Patient Visits Another Medical Doctor for a Routine Health Problem**

Although rostered with Dr. G., patient N.C., who is experiencing extreme stress, has started going to see Dr. P., a family physician who exclusively offers counselling services and psychotherapy twice a week. Dr. P. submits their fee-for-service bill for each of N.C.'s visits to the province at the end of each bill submission cycle. Dr. G., as N.C.'s primary care physician, may have the amount Dr. P. submitted to the ministry deducted from the amount of money the province pays them.

Being rostered is probably not appropriate for a person living in a temporary residence (e.g., a college student living away from home to attend school) because they may need to seek health care elsewhere.

### Payment Mechanisms

Fee-for-service was the most prevalent payment mechanism for physicians prior to the formation of primary care groups. Within these groups, capitation-based funding and blended funding (see Chapter 4) are most popular. There are also billing opportunities for milestones reached for certain services to encourage health care providers to improve patient care outcomes and lower costs. Incentive billing encourages preventive care within a practice. For example, in order to be paid, a physician must ensure that a given percentage of applicable patients have the suggested immunizations, colorectal screening, Pap smears, and mammograms. The higher the percentage of patients who receive the recommended services, the more the doctor is paid. Bonus payments may also be made when a doctor provides additional services, such as diabetic management, smoking cessation counselling, insulin therapy support, and fibromyalgia or chronic fatigue syndrome management. Collectively, these services are referred to as a "basket" of services associated with medical incentives.

### THINKING IT THROUGH

#### *Primary Health Care Group versus a Physician in a Solo Practice*

You move to a new town and set out to find a family doctor. You find one physician in solo practice who agrees to take you as a patient because they care for friends of yours. However, you also find a newly formed primary health care group with two physicians taking new patients.

  Consider the benefits that the primary health care group offers versus the close relationship you would likely develop with the physician in solo practice. Which would you choose?

### DID YOU KNOW?

#### *Telehealth*

Registered nurses and other health professions, when responding to a call on a telehealth line, use algorithms when responding to a caller's health concerns. These algorithms are constructed on the basis of best practices, evidence-informed information to direct the advice given to a caller.

### Virtual and Telephone Access to Care

All jurisdictions offer confidential telephone help assistance free of charge to those who need it. Helpline names vary, for example **Telehealth** in Ontario, Healthline in Newfoundland and Labrador, and Health Link in Alberta. Helplines offer callers advice from health care providers (usually registered nurses), 24 hours a day, 7 days a week. Nurses will not provide callers with a diagnosis, but will answer questions and, if needed, direct the caller to the appropriate resource or level of care, ranging from the person's primary care provider to a clinic or emergency department. Alternatively, the nurse may provide advice to callers on how to handle a situation themselves. In addition to provincial and territorial helplines, some primary care groups have their own helplines. See Case Example 5.9.

Telehealth and virtual visits (e.g., via Zoom) with physicians increased exponentially during the COVID-19 pandemic. The primary reason was to minimize the spread of the virus for the sake of health care providers as well as patients. Virtual and telephone visits are still in place, although to what extent varies with each jurisdiction. Some jurisdictions have removed or are considering removing or adjusting some of the billing codes that physicians can use or submit for remuneration resulting from a telephone or virtual visit. This move is to encourage providers to begin seeing more patients in person.

Although most helplines have follow-up procedures, these are not always foolproof. If a helpline responder does not diligently obey such rules, using telephone helplines can result in a breakdown in communication and continuity of care, as demonstrated in a rather extreme but not entirely unheard-of circumstance in Case Example 5.10. A helpline responder should never assume that the person calling in will follow, or is capable of following, instructions. The responsibility for reporting calls and following up properly lies with the responder.

---

### CASE EXAMPLE 5.9 Using a Helpline

H.W. lives in British Columbia and has a 3-year-old daughter, G.W. G.W. wakes up at 2:00 a.m. She is warm, crying, and has diarrhea. H.W. is not sure what to do. Should she take the child to the emergency department, or is it something that can wait until morning? H.W. calls HealthLink BC, which offers British Columbians health information and advice from a registered nurse around the clock. The nurse gives H.W. some advice on how to care for the little girl, feeling it is nothing serious enough to warrant a visit to the ED. She tells H.W. to call their family doctor in the morning if they are still concerned about their daughter, which H.W. does. In the meantime, HealthLink BC transmits an electronic report of the occurrence to the family doctor's office.

---

### CASE EXAMPLE 5.10 Helpline Follow-up

T.M. called a telephone helpline at 2:00 a.m. on Monday. T.M. said they had tried to commit suicide by taking a bottle of Aspirin and half a bottle of sleeping pills. The pills had only made T.M. slightly drowsy. With a change of heart, T.M. wondered what to do. The nurse advised T.M. to go to the nearest emergency department and offered to call an ambulance for them. T.M. responded that they would have someone drive them to the hospital. Normally, a summary of the incident would be entered into T.M's electronic health record and their doctor's office would be notified electronically or by phone, which their physician would receive the next morning. For some reason, this did not happen.

The helpline did not follow up with T.M.'s family doctor about this call. At 3:00 p.m. on Wednesday, a family friend found T.M. semiconscious and dehydrated on the floor of their kitchen and called 911. T.M.'s kidneys had failed. Today T.M. is alive but on dialysis awaiting a transplant. If T.M.'s doctor had been notified of the event Tuesday morning, the doctor could have arranged for follow-up immediately and perhaps minimized the kidney damage.

## Primary Care in Northern Regions

Primary care in Canada's northern regions is delivered by nurse practitioners and other health care providers from a centralized nursing station or clinic. Nurses are available 24/7, meaning they are on call outside of regular clinic hours. A number of nurses in the north have specialized training beyond that of a nurse practitioner. Aurora College in Yellowknife, for example (affiliated with the University of Victoria), offers a 1-year postgraduate certification in remote nursing. It involves intensive advanced assessment and clinical skills and also advanced pharmacokinetics. In most cases, these nurses have a broader scope of practice than nurse practitioners (although nurse practitioners are present in many northern communities). Nurses assess patients and diagnose conditions; order, run and interpret routine laboratory tests (done on site); and prescribe and dispense medication. They respond to routine, acute, and emergency situations. Sometimes the care provided in these communities is referred to as "cradle-to-death" care, meaning that care provided is continuous and meant to last throughout a lifetime. The number of nurses in a community is mostly determined by the size of the community, but also by the patient contact statistics. One community with 600 people and an average of 800–900 patient contacts a month will generally have three nurses; another community with the same population might have 1400 patient contacts in a month, which could justify having a fourth nurse.

Another consideration affecting the number of nurses assigned to a community is the mix of health problems, and sometimes employment. Norman Wells, in the Northwest Territories, for example, is a small community; however, with the ESSO petroleum base located here, more industrial accidents occur and will increase the patient contact hours. More nurses may be needed in this and similar communities.

Retaining medical and nursing staff is a challenge, and turnover is high. Living in an isolated area is a significant deterrent, especially when they are away from their families. Access to ongoing education and professional development is a concern, although there are increasingly more educational opportunities available online.

In an effort to retain practitioners in northern regions, provincial and territorial governments offer financial, tax, and other benefits as incentives (e.g., longer paid vacations, living allowances, educational opportunities). Nurses usually work in remote communities on a rotational basis, which can vary. For example, short rotations of 3 weeks in and out of communities are managed by Indigenous Services Canada. Otherwise, 1 to 3 months per rotation is the usual pattern with nurses, although at times a nurse may be asked to stay longer if there are staffing shortages. Nurses often establish bonds with individuals in their community, which draws them back.

Nurses are provided with accommodation, usually apartments of their own, although this will vary. The health centres (replacing nursing stations) typically have one or two examination rooms, a treatment room, and two or three beds in case a patient requires a short-term stay or must wait for air ambulance transport to a larger centre. Although health centres, nursing stations, and clinics they facilitate tend to be well equipped by most standards, the extent of care provided is limited to less serious conditions and trauma cases.

Physicians visit at designated intervals, for example, once a month for several days. Nurses keep a list of people within the community who feel they need to see the doctor. A patient must be referred by the nurse. Appointments with the doctor are reserved for cases that the nurses feel they cannot manage or that require a second opinion. Nurses have 24-hour access to a regional physician whom they can call for guidance as the need arises. Nurses make use of teleconferencing and virtual conferencing. Likewise, physicians will conduct patient consultations remotely.

## SUMMARY

5.1  Complementary or alternative medicine includes all health care practitioners not considered mainstream. Although the terms are sometimes used interchangeably, there are differences: complementary medicine supports, or complements, conventional medicine, whereas alternative medicine typically provides an option, or alternative, sometimes to the exclusion of conventional medicine. As the roles and responsibilities of many health care providers continue to evolve and with a greater emphasis on an interprofessional team approach to treatment, categorizing health professionals into these categories has become controversial. Even the names of the categories are fluid, as health care providers from various disciplines assume more autonomy and central roles in patient care.

5.2  Regulated professions provide the public with a choice of health care providers, with the assurances that the professional they choose meets legislated standards of education and practice. Although regulated professions offer support to practitioners, the emphasis is on providing safe and high-quality care to patients. Practitioners must be in good standing with their regulated body, and standards or practice must be maintained. Nonregulated health professions may still have a professional association, some providing their members with certification, which may require a written examination. Personal support workers represent one of the largest categories of nonregulated health care workers. Initiatives across the country are either experimenting with or have established registries to provide oversight to these workers with the goal of establishing provincial/territorial standards that are in the best interests of the workers and the public.

5.3  There is a large variety of health providers and practitioners in Canada in both regulated and unregulated professions. Many offer a variety of specialties within the profession, each requiring additional education, both in theory and clinical skills. Roles and scope of practice of various professions are changing to meet current and varied health care demands. Nurse practitioners function independently, assessing, diagnosing, and treating patients. The use of physician assistants is becoming more widespread, although they are not independent practitioners. Registered psychiatric nurses in the western provinces continue to provide invaluable support to the mental health community, advocating for their patients.

5.4  Practice settings range from hospitals and doctors' offices to primary health clinics or settings. Optimal primary care is centrally located, with a range of health care professionals in one building or close by. Several types of clinics offer primary care, including urgent care, walk-in, and ambulatory care clinics, most using an interprofessional team to provide care. Harm-reduction sites can be found in communities across Canada providing supervision and support services for individuals with addictions.

5.5  Provinces and territories continue to experiment with various models for delivering primary care. Presently, interprofessional health care teams appear to be the most effective approach to primary care delivery. Primary care groups differ in name, structure, services offered, and method of remuneration. A typical primary health care team, for example, might have seven or eight physicians, two or three nurse practitioners, a psychologist, a podiatrist, nutritionist(s), counsellors, and nurses. Nurses often operate as clinical specialists attending to individuals with a variety of health issues, including hypertension, diabetes, and other chronic diseases.

## REVIEW QUESTIONS

1. What are some of the concerns associated with categorizing health professionals as mainstream or conventional, complimentary, or alternative ? Discuss what you see as the rationale supporting assigning health professions into these categories.
2. What is the difference between a self-regulated profession and a regulated profession?
3. Explain the purpose of title protection.
4. What is a controlled act?
5. Who can perform controlled acts, and under what circumstances can an act be delegated to someone else?
6. Who is eligible for home and community care services?
7. What are the benefits of an interprofessional team approach to health care?
8. When would a midwife consult with an obstetrician regarding the care of a pregnant patient?
9. Either individually or in a small-group setting, design what you consider to be the "perfect" primary care organization. Consider such entities as the health care needs of your own community, professionals involved, access to care, hours of operation, and services provided.
10. How is communications technology contributing to better patient care?
11. What benefits do you see resulting from the expanded roles of pharmacists? What other responsibilities would you like to see assigned to pharmacists?
12. Explain three challenges facing home and community care services in your community before and as a result of the COVID-19 pandemic. If it were up to you, what changes would you make to deal with these challenges?

## REFERENCES

Canadian Association of Naturopathic Doctors. (n.d.) *Executive summary*. https://www.ourcommons.ca/Content/Committee/421/FINA/Brief/BR9073202/br-external/CanadianAssociationOfNaturopathicDoctors-e.pdf.

Canadian Dental Assistants Association. (2017, August). *Dental assisting across Canada: An overview of the organization of the profession of each region of Canada. CDAA Research Series Papers*. https://www.cdabc.org/media/22240/dental-assisting-across-canada-2017.pdf.

Canadian Institute for Health Information (CIHI). (2021a, August 19). *Registered nurses*. https://www.cihi.ca/en/registered-nurses.

Canadian Institute for Health Information (CIHI). (2021b, August 19). *Licensed practical nurses*. https://www.cihi.ca/en/licensed-practical-nurses.

Canadian Institute for Health Information (CIHI). (2021c, August 19). *Registered psychiatric nurses*. https://www.cihi.ca/en/registered-psychiatric-nurses.

Canadian Nurses Association. (2019). *Nursing statistics*. https://www.cna-aiic.ca/en/nursing/regulated-nursing-in-canada/nursing-statistics.

College of Licensed Practical Nurses of Manitoba. (2022). *The Canadian practical nurse registration examination*. https://www.clpnm.ca/education/cpnre-2/#:~:text=The%20Canadian%20Practical%20Nurse%20Registration%20Examination%20(CPNRE)%20is%20the%20entry,(YAS).

College of Nurses of Ontario. (2021, December 1). *REX-PN: Frequently asked questions*. https://www.cno.org/en/become-a-nurse/entry-to-practice-examinations/rpn-exam/faq-rexpn/.

Desmarais, A. (2021). December 1. *Zero midwives in Yukon leads some expecting parents to make tough calls*. CBC News. https://www.cbc.ca/news/canada/north/yukon-midwife-update-1.6266705.

Esmail, N. (2017). *Complementary and alternative medicine: Use and public attitudes 1997, 2006, and 2016*. Fraser Institute. https://www.fraserinstitute.org/sites/default/files/complementary-and-alternative-medicine-2017.pdf.

Glauser, W. (2019). Lack of interest in geriatrics among medical trainees a concern as population ages. *Canadian Medical Association Journal, 191*(20), E570–E571. https://doi.org/10.1503/cmaj.109-5752.

Immigration Canada. (2022). *British Columbia recruiting foreign-trained nurses with $12M funding boost.* https://www.immigration.ca/british-columbia-recruiting-foreign-trained-nurses-with-12m-funding-boost/.

Khaira, M., Mathers, A., Benny Gerard, N., et al. (2020). The evolving role and impact of integrating pharmacists into primary care teams: Experience from Ontario, Canada. *Pharmacy, 8*(4), 234. https://doi.org/10.3390/pharmacy8040234.

Ordre des infirmieres et infirmiers du Québec. (n.d.). *Becoming a nurse in Québec.* https://www.oiiq.org/en/acceder-profession/exercer-au-Québec/infirmiere-diplomee-hors-canada#:~:text=Everyone%20who%20wishes%20to%20practice,nurse%E2%80%9D%20is%20a%20reserved%20title.

Statistics Canada. (2020, January 22). *Care receivers in Canada, 2018.* The Daily. https://www150.statcan.gc.ca/n1/daily-quotidien/200122/dq200122e-eng.htm.

Truth and Reconciliation Commission of Canada. (2015). *Calls to action.* https://www2.gov.bc.ca/assets/gov/british-columbians-our-governments/indigenous-people/aboriginal-peoples-documents/calls_to_action_english2.pdf.

# 6

# Essentials of Population Health in Canada

## LEARNING OUTCOMES

6.1 Explain the concept of population health.
6.2 Summarize the events leading to the use of a population health approach in Canada.
6.3 Describe the effects the determinants of health on a population.
6.4 Explain the eight key elements in the Public Health Agency of Canada's population health framework.
6.5 Discuss the principles of population health promotion.
6.6 Summarize the current status of the population health approach in Canada.

## KEY TERMS

Disease prevention
Ethnicity
Health indicators
Health promotion
Inequities in health
Precarious worker

Population health
Primary care
Primary health care
Public health
Qualitative research

Quantitative research
Racism
Upstream investments

How healthy are Canadians? What is most affecting their health? What must we do to prevent illness in ourselves and in our children? How can we best implement population health and health promotion initiatives within our communities or within our provinces or territories? Do we know enough about the profound effects of the socioeconomic determinants of health on individuals and population groups? Are we able to identify and address inequities in health care, especially for marginalized Canadians? What barriers do newcomers to Canada face with respect to the determinants of health and access to equitable health care?

The answers to these questions are found in a population health approach to health care. These approaches involve all levels of government, communities, individuals, and other stakeholders.

## POPULATION HEALTH EXPLAINED

**Population health** refers to the health outcomes of a population group and the equitable sharing of those outcomes with that group. An entire population or a population group can be defined by its ethnicity, geography, nationhood or other jurisdictional nature (e.g., a province or territory), sense of community, or setting (e.g., within schools or in the workplace).

---

**BOX 6.1   Population Health Approach versus Public Health**

| Population Health Approach | Public Health |
| --- | --- |
| Gathers data about the health of a population | Uses health information to prevent disease and promote health in groups of people or the entire country |
| Analyzes the information gathered | Applies strategies to improve health rather than analyzing and researching strategies |
| Makes recommendations to improve good health or prevent disease | Carries out recommendations derived from population health studies |

---

A population health approach looks at health in broad terms. The approach considers health to be a resource influenced by numerous factors—physical, biological, social, and economic. The aim of a population health approach is to improve the health status of a targeted population, rather than that of the individual. A framework needs to be in place to gather and analyze data around related factors that affect a population's health. This analysis of the data helps identify the reasons why some groups are healthier than others, and subsequent actions are taken to look for ways to improve health. A population health approach also helps to build a sustainable and integrated health care system that is flexible, effective, and equitable, even in the face of the current challenges facing our health care system.

The terms *population health* and *public health* are often used interchangeably, but they are different entities with a common denominator—health information. Population health integrates public health initiatives such as **health promotion** and **disease prevention**. **Public health** transforms the recommendations from population health research into action (e.g., administering recommended vaccines, implementing health education initiatives). Public health strategies are federal, funded and implemented by provincial, territorial and municipal governments, and involve collaboration with health care providers, industry, and community agencies (Box 6.1).

## THINKING IT THROUGH

### Childhood Vaccinations

Until recently, many childhood diseases in North America were thought to be either well controlled or eradicated as a result of vaccination programs (e.g., with vaccines against polio, measles, diphtheria, pertussis [whooping cough], rubella, mumps, tetanus, rotavirus, and *Haemophilus influenzae* type b). However, some of these diseases are reappearing because of low vaccination rates in some regions. The proportion of children who are vaccinated varies across the country, although exact numbers are not known because Canada has no national protocol for gathering this type of information.

Although it is highly recommended that all children attending school complete the recommended vaccination regimens, only Manitoba, Ontario, and New Brunswick have legislated vaccination policies, applying only to schoolchildren. In these provinces, children who are not vaccinated must present a certificate from a medical authority stating they cannot be vaccinated (the reason remains confidential). Guardians can also exempt their children from vaccination, based on religious or conscientious grounds. In Ontario, under the *Immunization of School Pupils Act*, if the school does not have a completed immunization report, a student can be suspended for up to 20 days (or until such time as the proper documentation has been submitted).

Alberta has legislation in place that enables school officials to cross-reference immunization records from school enrollment lists with Alberta Health's vaccination records to identify children who are not immunized. With this information to hand, school officials can contact families to ask that their unimmunized children stay home if there is an outbreak of a communicable disease in the school. The Alberta law also allows health officials to contact the parents or guardians of unvaccinated children to provide information on the benefits of immunization.

COVID-19 and influenza vaccinations are not included in recommended vaccination protocols for school-aged children.

1. What are your own thoughts about mandatory vaccination protocols?
2. Do you believe the risks of not vaccinating a child outweigh the benefits? Support your answer.
3. In your opinion, should the influenza, COVID-19, or both vaccinations be mandatory? Explain your answer.

## INTRODUCTION OF POPULATION HEALTH TO CANADA

The reports and conferences discussed in this section have been instrumental in introducing the concepts and development of population health in Canada.

### The Lalonde Report, 1974

In *A New Perspective on the Health of Canadians*, Marc Lalonde, then the Minister of National Health and Welfare (which became Health Canada in 1993), introduced the concept of population health to Canada (Lalonde, 1981; Public Health Agency of Canada [PHAC], 2001). Informally called the "Lalonde Report," this is the first document acknowledged by a major industrialized nation to state that health is determined by more than biology and that improved health could be achieved through changes in environment, lifestyle, and health care organization—"the quantity, quality, arrangement, nature and relationships of people and resources in the provision of health care."

### Declaration of Alma-Ata, 1978

In September 1978, the World Health Organization (WHO) convened an international conference in Almaty (formerly Alma-Ata), Kazakhstan, to address the need for global cooperation on health issues and in health care reform. The slogan that emerged from that conference, "Health for All—2000," reflected the shared goal to reduce **inequities in health**—unfair and unequal distribution of health resources—across the globe by emphasizing primary health care. **Primary health care**, as defined by the conference attendees (Box 6.2), encompasses a broad range of concerns that parallel those of the population health approach. Primary health care that emphasizes individuals and their communities includes essential medical and curative care that extends when necessary to secondary or tertiary levels and involves health care that is cost-effective, comprehensive, and collaborative.

The 10-point Declaration of Alma-Ata states that health is a fundamental human right and that all nations should prioritize attaining an optimum level of health. The declaration calls for the right of people and communities to be involved in planning their own health care and challenges governments to develop strategies to improve primary health care. See the Declaration of Alma-Ata on the Evolve site.

---

BOX 6.2   **The Alma-Ata Definition of Primary Health Care**

"Primary health care is essential health care based on practical, scientifically sound, and socially acceptable methods and technology made universally accessible to individuals and families in the community through their full participation, and at a cost that the community and country can afford to maintain at every stage of their development in the spirit of self-reliance and self-determination."

Source: Reproduced, with the permission of the publisher, from Declaration of Alma-Ata: International conference on primary health care. Alma-Ata, USSR, 6–12 September 1978. World Health Organization.

## Ottawa Charter for Health Promotion

The first International Conference on Health Promotion, in 1986 in Ottawa, was convened to review and expand on the proposals put forward at the 1978 Conference on Primary Health Care, at Alma-Ata, and to determine what progress had been made toward assuring health for all by the year 2000 (World Health Organization, 1986).

The factors affecting health outlined in the Lalonde Report were expanded and termed "health prerequisites," and the need for a collaborative approach to addressing health-related problems was reinforced. Five principles emerged from the conference, including the need for all levels of government to become involved in health promotion and for individuals to assume some responsibility for their own health (not just seeing the doctor when sick and expecting the doctor to make them well). The Ottawa Charter for Health Promotion also looked at community-level strategies to enhance health; for example, government-funded day care was cited as ultimately benefitting the health and well-being of both children and their parents or guardians. A national day care program initiated by the federal government in 2021 has been implemented in stages.

## The Epp Report, 1986

*Achieving Health for All: A Framework for Health Promotion*, known as the Epp Report, after the then-Minister of Health and Welfare Jake Epp, was released at the 1986 Ottawa conference. It focused on proposals to reduce inequities for disadvantaged groups, to better manage chronic diseases, and to prevent disease. The report recommended that these initiatives have financial support from all levels of government (Health and Welfare, 2006).

## Toward a Healthy Future: The First Report on the Health of Canadians, 1996

The *Report on the Health of Canadians* was released in September 1996 for the Meeting of Ministers of Health. Its recommendations carried forward the proposals made by the Canadian Institute for Advanced Research (CIFAR) in 1989. This report was the first to officially recognize and incorporate the determinants of health into its findings and recommendations.

Although the report concluded that Canadians were among the healthiest populations in the world, it emphasized that collaboration among all levels of government, industry, and the private sector must be intensified to improve our health. Box 6.3 lists strategies specified by the report to improve or maintain the health of Canadians, a further endorsement of the principles of the population health approach.

## National Forum on Health, 1994–1997

The National Forum on Health was the blueprint for current Health Canada initiatives. The forum was launched by the then Prime Minister Jean Chrétien in 1994 and wrapped up in 1997. An integral part of this forum was public input—the beliefs and values of people across

BOX 6.3    Report on the Health of Canadians

**Strategies for Improving the Health of Canadians, 1996**
*Living and Working Conditions*
- Create a thriving, sustainable economy, with meaningful work for all.
- Ensure an adequate income for all Canadians.
- Reduce the number of families living in poverty.
- Achieve an equitable distribution of income.
- Guarantee healthy working conditions.
- Encourage life-long learning.
- Foster friendship and social support networks, in families and communities.

*Physical Environment*
- Foster a healthy and sustainable environment for all.
- Build suitable, adequate, and affordable housing.
- Create safe and well-designed communities.

*Personal Health Practices and Coping Skills*
- Foster healthy child development.
- Encourage healthy life-choice decisions.

*Health Services*
- Ensure appropriate and affordable health services, accessible to all.
- Reduce preventable illness, injury, disability, and death.

Source: Federal, Provincial, and Territorial Advisory Committee on Population Health. (1996, September). *Report on the health of Canadians.* https://publications.gc.ca/collections/Collection/H39-385-1996-1E.pdf

the country were sought through public discussion groups, conferences, meetings with experts, commissioned papers, letters, and briefs.

In February 1997, the forum published two final reports: *Canada Health Action: Building on the Legacy, Volume I: Final Report* and *Canada Health Action: Building on the Legacy, Volume II: Synthesis Reports and Issue Papers.* One of the key recommendations that emerged was the need for more analysis and concrete evidence (i.e., an evidence-informed approach) to support initiatives for improving health.

All of these reports, beginning with the Lalonde Report, were significant in initiating a united population health approach to achieving better health for Canadians. Subsequent reports—including *Toward a Healthy Future: The Second Report on the Health of Canadians*, published in 1999; *The Future of Health Care in* Canada, 2001; *The Health of Canadians—The Federal Role: Final Report, Volume 6*, published in 2002 (also known as the Kirby Report); and *Building on Values: The Future of Health Care in Canada*, published in 2002 (also known as the Romanow Report) (see Chapter 1)—have analyzed the health of Canadians using a population health approach and offered recommendations for action.

## THE DETERMINANTS OF HEALTH

How people look at health care (their worldviews) is shaped by their **ethnicity** (which refers to their place of origin or ancestry and may be shaped by the languages they were brought up using, and their religion); culture (which takes into account beliefs, values, norms, practices and customs, behaviours, and attitudes); language; sex and gender; age; and previous experiences with the health care system. Any of these factors can have a significant impact on a person's interactions and experiences with health care and, in turn, health outcomes (Government of Canada, 2022a).

A health provider's worldview may also affect how they respond to people seeking treatment, the type and quality of the care they deliver, and the trust they build with their patients. The beliefs and values of both patients and health care providers can lead to health disparities. This situation can be compounded if there is lack of cultural competence on the part of health care providers, leading to a lack of understanding and trust and to intolerance (on the part of both the person seeking treatment and the health care provider). For example, some people's outlook on health and health care is linear (e.g., believing only in genetics, biology, and disease), while others view health and health care from a holistic perspective.

First Nations peoples look at health and wellness from a holistic perspective, using, for example, the medicine wheel to emphasize the balance between physical, mental, emotional, and spiritual components of health (First Nations Health Authority, n.d.). When these components are integrated and nurtured, they promote health and well-being. The health traditions and customs of Indigenous people are being increasingly integrated into health care delivery models across Canada (see Chapters 1 and 7).

Respecting health-related customs and traditions is essential, as is adapting practices so that the delivery of health care is sensitive and appropriate to people's cultures. Only then will disparities and gaps in health care delivery begin to close; this, in turn, will have a positive impact on the determinants of health.

Public health in Canada typically addresses health promotion, disease and injury prevention, and behavioural risks that can affect a person's health. The profound effect of economic, social, personal, and environmental factors on the health of Canadians is also recognized.

The health of a population and of individuals depends on a combination of factors that go beyond genetics, biology, and disease and cannot be addressed by health care interventions alone. By and large, the social determinants of health are within societal control, even if solutions are complicated (Government of Canada, 2022a).

Health Canada has identified 12 determinants of health (Government of Canada, 2022a). Health Canada and the Public Health Agency of Canada (PHAC) also refer to these determinants as the "social determinants of health," namely social and economic factors having to do with a person's place in society that affect all aspects of a person's health and health outcomes. The determinants of health and their descriptions can vary among population groups, as is seen with Indigenous people in Canada (Assembly of First Nations, n.d.). For example, the determinants of health identified for Inuit people were initially drafted and subsequently updated by Inuit Tapiriit Kanatami (meaning "Inuit are united in Canada," also known as "ITK") (Inuit Taprit Kanatami, 2014). The Inuit determinants of health highlight the key social determinants of health that are relevant to Inuit populations in Canada today (Fig. 6.1).

## THINKING IT THROUGH

### Comparing the Determinants of Health

Health Canada's 12 determinants of health are similar to the 11 determinants of health identified by the Inuit people, but differences are also evident, including in the hierarchy of the determinants listed. Compare Health Canada's list with the social determinants of Inuit health shown in Fig. 6.1a and b. Answering and discussing these questions may be more meaningful if answered with another student or in small groups.

1. How do the two lists differ?
2. What do you think is the rationale behind the different determinants in the social determinants of Inuit health?

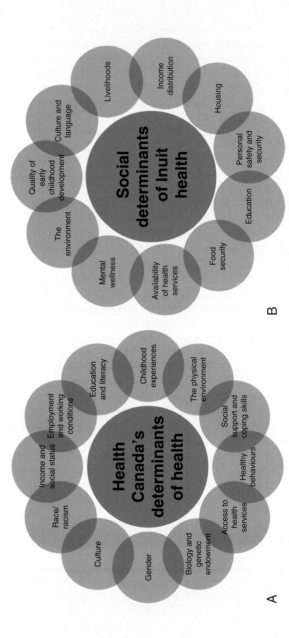

**Fig. 6.1** (a) Health Canada's determinants of health. (b) Social determinants of Inuit health. (Source: Inuit Tapiriit Kanatami. (2014). *Social determinants of Inuit health in Canada.* https://www.itk.ca/wp-content/uploads/2016/07/ITK_Social_Determinants_Report.pdf)

## 1. Income and Social Status

Income and social status are one of the most important determinants of health. Lower socioeconomic status (SES; or a lower position on the SES gradient) is associated with poorer health and an early death, while a higher socioeconomic status is associated with better health (Box 6.4).

In 2020, Canada's median household income, after taxes, was $66,800, an increase of 4% over the previous year (Statistics Canada, 2022a). This increase was larger for lower-income families, likely driven by income support provided by the government during the COVID-19 pandemic. Anyone whose household income is less than half the national median is considered to be living below the poverty line. This calculation is referred to internationally as "low-income measure, after tax" (LIM-AT). In 2019, the poverty line in Canada was approximately $31,459; in 2021, it was an estimated $32,996 (Statistics Canada, 2022a). In 2020, approximately 6.4% of the Canadian population was living below the poverty line, a decrease from 10.3% in 2019 (Statistics Canada, 2022a). This decrease was experienced by all types of families and was, at least in part, due to financial transfers from the federal government to assist individuals and families financially during the pandemic. Marginalized Canadians still experience much higher levels of poverty than nonmarginalized population groups (Employment and Social Development Canada, 2022a).

Almost one-fifth (17.4%) of newcomers 16 years of age or older and who arrived in Canada within the past 10 years live in poverty. Recent newcomers (with or without a skill set) face numerous barriers, including language (which makes it a challenge to find the appropriate information concerning jobs and, when indicated, related training); cost of skills upgrading as well as the time this upgrading takes; lack of bridging programs (to upgrade); as well as discrimination and bias (Ng & Gagnon, 2020).

### The Market Basket Measure

Canada's official measure of poverty was developed by Employment and Social Development Canada and is called the *Market Basket Measure* (MBM). This measure is based on the cost of specific goods and services that represent a basic standard of living for a family of four. The basket includes nutritious food (based on Health Canada's 2019 National Nutritious Food

---

### BOX 6.4 Socioeconomic Status Explained

Socioeconomic status (SES) is derived from combining a person's or a group's education, occupation, income, social status, and sometimes geography. The results are shown on a scale or gradient. This socioeconomic scale or gradient is widely used in population health studies. At one end of the socioeconomic scale are people who are living below the poverty line, are unemployed or underemployed, and living in substandard housing; they are at greater risk for poor health. As socioeconomic status improves, so does an individual's or group's health.

Socioeconomic studies usually examine and compare several population groups. A single socioeconomic indicator can be used for measurement (e.g., occupation) or multiple indicators can be grouped together (e.g., by income, education, geography, ethnicity, gender/sex, or sexuality). The goal is to determine gaps in health across the population groups and identify what actions are needed to narrow the gaps.

In Canada, poverty, unemployment, and substandard housing are not uncommon on First Nations reserves and in many Indigenous communities. If you review the determinants of health as applied to large portions of this population group, you will see how broadly Indigenous people are affected.

Basket), clothing, shelter (e.g., a three-bedroom apartment including utilities), transportation (a basic vehicle and some public transportation), as well as other goods and services (Djidel et al., 2020).

The MBM incorporates the fact that income, circumstances, and the cost of goods and services vary with the size and demographic makeup of communities, the jurisdiction, and geography, all of which are important to consider when researchers and policymakers are making assessments and recommendations. A family or an individual who has a disposable income (after taxes) that is lower than the MBM adjusted for the size of the family and geographic location would be considered to be living in poverty. This definition may differ from the LIM-AT.

The MBM is only applicable to the provinces. The Northern Market Basket Measure (MBM-N) is being developed for Nunavut, Yukon, and the Northwest Territories, based on similar criteria. Because economic realities and the cost of living change with time, the MBM-N is reviewed at designated intervals of approximately 5 years.

### Food Insecurity

Moderate or severe food insecurity affected about 10% of households in 2018 and 2019 across the provinces (Statistics Canada, 2022a). The financial constraints caused by the COVID-19 pandemic economic shutdown further affected Canada's working poor, influenced quality of food intake, and increased physical and mental health problems (Polsky & Gilmour, 2020). The rising inflation rate that began in 2022 was another concern, particularly for lower-income and **precarious workers** earning minimum wage (versus those earning a living wage). In general, families and individuals experienced a decrease of approximately 3% in income, reducing the average income to $55,700 from $57,600 as a result of COVID-19 restrictions and the related impact on the Canadian economy.

Table 6.1 illustrates the median after-tax income in Canada, across provinces, for 2019 and 2020.

### Indigenous People's Incomes

At over $93,000, the 2019 median after-tax incomes in the Northwest Territories and Nunavut were higher than Yukon's, at $77,800. This was also higher than in any of the provinces, where the median after-tax income was about $62,000 (Statistics Canada, 2022a). Indigenous families living off-reserve in the three territories had a median after-tax income of $71,900 (Statistics Canada, 2021).

The Canadian Income Survey: Territorial Estimates, 2019, released in November 2021, shows that almost 12% of the total population of the territories live in low income, despite the reasonably high median after-tax incomes. At almost one-fifth of the population, Nunavut had the highest number of individuals living in low-income households.

In 2019, 16.5% of Indigenous people aged 16 and older living off-reserve in the three territories were living in low income. The proportion was even higher in the provinces, at 20.7%. Across Canada, in 2019, almost one-fifth of Indigenous people living off-reserve lived below the poverty line (Employment and Social Development Canada, 2021; Statistics Canada, 2021). Income disparities for First Nations people living on-reserve and in isolated communities are accentuated by geographic isolation, limited employment opportunities, limited or no access to secondary and post-secondary education, and the traumatic effects of intergenerational trauma caused by colonialism and residential schools.

### 2. Employment and Working Conditions

Unemployment is considered to be one of the biggest stressors that a person or family can face. People who are precariously employed, underemployed, or unemployed and who work

TABLE 6.1 Median After-Tax Income, Canada and Provinces, 2019 and 2020

| | 2019 | 2020 |
|---|---|---|
| | *(2020 constant dollars)* | *(2020 constant dollars)* |
| Canada | $62,400 | $66,800 |
| Newfoundland and Labrador | $55,900 | $59,300 |
| Prince Edward Island | $57,200 | $59,400 |
| Nova Scotia | $53,300 | $57,500 |
| New Brunswick | $54,800 | $56,900 |
| Québec | $55,400 | $59,700 |
| Ontario | $65,100 | $70,100 |
| Manitoba | $60,600 | $63,000 |
| Saskatchewan | $64,400 | $67,700 |
| Alberta | $74,400 | $77,700 |
| British Columbia | $63,000 | $67,500 |

**Source:** Statistics Canada. (2022, March 23). *Table 2 median after-tax income, Canada and provinces, 2016 to 2020*. Table 11-10-0190-01 (Formerly CANSIM table 206-0011). https://www150.statcan.gc.ca/n1/daily-quotidien/220323/t002a-eng.htm

in low-satisfaction or high-stress jobs tend to have poorer health. The prevalence of low self-rated mental health, a subjective measure of overall mental health status, is almost eight times higher among adults permanently unable to work than among those who are employed, and it is over two times higher among people working in unskilled occupations than those in professional occupations (PHAC, 2018a; Russell, 2020; Russell & Parker, 2020). These people have a higher mortality rate at a younger age and higher morbidity rates from chronic diseases (e.g., cardiorespiratory disease). Families of unemployed or underemployed people also have poorer health, likely because of the resulting high stress, related emotional problems, poverty, and a lower socioeconomic status that affects their ability to buy prescription drugs and afford dental services.

### Unemployment Rates

The unemployment rates in Canada in 2020 to 2022 ran at almost 10% (Statistics Canada, 2022b). The people most affected during the periods of lockdown imposed to try and control the spread of COVID-19 were those working in hotels, restaurants, bars, gyms, and retail and personal services. By June 2022, the unemployment rate had dropped to 4.2% in the face of an immense shortage of people available to fill a wide range of mostly blue-collar jobs across the country. Unemployment rates are predicted to hover at about 5% for the next 5 years (O'Neill, 2022).

### Wage Gap

Canadian women in full-time positions in the core age category earn, on average, about 89 cents for every dollar men make (Canadian Women's Foundation, 2022; Pelletier et al., 2019). This difference, or wage gap, typically widens for women with disabilities, Indigenous and racialized people, and newcomers to Canada.

August 2021 saw the federal *Pay Equity Act* come into effect. The Act affects those working in federally regulated public and private workplaces and addresses the government's commitment to workers receiving equal pay for work of equal value (Boisvert, 2021).

Other jurisdictions also have payment equity acts to address the problem of gender wage discrimination. Human rights legislation in British Columbia, Alberta, Ontario, and Saskatchewan prohibits payment discrimination based on gender, and equal pay for same or similar work is a requirement of employment standards legislation in Ontario, Manitoba, Saskatchewan, Yukon, Newfoundland and Labrador, and the Northwest Territories (Pay Equity Office, 2022).

Pay equity is legally required in separate pay equity legislation for the public sector in Manitoba, Nova Scotia, New Brunswick, and Prince Edward Island and for the public and certain private sectors in Québec and Ontario.

## 3. Education and Literacy

A higher level of education widens people's knowledge base and ability to think logically and problem solve. Having a higher education often motivates people to engage in meaningful relationships and become involved in the community, resulting in greater life satisfaction overall. Higher levels of education also typically lead to better-paying jobs with a higher standard of living and social status. Associated financial security increases the opportunities for a person or a family on many levels, and advantages can accumulate over generations: how our parents and grandparents lived influences our opportunities and outcomes. In addition, early childhood education programs have long-term effects on social-emotional skills and academic and social outcomes and are associated with significant gains in adult employment, earnings, and other outcomes.

### Newcomer Job Prospects

Newcomers to Canada with certain occupations or professions often find that their educational qualifications are not recognized in Canada. To qualify to work in their field, they may have to complete foreign credential recognition programs. Gaining the specific professional licenses or certifications to work may be too much to overcome as a recent newcomer, and individuals often end up looking for any job that provides them with an immediate income. There are doctors and dentists, engineers and architects working in factories or driving taxicabs. Individuals in such situations often decide to work in areas that are similar but less challenging to qualify in (see Case Example 6.1). That said, as a result of the current acute shortage of health human resources in Canada, the federal, provincial and territorial governments are investing in projects and initiatives to reduce barriers for internationally educated health professionals to qualify to practise in the country.

## 4. Childhood Experiences

The experiences a child has throughout their formative years has a significant and lasting impact on their cognitive, emotional, and physical development and general health—effects that last into adulthood. From infancy, a baby's surroundings and the type of care and love they receive affect their outlook on the world, their ability to develop meaningful relationships,

### CASE EXAMPLE 6.1   P.V.'s Nursing Career

P.V. was enrolled in a program to train to be a licensed practical nurse (LPN). P.V. was working on a pediatric unit as part of the required clinical practice experience. An alarm went off in the neonatal intensive care unit. Without hesitation, P.V. ran to the baby that was in distress and dealt with the emergency. An astonished clinical instructor learned that P.V. was a pediatric cardiologist from Beijing, China. P.V. simply could not afford the cost of going back to university for several years to qualify as a pediatric cardiologist in Canada. (This case is from the author's personal experience.)

and their ability or inability to trust others (experienced, for example, by many Indigenous people in Canada as a result of intergenerational trauma) (Childwatch, 2019; Cowan, 2020; Limmena, 2021).

Stress in a child's life—due to physical or emotional abuse, poverty reflected in food insecurity and living in precarious housing or unsafe neighbourhoods, and discrimination—can impede the development of adaptive coping skills, result in difficulty in controlling emotions, and impair social function (Kronstein, 2017). Children who live in poverty for extended periods of time are at a higher risk of developing chronic diseases as well as cognitive and emotional challenges, which may in turn contribute to poor academic outcomes. This affects a person's ability to find stable employment and financial security, factors that further contribute to poor physical and mental health. Parenting skills may be compromised, and the cycle repeats itself.

### Child Poverty in Canada

In 2020, a decrease in the poverty rate of 4.7% was experienced by children in all age categories, reducing the number of children in poverty by half (Statistics Canada, 2022a). This decrease occurred in every province. The largest decreases were in Saskatchewan (down 5.2%), Prince Edward Island (down 4.7%), and Manitoba (down 4.7%). These decreases in poverty rates are likely temporary and, as with other income-based statistics for the same time frame, are affected by income support provided by various levels of government in 2020.

### Government Assistance

For the 2021—2022 benefit year, the maximum annual child benefit payout was $6833 per child under age 6 and $5765 for children between the ages of 6 through 17 years. The maximum benefit payout for a child with a disability is $2915 annually ($248.75 per month) (Employment and Social Development Canada, 2021; Government of Canada, 2022b). Although the goal of this tax-free payment and other benefits is to reduce or eliminate child poverty, they fall short of providing financial security for children and their families living in low income. For the 2021—2022 benefit year, the maximum annual benefit was set at $6833 per child under age 6 and $5765 per child aged 6 through 17 years (Macdonald & Friendly, 2020). That's over $350 more per child than when the Canada child benefit was first introduced.

### Day Care

The variety of day care options available to choose from ranges from home day care (where a child goes to someone's home) and nannies (where a carer comes into the child's home), to child care centres. Only some child care programs are regulated. Registered day care facilities are licensed and monitored by the provincial/territorial government.

The cost of day care relative to the family's income affects the choices parents and guardians make. Prices range from under $200 to over $2000 per month for one child. Two provinces, Québec and Manitoba, have preset prices for child care. Monthly costs of regulated child care centres are highest in Nunavut and the Northwest Territories (Arrive, 2020).

About 60% of Canadian children are enrolled in some type of day care (Klukas, 2021). In 2021, the federal government introduced a nationwide early learning and child care agreement which, at least in theory, will bring the cost of day care in all jurisdictions down to $10 per child per day within 5 years by 2025. The federal government has agreed to assume half of the cost of the program. As of March 2022, all the provinces had signed on to the national child care plan. Although the plan sounds effective, numerous concerns exist among jurisdictions, including finding qualified individuals to work in child care facilities and the funding to pay them adequately. In addition, not all day care organizations are likely to participate in the agreement.

**THINKING IT THROUGH**

*Day Care in Other Countries*

In Iceland, day care is considered an essential part of a child's education and early development, and every child under 6 years of age has the opportunity to attend what is called play school, although it is not mandatory. Norway regards child care as a "statutory right," and every child has a guaranteed spot in a day care facility after their first birthday.

1. Do you think that funding day care for every child would be cost-effective in Canada?
2. What impact do you think licenced day care and guaranteed spaces have on children's physical and mental or emotional development?
3. How might day care affect the social determinants of health in terms of early childhood experiences?

## 5. The Physical Environment

The physical environment consists of natural and manufactured environments. The natural environment includes the food people eat, the water they drink, the air they breathe, and the places they live—the outside or physical world.

The "built" environment refers to the parts of the physical environment produced by people—public spaces, parks, buildings (houses, schools, shops, offices, for example)—and the transportation infrastructure (e.g. streets, cycle paths, sidewalks). How this built environment is structured and constructed affects health status.

### Living with Disabilities

Nearly one-third of people with disabilities are not provided with the accommodations they ask for in their workplace. A similar proportion reported that their disability hinders them from advancing in their careers or changing jobs (Canadian Human Rights Commission [CHRC], 2018). For the 10% of students aged 15 to 24 years who require accessible buildings, classrooms, or washrooms to attend school, up to one-third reported that these were made available to them (Brown & Emery, 2009; Canadian Association for Community Living [CACL], 2013; CHRC, 2012; Choi, 2021; Turcotte, 2014).

These factors, plus the lack of social and structural supports and networks, contribute to higher unemployment rates among people with disabilities than among people who do not have disabilities, and increase the likelihood that they live in isolation and below the poverty line.

### Housing Costs

The Canada Mortgage and Housing Corporation (CMHC) defines housing as affordable only if a person or family is spending less than 30% of their income (before taxes) on housing.

Over the past 20 years, the price of a home has increased by 375%, on average, and by up to 450% in Toronto and Vancouver (Schwartz, 2022). Despite a decrease in the cost of housing in late 2022, owning a home remains out of reach of many. The cost (average, all rental properties) of renting also increased in 2022, on average by 6.6% over the previous year. The highest rental rates were in British Columbia and Ontario, and the lowest in Newfoundland and Labrador (Fawcett, 2022; To Do Canada, 2022).

The need for adequate and affordable housing in Canada has been described as a national emergency, particularly for people living in low income, newcomers, and racialized people. Housing for low-income population groups is below standard 7.5 times as often as for those in high-income groups (PHAC, 2018a). Twice as many newcomers live in housing that is substandard. This trend is accentuated among racialized newcomers compared with racialized nonimmigrants.

In 2020, acting on the commitment that everyone has the right to affordable housing, the federal government, through the CMHC, launched the Rapid Housing Initiative (RHI) to create new affordable housing for vulnerable people and populations. The initial funding for this initiative was $1 billion to help address urgent housing needs of vulnerable Canadians, especially in the context of COVID-19. Over 3000 units were constructed in 2020–2021 and an additional 4000 in 2022.

---

**DID YOU KNOW?**

### *Availability of Housing Units*

At 424 housing units per 1000 residents in 2020, Canada has the lowest ratio of housing units per population of any G7 country. To accommodate the number of individuals requiring housing units between 2016 and 2021, as many as 100,000 dwellings would have been needed—and this number does not take into account the sharp rise in population growth due to immigration.

Source: Perrault, J-F. (2021, May 12). *Estimating the structural housing shortage in Canada: Are we 100 thousand or nearly 2 million units short?* https://www.scotiabank.com/ca/en/about/economics/economics-publications/post.other-publications.housing.housing-note.housing-note--may-12-2021-.html

---

### Housing for Indigenous People

Housing for First Nations people living on-reserve and Inuit is precarious at best. Overcrowding is rampant—seven times greater than for the non-Indigenous population—and it is not unusual for 18 people to be living in a small dwelling. Many homes are constructed using substandard materials and do not comply with building codes, thus deteriorating more quickly than other homes. About 40% of homes on-reserve are in need of major repairs because of insufficient funding, poor-quality materials to maintain homes, or a lack of skilled labour to complete necessary repairs (Senate of Canada, 2015). These conditions are worse on reserves that are geographically isolated.

Housing inequities and crowded conditions contribute to numerous health problems for adults and children. Health issues include the spread of infectious diseases, such as tuberculosis, bronchitis, influenza, and, recently, COVID-19.

Poor housing conditions also contribute to injuries and death. Many on-reserve communities have woefully inadequate resources to respond effectively to fires, and First Nations people living on-reserve are 10 times more likely to die in a house fire than non-Indigenous people (Canadian Institute of Child Health [CICH], 2022).

In 2020, the First Nations Information Governance Centre reported that over 34,000 housing units were required to meet housing needs across First Nations communities. On average, each community currently needs over 80 additional housing units (First Nations Information Governance Centre, 2020). Funding programs in place to address the housing needs of First Nations across Canada, for example, the First Nations On-Reserve Housing Program, are available through Indigenous Services Canada. In British Columbia, this support is provided through the British Columbia Housing Support Program.

Indigenous Services Canada provides various funding programs for housing on reserves in addition to annual targeted funding (for housing). However, the ministry does not cover the full cost of housing: First Nations communities are expected to share the housing costs, finding additional funding from other sources (e.g., private loans). Local authorities can use the annual funding for the construction and maintenance of homes and insurance, and to plan and manage other housing-related needs.

### Climate Change and Disease

Aside from the tragic and often deadly effects of catastrophic weather events on people and communities around the world, climate change has resulted in an increase in disease spread by insects and other animal vectors as warmer temperatures have made it easier for carriers of, for example, Lyme disease, eastern equine encephalitis, and West Nile disease to expand their range and their active periods each year (Health Canada, 2022). The risk of importing climate-sensitive diseases from further afield may also increase for Canadians. Fungi in soils may directly affect humans and animals as well as our food sources. A warming climate is also expected to worsen air pollution levels in Canada. Exposure to some air pollutants, including fine particulate matter and ozone, increases the risk of respiratory illnesses, the development of disease, and premature death (Health Canada, 2022) (see Chapter 10).

## 6. Social Support and Coping Skills

The social environment is constructed by how people behave; their relationships with others and their community (including a person's level of attachment and social comfort in terms of feeling they belong and their relationships); their sex or gender; their culture and ethnicity; their education and roles in the workforce; the conditions and communities in which they live; and how they feel about themselves. Individuals in the same or similar social environments have been shown to demonstrate similar values, outlook on life, and ways of thinking.

The more tightly knit and organized a community is, and the more involved its members are with activities within the community, the stronger the health of that community. Keep in mind that the makeup of a community and how it impacts the health of its population can vary. For example, individuals or families living in a condominium may not know their immediate neighbours, but they may be involved via various group activities or organizations or a volunteering team. Remote communities, such as those in the northern parts of Canada, are usually close-knit, but they lack access to the variety of services and activities available in more populated regions.

Newcomers to Canada may be subject to social isolation if they left their families, friends, and support networks behind and are trying to adapt to a new culture and environment. Newcomers who are sponsored by, for example, a church group, have more support than those that are not similarly sponsored.

### Social Isolation

*Social isolation* is often defined as reduced contact with other people, in terms of both the amount and quality of contact (e.g., brief interactions with individuals one doesn't know well instead of longer, more meaningful communication with family, friends, and others who are part of a supportive social network) (Employment and Social Development Canada, 2022a). Social isolation can have a profoundly negative effect on a person's physical, emotional, and mental health. Social isolation as such is a complex issue, rarely resulting from one or two isolated circumstances.

The opportunity to share feelings, discuss problems, and receive the support of others can relieve stress and enhance a sense of well-being. It promotes the feeling of being wanted and valued and improves a person's physical and emotional health.

---

**CASE EXAMPLE 6.2** **J.R. and the Benefits of Support**

J.R. is 50 years old and has been married to R.O. for 15 years. They have been having marital problems for some time. J.R is uncomfortable voicing personal problems and does not have a close friend with whom he could discuss personal issues. He bottles up his feelings and, as a result, is argumentative, critical, and bad-tempered most of the time. His mood affects his family, friends, and colleagues. He has trouble sleeping, and he was diagnosed with high blood pressure in recent weeks. He has refused counselling. R.O., on the other hand, is able to reach out to close friends and family for support and has joined a meditation group.

---

Social support and a social network can come from family members, friends, or a community. Having close ties to a community—with work, religious groups, volunteer organizations, or even gym or cycling groups—provides a sense of belonging and security. The type and level of support a person has or seeks are influenced by age, sex or gender, culture, and many other factors. Typically, men are less likely to form supportive networks and share feelings, often because of societal pressures to avoid sharing personal feelings with others. Consider Case Example 6.2.

J.R's behaviour is not unusual for many men. This may be partly due to the inability (or reluctance) of some men to access a social network for support and advice. In fact, numerous source show a link (in general) between the social environment and the risks of morbidity and mortality, independent of the effects of other health determinants (Employment and Social Development Canada, 2022b; Government of Canada, 2022a). Findings also indicate that social environments can influence the course of a disease. For example, a person with cancer or cardiovascular disease is likely to survive much longer if they can access supportive social networks (Koven, 2013). This may relate to a reduction in stress and a positive, even optimistic, outlook generated by a loving and caring environment.

Restrictions limiting social contacts to limit contagion during the COVID-19 pandemic resulted in many people feeling isolated, lonely, and depressed. Even though most people could connect with others by telephone, video-conferencing tools, and online messaging apps, the physical component of getting together with friends and family, being able to touch and hug them, and have spontaneous, unplanned conversations was drastically missed. This social isolation proved to be particularly difficult for individuals with fewer social networks who were living alone or in long-term care facilities. Prolonged social isolation can lead to cognitive disorders, cardiac disease, and altered immune systems (Pietrabissa & Simpson, 2020).

## Older Canadians

Approximately 30% of older persons in Canada (over the age of 65) are at risk for being socially isolated. Statistics Canada reports that between 19 and 24% of individuals in this age group feel isolated from others, wanting to participate in more social activities (Employment and Social Development of Canada, 2022b).

## Resilience

Adaptive coping skills are influenced by genetic makeup and socioeconomic factors. Some people are better able to deal with problems, stress, and daily challenges than others, even in the face of family disharmony, financial and employment insecurity, marginalization, and other challenges; they are simply more resilient.

Consider the challenges faced by refugees who recently arrived in Canada from war-torn countries. Cultural differences may affect health beliefs, practices, and expectations, and the new environment will have a profound effect on how they are able to adjust and cope in their new home. The more help and support an individual or family have when transitioning to their new life, the more positive the outcomes will be in terms of their health, ability to cope, and, in turn, contributions to society.

## 7. Healthy Behaviours

Unhealthy behaviours, such as cigarette smoking, poor diet, and lack of exercise, affect life expectancy. Personal health behaviours relate to experience of and beliefs about health and risk behaviours as well as societal organization and socioeconomic status. In turn, healthy behaviours impact our health and well-being (Health Canada, 2021).

### Cigarette Smoking and Vaping

The use of tobacco is the number 1 risk factor for preventable disease in Canada. Those individuals who smoke are approximately 20 times more likely to develop lung cancer than nonsmokers (Canadian Cancer Society, 2022).

Anti-tobacco campaigns have led to smoking being concentrated among marginalized Canadians, because those who are better educated and more affluent tend to have greater health literacy and more resources to act on smoking cessation (PHAC, 2018b).

E-cigarettes and other tobacco products are also carcinogenic, but almost one-third of current or former smokers have used e-cigarettes to help them stop cigarette smoking (Government of Canada, 2021). On the other hand, 15% of Canadians who used a vaping product said they had never smoked cigarettes. This is a disturbing trend, as vaping can increase the risk of nicotine addiction, alter brain development, and increase the likelihood of nonsmokers (including adolescents and young adults) starting smoking cigarettes (Government of Canada, 2021; Soneji et al., 2017). Aside from the unknown risk of exposure to the chemicals in e-cigarettes (including formaldehyde and metals, and diacetyl, a flavouring compound known to cause bronchiolitis), the risk of chronic bronchitis is higher among people who vape (Chun et al., 2017; McConnell et al., 2017).

In May 2022, the Canadian government proposed adding health risk information to each cigarette in a pack to target those who often "borrow" single cigarettes from a friend rather than buying their own pack (which have graphic images showing the harm caused by smoking-related cancers) (Thompson, 2022).

### Avoiding Vaccinations

It is debatable if actions (or inactions) involving vaccination and vaccine hesitancy can be considered health behaviours or not. That said, there is no doubt that not receiving recommended vaccinations can result in serious illness for the unvaccinated person and for others through the transmission of disease by those who are unvaccinated (e.g., not receiving childhood vaccinations, the seasonal flu vaccine, and vaccinations for COVID-19).

Vaccinations are regarded as one of the most important advances in preventing a number of serious diseases, particularly in childhood. People who choose not to get vaccinated or decide against their children being vaccinated do so for a variety of reasons. One is complacency—they consider the risks of contracting the vaccine-preventable disease and of developing serious illness to be low. Another involves health concerns; the ratio of risks to benefits may not be well communicated, which relates to culture and health literacy, or they are worried about the health risks of a vaccine, having heard varying views about it from individuals who do not agree with the science behind vaccines. Finally, individuals may lack confidence or trust in the effectiveness and safety of vaccines, in the people who administer the vaccines, in the system that delivers them, and in the reasons why policymakers and governments decide on a vaccine (Fieselmann et al., 2022; MacDonald, 2015, 2020).

## Substance Use

The use of substances such as alcohol and drugs is considered a risk behaviour because of the negative health outcomes linked to the use of these substances. Outcomes depend on the amount and frequency of the substance used and whether or not an individual develops a substance dependency. Alcohol, for example, is a level one carcinogen and one of the three leading causes of cancer. The risk of cancer increases with the amount of alcohol a person consumes. Moreover, alcohol consumption (as with drug use) leading to addiction is a disease in itself. Addiction can lead to physical, mental, and emotional trauma with devastating socioeconomic outcomes and can be a mediator to violence, injuries, and accidental deaths.

## 8. Access to Health Services

Disease diagnosis, treatment (both to maintain and restore health), and prevention as well as health promotion are pillars of the population health approach. The type of health care services offered and their method of delivery affect the health of a population. Greater availability of **primary care** services and of health promotion and disease prevention programs (e.g., immunizations, preventive care such as screening, prenatal care, and well-baby initiatives) can lead to a healthier population (with adequate resources). Equally important are community and long-term care services, which, at present, are stretched beyond capacity across the country.

Health services in Canada currently face multiple financial, logistic, and resource challenges. Years of chronic shortfalls in health care funding have adversely affected all aspects of the health care system at the federal, provincial, and territorial levels. Currently, the shortage of human health resources has had and continues to have perhaps the most dramatic impact on the availability of health care services across the country. This shortage has impaired prompt access to primary care, emergency care, and diagnostic, medical, and surgical procedures and prompted the (mostly intermittent) closure of emergency departments and ambulatory care clinics in many regions. The COVID-19 pandemic has had a devastating effect on the health of Canadians, exacerbating many of these shortfalls, most of which were evident before the pandemic began (Canadian Medical Association, 2021).

In short, the capacity of primary care and other health providers to deliver quality care to Canadians is currently inadequate (described by many as being critical). According to the Canadian Medical Association (2021), this demand for extra capacity poses a significant risk to the sustainability of the health care system itself.

## 9. Biology and Genetic Endowment

*Biology and genetic endowment* refers to the attributes that people inherit from their birth parents. These inherited attributes can make a person vulnerable to developing specific diseases and conditions. Genetic studies can help people understand their risk of developing certain diseases (e.g., Huntington's disease, cystic fibrosis, certain forms of cancer such as breast cancer, and Alzheimer's disease) and of passing certain conditions on to their children. How individuals use this information varies; some may choose not to know.

Socioeconomic and environmental influences can affect biology. If a person grows up and lives in ideal socioeconomic and environmental conditions, they are more likely to have good physical and mental health. An older person who is physically active and who has healthy behaviours, a strong social network, and easy access to medical care may never develop chronic diseases and musculoskeletal decline.

## 10. Gender, Sex, and Sexuality

### Gender versus Sex

Although the terms *sex* and *gender* are sometimes used interchangeably, they have different meanings. Most often categorized as male or female or intersex, the term *sex* typically refers to biological characteristics of a person, which include physical and physiological traits (e.g., chromosomes, hormone levels, and reproductive systems) (Treasury Board of Canada Secretariat, 2019). *Gender* relates to social identity, behaviours, expressions, roles, and other entities that identify males and females as well as other gender-diverse individuals (e.g., non-binary, Two Spirit) (Canadian Institutes of Health Research, 2020). Gender affects how a person perceives themselves and others as well as how they act and interact in society; it is not specific to any binary and may be fluid, thus subject to change over time.

## Gender Identity

There are many evolving terms to describe gender identity (Women and Gender Equality Canada, 2022). People are most likely to identify as *cisgender*, meaning that they identify with the gender they were assigned at birth.

- A *non-binary* person does not identify as either male or female. Their gender identity may include man and woman, androgynous, fluid, multiple, no gender, bigender, agender, or other components. Canadian society is adopting gender-neutral language to promote inclusivity for non-binary individuals. Societies that only recognize two genders (male and female) are referred to as *gender binary societies* (National Center for Transgender Equality, 2018).
- *Transgender* (or trans) describes a person whose gender identities and experiences do not align (fully or in part) with the gender they were assigned at birth.
- A *gender-diverse* (or gender-fluid) person's gender identity varies over time and may include male, female, and non-binary gender identities.
- A person who is *questioning* is unsure of or still exploring their sexual orientation or gender identity.

*Gender expression* is defined as how a person presents their gender identity in terms of their behaviour—the voice they use, the clothes they wear, and how they style their hair (Human Rights Campaign, n.d.). These may not conform to behaviours or expressions typically defined as masculine or feminine.

## Sexual Orientation

Sexual orientation is a fundamental part of a person's identity and not a choice. It is a person's physical or emotional attraction to people based on their sex, gender identity, or gender expression.

LGBTQ2 is the acronym used by the Government of Canada for lesbian, gay, bisexual, transgender, queer, and Two-Spirit. LGBTIQ2 is the internationally accepted acronym standing for lesbian, gay, bisexual, transgender, intersex, queer, and Two-Spirit.

- A *lesbian* is a woman who is sexually, emotionally, or romantically attracted to other women.
- Someone who is *gay* is sexually, emotionally, or romantically attracted to others of the same sex or gender identity. This term used to be used exclusively for men but has been adopted by other gender identities.
- A *bisexual* person is sexually, emotionally, or romantically attracted to people with either the same or different sex or gender.
- As defined previously, the adjective *transgender* (or trans) describes a person whose gender identities and experiences do not align (fully or in part) with the gender they were assigned at birth.
- *Queer* is an adjective reclaimed by the LGBTQ2 community to refer to the many identities not covered by lesbian, gay, bisexual, transgender, questioning, or Two-Spirit that indicates a person's sexual orientation or gender identity differs from the normative binary view.

- *Two-Spirit* (or Two-Spirited) is an English umbrella term used to capture concepts traditional to some Indigenous cultures where a person's gender identity, sexual orientation, or both has both male and female spirits. *Two-Spirit* can be used instead of or in addition to the terms *lesbian, gay, bisexual, trans,* and *queer* to reflect how all aspects of identity are interrelated (Egale Canada, 2022).
- *Intersex* people have "variations in their sex chromosomes, internal reproductive organs, genitalia, and/or secondary sex characteristics (e.g., muscle mass, breasts) that fall outside of what is typically categorized as male or female" (Women and Gender Equality Canada, 2022).

There are many other terms used to describe other identities. For example:
- *Asexual* typically refers to a person who lacks sexual attraction or sexual expression.
- A *demisexual* person is attracted to another person only after they have established an emotional bond. A demisexual person can belong to any sexual orientation.
- A person who is *pansexual* can be physically or emotionally attracted to a person regardless of their gender.
- The term *transsexual* is an adjective that is occasionally still used to describe a person whose gender identity does not correspond with the sex they were assigned at birth and who undertakes (or wants to undertake) gender-affirming surgery, hormone therapy, or both.

### Gender Identity and Sexual Orientation

As a determinant of health, gender identity poses many challenges. Gender expectations and internalized stress related to stigma, discrimination, and acceptance or rejection by friends, families, and the community can have a profound effect on well-being. For example, lesbian, gay and bisexual individuals are more likely to experience depression, anxiety, suicide, and suicide ideation and substance abuse than their heterosexual counterparts (Gilmour, 2019).

The medical community often fails to provide gender-sensitive and appropriate care, resulting in corresponding inequities. In addition, those persons transitioning face long wait times, emotionally exhausting physical and mental assessments, and uncertainty as to what procedures are covered under public health plans. The procedures collectively are called *sex reassignment, gender-affirming surgery,* or *gender-confirming surgery.* Criteria for coverage in most jurisdictions are based on standards determined by the World Professional Association for Transgender Health for gender dysphoria (discomfort and stress a person experience when their gender identity differs from their sex as assigned at birth). Surgery required because of this diagnosis is considered to be medically necessary. Several facilities in Toronto, Montreal, and Vancouver do genital surgery. Montreal has a private clinic.

### 11. Culture

*Culture* can be described as a way of life (e.g., behaviours, values, attitudes, and geographic and political factors) that is attributed to a group of people. *Ethnicity* refers to place of origin or ancestry, language, and religion. Culture and ethnicity are often linked—and both affect health, particularly in terms of health beliefs, health behaviours, and lifestyle choices.

Newcomers with social, religious, value, and belief systems that are different from those of others in their community are more likely to face inequities, marginalization, and isolation, which in turn can affect their health. As previously mentioned, new Canadians sponsored by individuals or groups have more support in adapting to life in their new country as their sponsors provide assistance with many aspects of resettlement, including finding a suitable place to live and connecting to and understanding the health care system. In most cases, the government provides newcomers with financial assistance for a year. Beyond that, if new Canadians don't find employment, they rely on provincial or territorial social assistance, which results in financial insecurity—affecting all aspects of daily living. People who have spent long periods of time in refugee camps may arrive with significant mental and physical health challenges that require specialized care that may not be covered by public health insurance.

As mentioned earlier, language can be a significant barrier to a newcomer finding employment. For most newcomers, access to learning English or French is provided within a certain time frame, but attending classes may be complicated; a parent may have to stay home with small children, or irregular hours of work may prevent a person from attending scheduled classes.

The Québec government has implemented its language Bill 96, an *Act respecting French, the official and common language of Québec* (Date of assent, June 1, 2022). The purpose of this Act is to affirm that the only official language of Québec is French. It also affirms that French is the common language of the Québec nation. Sections 22.3 and 22.4 of the Act require government officials to communicate with new immigrants exclusively in French, 6 months after their arrival—with no exceptions for refugees and asylum seekers. Exceptions are in place allowing the use of another language in situations where public safety is threatened or "the principle of natural justice so requires," such as matters relating to health care. Newcomers to Québec, in essence, have a 6-month grace period in which to learn to communicate in French. A link for two short videos on Evolve provide you with more information about Bill 96.

---

**THINKING IT THROUGH**

### Migrant Workers and Health Insurance

With Canada facing a critical labour shortage, thousands of seasonal migrant workers come to work on farms across the country through programs such as the Agricultural Worker Program. News of seasonal workers' living accommodations—often crowded, sometimes without adequate bathroom facilities or places to wash and prepare meals—came to light during the COVID-19 pandemic. Health coverage is precarious; the type and extent of the health insurance vary with jurisdiction and the employer. In some situations, if a worker is laid off (including because of injury or illness) they lose their health insurance. Human rights groups and other organizations, including the Canadian Medical Association and the College of Physicians and Surgeons of Canada, are advocating for extending public health coverage to everyone, regardless of their immigration status.

1. Do you think that employers should be responsible for seasonal workers' health insurance, or do you think that should be the responsibility of federal and provincial governments?
2. What are the consequences if a migrant worker contracts COVID-19 and becomes ill but is afraid to report it for fear of losing their job?
3. Should accommodations for migrant workers be subject to provincial standards and inspected regularly? What are the health implications when living conditions are crowded and substandard?

Source: Doyle, S. (2020). Migrant workers falling through cracks in health care coverage. *CMAJ,* *192*(28), E819–E820. doi: https://doi.org/10.1503/cmaj.1095882

---

## 12. Racism

The fundamental right to equal treatment is outlined in the *Canadian Human Rights Act.* Nevertheless, before the pandemic, according to a Statistics Canada survey, approximately 38% of respondents 15 years of age and older reported that they had experienced some form of discrimination at some point in their lives, with race and ethnicity being the most frequently cited reasons (Statistics Canada, 2022c).

**Racism** can affect all aspects of a person's life, influencing life expectancy, health status and outcomes, health behaviours, and health-seeking behaviours. Consider Joyce Echaquan (see Chapter 2), who died because she did not receive necessary care, as the hospital personnel assumed her agitation and heart palpitations were signs of withdrawal rather than symptoms of her medical condition and subjected her to abuse. Consider also Brian Sinclair (see Chapter 9), who died while waiting, for more than a day in an emergency department in a Manitoba hospital, to be seen by a health care provider.

The COVID-19 pandemic has affected racialized Canadians more than nonracialized population groups. Surveillance data from Toronto and Ottawa show that cases of COVID-19 are between 1.5 and 5 times higher among racialized than among nonracialized population groups in these two cities.

Indigenous communities, particularly on-reserve, have had COVID-19 infection rates that are an astonishing 60% higher than among the non-Indigenous population (PHAC, 2021). Moreover, the Statistics Canada survey noted above reported that, during the pandemic, the racial and ethnic discrimination increased most significantly among Asian population groups. During the first year of the pandemic, the Chinese population reported experiencing either ethnic or racial discrimination 10 times more than population groups not designated as a visible minority (Statistics Canada, 2022c).

The social determinants of health—including education (affecting job opportunities), employment (often precarious), housing (often overcrowded conditions), and, for some groups, intergenerational trauma—increase people's vulnerability to COVID-19 and other infections (PHAC, 2021). A significant risk is the physical inability to implement social distancing at home and at work. Many racialized population groups work in crowded factories, food services, and agriculture, not to mention the large number of individuals employed in long-term care facilities.

Strategies were developed to improve access to vaccinations for racialized and Indigenous groups during the pandemic. Public vaccine allocation was prioritized to Indigenous populations with the communities themselves managing supply and deciding who should receive the vaccine first (Indigenous Services Canada, 2021). Public health authorities in some jurisdictions (e.g., Manitoba and Saskatchewan) worked with Indigenous Knowledge Keepers to provide information about vaccines to communities along with opportunities to answer questions. In many communities, Indigenous Elders chose to receive the first vaccinations, to promote confidence and trust in the process.

The Health Association of African Canadians and the Association of Black Social Workers in Nova Scotia have held town hall meetings over the past few years in various communities to provide information about vaccines.

## THE POPULATION HEALTH APPROACH: THE KEY ELEMENTS

Implementing a population health approach to health care requires the collaboration and cooperation of a number of agencies, organizations, health professionals, policymakers, stakeholders, and volunteers. The Public Health Agency of Canada takes the lead role in this process. Other important partners include the Canadian Institute of Health Information, the Canadian Institutes for Health Research, and Statistics Canada (see Chapter 2), supported by public health organizations at all levels of government and by communities. Implementation of population health requires a formal plan to identify critical elements and the role of agencies or individuals and to ensure a coordinated process. The Public Health Agency of Canada has identified eight key elements that provide the framework for its population health approach.

The eight key elements outlined in the framework are required steps to develop and implement a population health approach. In Fig. 6.2, the key elements 1 and 2 are considered to be particularly important as they reflect the very definition of population health.

### Key Element 1. Focus on the Health of Populations

The target population or subpopulation can include individuals within the country, province or territory, city, community within a city, ethnic group, setting (e.g., school or workplace), or age. A study might be done on the general health of a target population, or it can be more specific, such as rates of specific cancers or of cardiovascular disease within a geographic area. Information can be gathered over a predetermined time frame (e.g., 6 months) and may include multiple health issues. A mix of selected **health indicators** are used as measurements, from morbidity, mortality, and hospitalization rates to aggregate indicators, which combine health information for comparative purposes. Contextual elements also affect this phase of the framework—for example, demographics of the selected population, physical character sites (e.g., rural or urban and the related built environment), and the willingness of levels of government to be involved (perhaps with funding)

### An Aging Population: An Example of Population-Based Surveillance

Canada's aging population is already stressing the health care system and the economy. According to Statistics Canada (Grenier, 2017), the percentage of older Canadians in the country accounts for 16.9% of the population (and is predicted to reach 21% in 10 years), for the first time exceeding the percentage of children (under the age of 14 years). If the pattern continues, there will be 12 million older Canadians and fewer than 8 million children by 2061. Because women live longer, those 65 years and older will outnumber their male counterparts by about

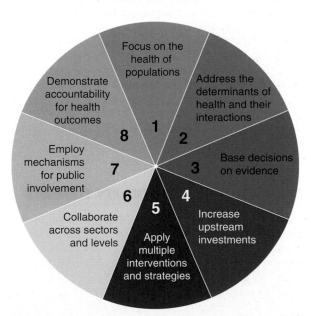

**Fig. 6.2** Population health approach: The organizing framework. (Source: Public Health Agency of Canada. (2013). *Population health approach: The organizing framework.* http://cbpp-pcpe.phac-aspc.gc.ca/population-health-approach-organizing-framework/)

20%. Reasons for a proportionately larger older population include the post—World War II baby boom (1946—1965), increased longevity, and lower birth rates (which started in the 1970s). Statistics Canada predicts that by 2056 older Canadians will account for at least a quarter of the population. In terms of demographics, this aging population has both social and economic consequences (Grenier, 2017). As older Canadians retire, fewer young people are moving into the workforce. As well as affecting the economy in general, this demographic shift will mean that fewer people are working to support Canada's social safety net, including seniors' pensions and health care benefits. Possible solutions that the government may consider include efforts to raise the birth rate and increase immigration.

### Key Element 2. Address the Determinants of Health and Their Interactions

Population health considers all of the factors (determinants) that affect health of the target population. As outlined in Fig. 6.2, these determinants are scrutinized in terms of how they interact with one another, and indicators are selected. This information then forms the basis for developing and implementing population health interventions.

Measuring and analyzing the determinants and how they are interrelated is complicated. One determinant rarely stands alone as a causative factor for a health problem. Diabetes, for example, is associated with obesity, which may be linked to inactivity, food insecurity, and poor nutrition.

### Key Element 3. Use Evidence-Informed Decision Making

All stages of a population health approach—selecting issues, choosing interventions, deciding to implement and continue these interventions—are supported by decisions based on the best evidence currently available, a process called *evidence-informed decision making*.

An evidence-informed approach uses the full range of qualitative and quantitative data available. **Qualitative research** examines the way a population group thinks, how it acts, and its health beliefs and health behaviours, and is conducted in a number of ways, including by administering surveys and holding open forums. **Quantitative research** deals primarily with numbers, which are interpreted most frequently as statistics. Data can be generated through epidemiological studies, databases, and surveys, such as the Census.

All evidence must be gathered in a predetermined and organized manner, with every step of the decision-making process examined and re-examined, and transparency assured to keep information current, relevant, and objective. Determining which interventions will be most effective and implementing them are complex endeavours. A number of stakeholders must be involved (including those who will be affected by policy changes and the application of interventions), in addition to contextual considerations. Ongoing evaluation of interventions and policy changes is essential with modifications made as indicated.

### Key Element 4. Increase Upstream Investments

**Upstream investments** refers to the process of making decisions that will benefit the health of a population group or community before a problem occurs. These investments typically address the root cause of a health problem and then work backward. Proactive investments are likely to address social, economic, and environmental health determinants and influence other community and regional resources. Politicians, community leaders, medical professionals, and other stakeholders must understand and be committed to any actions a population health program may propose.

Being proactive regarding health promotion and disease and injury prevention can save money and give a population a healthier future. Short-term and long-term goals are set and prioritized, and strategies are implemented on the basis of evidence—for example, introducing or reinforcing strategies encouraging Canadians to take responsibility for their own health (e.g., eating a healthy diet, exercising, reducing or eliminating risk behaviours, and partnering with their primary care provider to participate in both routine and disease-specific screening initiatives, when needed). Upstream investments and interventions must be re-evaluated periodically and necessary adjustments made. The principle of cost—benefit analysis is always considered—applying the best possible set of interventions and actions in a cost-effective manner to achieve the best possible outcomes.

### Key Element 5. Apply Multiple Strategies

Once a population health goal is set, the next step is to introduce interventions to achieve the goal. As no single action is likely to accomplish this, a multifaceted approach should be taken. Actions must relate directly to the situation; suit the age range, health status, and environment of the target population; and be implemented over a chosen time frame. Such interventions must also address all of the health determinants involved across the health care continuum, recognizing that they are interrelated.

Those involved in implementing a population health strategy must accept both the goal and the plan of action. Collaboration is essential. It is up to the government to work with all sectors that have an influence on the success of the interventions (e.g., the individuals, the community, industry, related agencies, and local, provincial, and territorial governments).

### Key Element 6. Collaborate Across Sectors and Levels

Intersectoral collaboration involves developing partnerships between different segments of society—private citizens, community groups, industry, health and educational agencies, and various levels of government—to improve health. Each group comes to the table with its own values, outlooks, opinions, agendas, and action plans. Harmonizing these variables is a challenge, but the benefits are profound: a commitment to common goals, and an assurance that plans are implemented to meet these goals. For such partnerships to work, sharing basic ideals and working toward improving health outcomes are essential.

The Pan-Canadian Public Health Network brings together individuals, public and private organizations, politicians, policy advisers, writers from all levels of government, and scientists from across the country. An excellent example of intersectoral collaboration, this network works together discussing health concerns and strategies for intervention. As part of its mandate, the Network shares public health best practices that are province or territory specific, while respecting the autonomy of each jurisdiction to implement actions suited to their own needs. Between 2014 and 2017, the organization's plans included working with all levels of government to develop a framework and create a list of priorities relating to mental health and to create a framework to promote healthy weight, prompted by the alarming rises in childhood obesity and type 1 diabetes.

Intersectoral collaboration at an international level is ongoing. The WHO and numerous countries worked together to contain disease and treat world populations when the Ebola outbreak occurred, for example, and more recently, the COVID-19 pandemic. Any disease outbreak that poses an international threat requires international cooperation with respect to tracking and containing the outbreak, and sharing best practices for infection control and treatments.

### Key Element 7. Engage the Public

Without public support, most health care—related implementations will fail, in part because it is the public's health at issue, and primarily its tax dollars that fund implementation. Public involvement increases the likelihood that citizens will embrace a plan in a meaningful way. The key is to capture the public's interest early and in a positive manner. Plans to achieve positive public interest must be carefully considered and executed so as not to turn public opinion against the plan—attempting to reverse public opinion can be difficult, if not impossible. Engaging the public requires the establishment of trust and an open process of decision making and implementation. Questions must be addressed promptly, properly, and persuasively. Take the opioid crisis as an example, which was compounded by the COVID-19 pandemic. Across the country, politicians at every level of government, health organizations, and the public at large were involved in determining the best course of action to deal with this problem.

In the context of the COVID-19 pandemic, bringing the public on board with respect to abiding with public health restrictions to minimize the spread of the infection, protect the health of Canadians, and support the capacity of the health care system to treat individuals as required, has, overall, been effective. However, for some population groups, opposition to public health regulations at the national, provincial, and municipal levels has been fierce (e.g., the convoy of protesters that converged on Parliament Hill in Ottawa in January 2022). Some feel that these regulations have infringed on their rights and freedoms (freedom of movement, mandatory closures of businesses, and restrictions imposed on those refusing to become vaccinated).

### Key Element 8. Demonstrate Accountability for Health Outcomes

A population health approach emphasizes the accountability for health outcomes—that is, the ability to determine if any changes in health outcomes can actually be attributed to specific policies or programs. The concept of accountability has an impact on planning and goal setting since it encourages the selection of interventions or strategies that produce the greatest health results.

Important steps in establishing accountability include determining baseline measures (i.e., a standard against which to gauge progress), setting targets, and monitoring progress so that a thorough evaluation can be done. Evaluation tools provide criteria for determining the impact of policies or programs on population health. Finally, publicizing evaluation results is critical for gaining widespread support for successful population health initiatives. For example, the reduction in infections from the SARS-CoV-2 (COVID-19) virus, the decrease in morbidity and mortality rates, and the decrease in hospitalizations were evident after each "wave" of the virus, clearly showing evidence-informed results that public health restrictions are effective.

## POPULATION HEALTH PROMOTION MODEL

A newer concept of population health promotion looks at population health and population health promotion as an integrated model that is, in part, based on the knowledge that many factors affect both the health of a population and that of an individual. From the perspective of an integrated model of population health and health promotion (IMPHHP), health status is influenced by a wide range of health determinants. This integrated model draws heavily on information from past policies, documents, and health promotion programs. The model organizes population health into three areas:
1. What—looking to the health determinants to measure the health of populations
2. How—creating and implementing prioritized strategies to improve health
3. Who—engaging multiple stakeholders to participate in health improvement strategies

The population health promotion model demonstrates the complexity of health promotion. The model emulates the population health approach by using the determinants of health as indicators to measure health and to gather information for health promotion initiatives.

Decisions about health promotion policies are made using three sources of evidence:
1. Research studies on health issues (i.e., the underlying factors, the interventions, and their impact)

2. Knowledge gained through experience

3. Evaluation of current programs to anticipate strategies needed in the future—in other words, upstream investments in health promotion

Collectively, stakeholders should address the full range of health determinants when adopting a population health promotion approach. Particular organizations, however, may wish to focus on specific determinants.

The population health promotion model can be used by any level of government, community agency, or group and can be accessed from any point of entry, depending on the health issue. The model can be altered or updated as determined by the user. Consider current issues facing Canadians in terms of mental health issues, including the use of opioids. All levels of government, including municipalities, are involved in a variety of actions to reduce deaths attributed to overdoses (largely from contaminated drugs), provide rehabilitation opportunities, and keep communities safe.

## POPULATION HEALTH IN CANADA AND ABROAD

The population health approach has been relatively successful in most regions in Canada, but it requires ongoing research, strategizing, funding, and commitment from all levels of government to have a truly positive impact on the health of Canadians. All provinces and territories have agencies that address their own population health needs and also work collaboratively with organizations at the federal level.

Information gathered by the Public Health Agency of Canada and other departments at the federal level may have similar implications for all jurisdictions, but differences may arise in how each province or territory deals with any given issue (e.g., planning for more hospital and long-term care beds as their population ages). Developing initial plans for national strategies for mental health, pharmacare, and home care, for example, depend on information gathered from provinces and territories to begin planning approaches, policies, and guidelines to move forward. Policies and guidelines are adjusted in accordance to ongoing feedback from all jurisdictions.

Guidance for certain strategies may contain general guidelines and recommendations that are adjusted by each jurisdiction to meet the needs of various population groups. The following are some examples of jurisdictional population health management.

In British Columbia, Population and Public Health collaborates with stakeholders and partners across the province, including the Ministry of Health, the regional health authorities, and nongovernment organizations to initiate and promote population health strategies to prevent chronic disease and preventable injury, promote health equity, and address key population health areas (BC Centre for Disease Control, 2022).

In Alberta, the Population, Public and Indigenous Health Strategic Clinical Network (SCN) is responsible for population health initiatives with a commitment to work with Indigenous people. The Network works collaboratively with SCNs across the province as well other stakeholders and organizations (Alberta Health Services, n.d.). The Network is comprised of two main committees, one assuming responsibility for population and public health, and the other prioritizing Indigenous health in the province.

Saskatchewan's Population and Public Health oversees several program areas, including disease control, environmental public health, healthy families, and health promotion.

In Ontario, the Ministry of Health, in collaboration with Public Health Ontario, determines and oversees strategies related to population health initiatives (for example, decisions regarding when the next booster vaccination is available, and what population groups are eligible) (Public Health Ontario, 2020). Booster vaccines are currently available within designated time frames and adjusted as much as possible to be effective against circulating (and evolving) variants.

Québec's Population Health Research Network (QPHRN/RRSPQ) is funded by the Fonds de recherche du Québec-Santé (FRQS). This organization conducts ongoing research and networking related to population health.

New Brunswick has adapted a populational health model to suit the province from one used by the University of Wisconsin, keeping a Canadian perspective by incorporating the determinants of health laid out by the Public Health Agency of Canada (New Brunswick Health Council, 2022).

## SUMMARY

6.1  Population health refers to the identification of the health outcomes of a population group and the equitable sharing of those outcomes with that group. The definition of a group varies and can be determined and defined by ethnicity, geography, a nationhood or allegiance to a province or territory or community, or a setting (e.g., within schools or the workplace). A population health approach (overseen by the Public Health Agency of Canada [PHAC]) considers health to be a resource influenced by numerous factors identified in the determinants of health. The population health framework considers health promotion, disease prevention, diagnosis and treatment of diseases, and treatment intervention. The aim is to improve the health of all Canadians.

6.2  Several reports and conferences were instrumental in the introduction and development of population health in Canada. The 1974 report *A New Perspective on the Health of Canadians* is considered to be the first to state that health is determined by more than just biology and to identify the significant roles that the environment, lifestyle, and health care organizations have in our health and well-being. Other reports include the *Ottawa Charter for Health* Promotion, 1986; the Epp Report, 1986; and *Toward a Healthy Future: The First Report on the Health of* Canadians, 1996. All the reports discussed in this chapter were significant in initiating a united population health approach to achieve better health for Canadians.

6.3  The health of a population, population groups, and individuals is dependent on a combination of factors, some of which may be beyond individuals' control. All people are affected, sometimes profoundly, by these factors, which go beyond genetics and biology to include the determinants of health. There are 12 generally accepted health determinants, the most significant of which appear to be those that affect the socioeconomic factors of people's lives and health. These determinants in isolation are unlikely to have a great effect on the health of either an individual or a population group but rather by the interconnectivity of numerous determinants.

6.4  Effectively implementing population health measures across Canada requires the collaboration of organizations, health professionals, volunteers, policymakers, and other stakeholders spearheaded by the PHAC. The PHAC framework for implementing population health includes eight key elements, which provide guidance for the process ranging from how to focus on a target population group to engaging the public in the process and assuming accountability for health outcomes.

6.5  A newer concept of population health promotion looks at population health and population health promotion as an integrated model, based on the knowledge that many factors affect both the health of a population and that of an individual. The population health promotion model arranges population health into three segments: what, how, and who, through which it identifies what the problem is, how it can best be dealt with, and whom it affects. Evidence-informed decision making is a critical component for making strategies effective.

6.6 A population health approach at the federal and provincial and territorial levels requires ongoing funding, research, strategizing, and commitment from all levels of government to have a truly positive impact on the health of Canadians. All provinces and territories have agencies that address their own population health needs and also work collaboratively with organizations at the federal level. National strategies for such entities as mental health, home and community care, and pharmacare (some of which are in the planning phases) provide guidelines for all jurisdictions. Precisely how these strategies are implemented at the provincial or territorial level is up to each jurisdiction, but they are best implemented when information and best practices are shared and transparency is maintained. Information gathered by various organizations at the federal level is available to all provinces and territories across Canada. Each jurisdiction may use the information differently, tailoring it to the specific needs of its population.

## REVIEW QUESTIONS

1. Compare and contrast the principal elements of population health, population health promotion, and public health.
2. What role did the Declaration of Alma-Ata play in developing population health initiatives?
3. Explain the purpose of the Public Health Agency of Canada's population health template.
4. Compare and contrast the 11 Inuit determinants of health with the 12 determinants of health identified by Health Canada.
5. Explain how education can impact the health of an individual or a family.
6. What is meant by the SES gradient, and how does a position on the gradient effect the health of an individual or a population group?
7. What impact does racism as a determinant of health have on a population group?
8. What are inequities in health?
9. State the advantages of engaging the public in developing population health initiatives.
10. How does the population health promotion model differ from population health itself?
11. What might make the population health needs of one province or territory different from those of another?
12. Research how health care is distributed in your jurisdiction. Who makes decisions about health care needs locally?
13. What elements of rationalization of care do you see in your area? Have hospitals merged and redistributed services? Explain how. What do you see as the benefits and drawbacks? Do you see the manner in which services are accessed and distributed as equitable? Cost-saving? What would you change?

## REFERENCES

Alberta Health Services. (n.d.a). Population, public & Indigenous health: Strategic clinical network. https://www.albertahealthservices.ca/assets/about/scn/ahs-scn-ppih-quick-facts.pdf.

Arrive. (2020, September 10). *Child care in Canada: Types, cost, and tips for newcomers.* https://arrivein.com/daily-life-in-canada/child-care-in-canada-types-cost-and-tips-for-newcomers/.

Assembly of First Nations. (n.d.). Social determinants of health. https://www.afn.ca/social-determinants-of-health-sdoh/.

BC Centre for Disease Control. (2022). *Population and public health.* http://www.bccdc.ca/our-services/service-areas/population-public-health.

Boisvert, N. (2021, July 11). *Canadian women make 89 cents for every dollar men earn. Can new federal legislation narrow that gap? CBC news.* https://www.cbc.ca/news/politics/pay-equity-legislation-1. 6097263#:~:text=Women%20in%20Canada's%20workforce%20earn,every%20dollar%20earned% 20by%20me.

Brown, C. L., & Emery, J. C. H. (2010). The impact of disability on earnings and labour force participation in Canada: Evidence from the 2001 PALS and from Canadian case law. *Journal of Legal Economics, 16*(2), 19—59.

Canadian Association for Community Living (CACL). (2013). *Assuring income security and equality for Canadians with intellectual disabilities and their families.* https://www.ourcommons.ca/Content/ Committee/411/FINA/WebDoc/WD6079428/411_FINA_IIC_Briefs/ CanadianAssociationforCommunityLivingE.pdf.

Canadian Cancer Society. (2022). *Cigarettes: The hard truth.* https://cancer.ca/en/cancer-information/ reduce-your-risk/live-smoke-free/cigarettes-the-hard-truth#:~:text=Lung%20cancer%20is%20the% 20leading,the%20more%20their%20risk%20increases.

Canadian Human Rights Commission (CHRC). (2012). *Report on equality rights of people with disabilities.* https://www.chrc-ccdp.gc.ca/sites/default/files/rerpd_rdepad-eng.pdf.

Canadian Human Rights Commission (CHRC). (2018). *Roadblocks on the career path: Challenges faced by persons with disabilities in employment.* https://publications.gc.ca/collections/collection_2019/ccdp-chrc/HR4-43-2018-eng.pdf.

Canadian Institute of Child Health (CICH). (2022). *4.4.2 First Nations housing on reserve. The health of Canada's children and youth.* https://cichprofile.ca/module/7/section/4/page/first-nations-housing-on-reserve/#:~:text=More%20than%20a%20quarter%20of,to%207%25%20of%20Canadian%20houses.

Canadian Institutes of Health Research. (2020). *What is gender? What is sex?* https://cihr-irsc.gc.ca/e/ 48642.html.

Canadian Medical Association. (2021, November). *A struggling system: Understanding the health care impacts of the pandemic.* https://www.cma.ca/sites/default/files/pdf/health-advocacy/Deloitte-report-nov2021-EN.pdf.

Canadian Women's Foundation. (2022). *The facts about the gender pay gap.* https://canadianwomen.org/ the-facts/the-gender-pay-gap/.

Childwatch. (2019, December 10). *Creating a sense of belonging for children.* https://childwatch.com/blog/ 2019/12/10/creating-a-sense-of-belonging-for-children/.

Choi, R. (2021). *Canadian survey on disability reports: Accessibility findings from the Canadian survey on disability, 2017.* Statistics Canada. https://www150.statcan.gc.ca/n1/pub/89-654-x/89-654-x2021002-eng.htm.

Chun, L. F., Moazed, F., Calfee, C. S., et al. (2017). Pulmonary toxicity of e-cigarettes. *American Journal of Physiology - Lung Cellular and Molecular Physiology, 313*(2), L193—L206. https://doi.org/10.1152/ ajplung.00071.2017.

Cowan, K. (2020). How residential schools led to intergenerational trauma in the Canadian Indigenous population to influence parenting styles and family structures over generations. *Canadian Journal of Family and Youth, 12*(s), 26—35. https://www.researchgate.net/publication/338424698_How_Residen tial_Schools_led_to_Intergenerational_Trauma_in_the_Canadian_Indigenous_Population_to_Influen ce_Parenting_Styles_and_Family_Structures_over_Generations.

Djidel, S., Gustajtis, B., Heisz, A., et al. (2020, February 24). *Report on the second comprehensive review of the market basket measure.* https://www150.statcan.gc.ca/n1/pub/75f0002m/75f0002m2020002-eng. htm.

Egale Canada. (2022). *2SLGBTQI Glossary of terms.* http://www.cglcc.ca/uploads/2/5/2/3/25237538/lgbtq_ terminology_-_echrt.pdf.

Employment and Social Development Canada. (2021, July 20). *Canada Child Benefit increases once again to keep up with the cost of living.* https://www.canada.ca/en/employment-social-development/news/ 2021/07/canada-child-benefit-5th-anniversary—indexation0.html.

Employment and Social Development Canada. (2022a). *Understanding systems: The 2021 report of the national advisory Council on poverty.* https://www.canada.ca/en/employment-social-development/ programs/poverty-reduction/national-advisory-council/reports/2021-annual.html.

Employment and Social Development Canada. (2022b). *Social isolation of seniors—Volume 1: Understanding the issue and finding solutions.* https://www.canada.ca/en/employment-social-development/corporate/partners/seniors-forum/social-isolation-toolkit-vol1.html.

Fawcett, M. (2022, January 10). We can't leave Canada's housing crisis up to the provinces. *Canada's National Observer.* https://www.nationalobserver.com/2022/01/10/opinion/we-cant-leave-canadas-housing-crisis-provinces.

Fieselmann, J., Annac, K., Erdsiek, F., et al. (2022). What are the reasons for refusing a COVID-19 vaccine? A qualitative analysis of social media in Germany. *BMC Public Health, 22*(846). https://doi.org/10.1186/s12889-022-13265-y.

First Nations Health Authority. (n.d.). First Nations perspective on health and wellness. https://www.fnha.ca/wellness/wellness-for-first-nations/first-nations-perspective-on-health-and-wellness.

First Nations Information Governance Centre. (2020, July). *First Nations on-reserve housing and related infrastructure needs (draft): Technical report.* https://www.afn.ca/wp-content/uploads/2021/01/res-1270-5648.pdf.

Gilmour, H. (2019, November 20). *Sexual orientation and complete mental health.* Statistics Canada. https://www150.statcan.gc.ca/n1/pub/82-003-x/2019011/article/00001-eng.htm.

Government of Canada. (2021, August 12). *Canadian tobacco, alcohol and drugs survey (CTADS): Summary of results for 2017.* https://www.canada.ca/en/health-canada/services/canadian-alcohol-drugs-survey/2017-summary.html.

Government of Canada. (2022a). *Social determinants of health and health inequalities.* https://www.canada.ca/en/public-health/services/health-promotion/population-health/what-determines-health.html.

Government of Canada. (2022b). *Child disability benefit (CDB).* https://www.canada.ca/en/revenue-agency/services/child-family-benefits/child-disability-benefit.html.

Grenier, E. (2017). *Canadian seniors now outnumber children for 1st time, 2016 Census shows. CBC News.* https://www.cbc.ca/news/politics/2016-census-age-gender-1.4095360.

Health and Welfare Canada. (2006). *Achieving health for all: A framework for health promotion.* http://www.hc-sc.gc.ca/hcs-sss/pubs/system-regime/1986-frame-plan-promotion/index-eng.php.

Health Canada. (2021). *Healthy living.* https://www.canada.ca/en/health-canada/services/healthy-living.html.

Health Canada. (2022). *Health of Canadians in a changing climate: Advancing our knowledge for action.* https://changingclimate.ca/site/assets/uploads/sites/5/2022/02/CCHA-REPORT-EN.pdf.

Human Rights Campaign. (n.d.). Sexual orientation and gender identity definitions. https://www.hrc.org/resources/sexual-orientation-and-gender-identity-terminology-and-definitions.

Indigenous Services Canada. (2021). *Lessons learned: Vaccine roll-out for Indigenous communities.* https://www.afn.ca/wp-content/uploads/2021/10/Dr.-Valerie-Gideon-Presentation_EN.pdf.

Inuit Tapirit Kanatami. (2014). *Social determinants of Inuit health in Canada.* https://www.itk.ca/wp-content/uploads/2016/07/ITK_Social_Determinants_Report.pdf.

Klukas, J. J. (2021 June 9). *Canada has child-care problems—but we can solve them. The Tyee* (p. 3). https://childcarecanada.org/documents/child-care-news/21/06/canada-has-child-care-problems-%E2%80%94-we-can-solve-them#:~:text=But%20Statistics%20Canada%20reports%20that.

Kronstein, A. (2017, May 30). Education and early childhood development—the social determinants of health, part 3. *The Nova Scotia Advocate.* https://nsadvocate.org/2017/05/30/education-and-early-childhood-development-the-social-determinants-of-health-part-3/.

Lalonde, M. (1981). *A new perspective on the health of Canadians: A working document.* Government of Canada. https://www.phac-aspc.gc.ca/ph-sp/pdf/perspect-eng.pdf.

Limmena, M. R. (2021, July 26). How intergenerational trauma affects Indigenous communities. *Science Borealis.* https://blog.scienceborealis.ca/how-intergenerational-trauma-affects-indigenous-communities/.

Macdonald, D., & Friendly, M. (2020). In progress: Child care fees in Canada, 2019. *Canadian Centre for Policy Alternatives.* https://policyalternatives.ca/sites/default/files/uploads/publications/National%20Office/2020/03/In%20progress_Child%20care%20fees%20in%20Canada%20in%202019_march12.pdf.

MacDonald, N. E. (2015). Vaccine hesitancy: Definition, scope, and determinants. *Vaccine, 33*(34), 4161–4164. https://doi.org/10.1016/j.vaccine.2015.04.036.

MacDonald, N. E. (2020). Fake news and science denier attacks on vaccines What can you do? *Canadian Communicable Disease Report, 46*(11/12), 432–435. https://doi.org/10.14745/ccdr.v46i1112a11.

McConnell, R., Barrington-Trimis, J. L., Wang, K., et al. (2017). Electronic cigarette use and respiratory symptoms in adolescents. *American Journal of Respiratory and Critical Care Medicine, 195*(8), 1043—1049. https://doi.org/10.1164/rccm.201604-0804OC.

National Center for Transgender Equality. (2018). *Understanding non-binary people: How to be respectful and supportive.* https://transequality.org/issues/resources/understanding-non-binary-people-how-to-be-respectful-and-supportive.

New Brunswick Health Council. (2022). *Population health model.* https://nbhc.ca/population-health-model.

Ng, E., & Gagnon, S. (2020, January 24). More research needed to break down job barriers for racialized Canadians. *Policy Options.* https://policyoptions.irpp.org/magazines/january-2020/more-research-needed-to-break-down-job-barriers-for-racialized-canadians/.

O'Neill, A. (2022, May 6). *Canada: Unemployment rate from 2017 to 2027.* Statista. https://www.statista.com/statistics/263696/unemployment-rate-in-canada/.

Pay Equity Office. (2022). *An overview of pay equity in various Canadian jurisdictions.* https://www.payequity.gov.on.ca/en/LearnMore/GWG/Documents/2022-04-27%20An%20Overview%20of%20Pay%20Equity%20in%20Various%20Canadian%20Jurisdictions%20-%20ENG.pdf.

Pelletier, R., Patterson, M., & Moyser, M. (2019, October 11). *The gender wage gap in Canada: 1998 to 2018.* Labour Statistics: Statistics Canada. Research Papers. https://www150.statcan.gc.ca/n1/pub/75-004-m/75-004-m2019004-eng.htm

Pietrabissa, G., & Simpson, S. G. (2020, September). Psychological consequences of social isolation during COVID-19 outbreak. *Frontiers in Psychology, 11,* 2201. https://doi.org/10.3389/fpsyg.2020.02201.

Polsky, J. Y., & Gilmour, H. (2020, December 16). *Food insecurity and mental health during the COVID-19 pandemic. Catalogue no. 82-003-X.* https://www150.statcan.gc.ca/n1/pub/82-003-x/2020012/article/00001-eng.htm.

Public Health Agency of Canada (PHAC). (2001). *A new perspective on the health of Canadians.* https://www.canada.ca/en/public-health/services/health-promotion/population-health/a-new-perspective-on-health-canadians.html.

Public Health Agency of Canada (PHAC). (2018a). *Key health inequalities in Canada: A national portrait.* https://www.canada.ca/content/dam/phac-aspc/documents/services/publications/science-research/key-health-inequalities-canada-national-portrait-executive-summary/key_health_inequalities_full_report-eng.pdf.

Public Health Agency of Canada (PHAC). (2018b). *Key health inequalities in Canada: A national portrait—Executive summary.* https://www.canada.ca/en/public-health/services/publications/science-research-data/key-health-inequalities-canada-national-portrait-executive-summary.html.

Public Health Agency of Canada (PHAC). (2021, February 21). *CPHO Sunday edition: The impact of COVID-19 on racialized communities.* https://www.canada.ca/en/public-health/news/2021/02/cpho-sunday-edition-the-impact-of-covid-19-on-racialized-communities.html.

Public Health Ontario. (2020, June 16). *Ontario public health system.* https://www.publichealthontario.ca/en/About/news/2020/Ontario-Public-Health-System#:~:text=Ministry%20of%20Health&text=The%20Ministry%20monitors%20and%20reports,educate%20Ontarians%20about%20health%20decisions.

Russell, E. (2020, September 17). *How have past pandemics affected business?* https://www.economicsobservatory.com/how-have-past-pandemics-affected-business.

Russell, E., & Parker, M. (2020, July 9). *How pandemics past and present fuel the rise of large companies.* The Conversation. https://theconversation.com/how-pandemics-past-and-present-fuel-the-rise-of-large-companies-137732

Schwartz, J. (2022, January 31). *Canadian housing bubble growing. Consolidated Credit Canada.* https://www.consolidatedcreditcanada.ca/financial-news/housing-bubble/.

Senate of Canada. (2015). *On-reserve housing and infrastructure: Recommendations for change.* https://sencanada.ca/en/content/sen/committee/412/appa/rms/12jun15/home-e.

Soneji, S., Barrington-Trimis, J. L., Wills, T. A., et al. (2017). Association between initial use of e-cigarettes and subsequent cigarette smoking among adolescents and young adults: A systematic review and meta-analysis. *JAMA Pediatrics, 171*(8), 788—797. https://doi.org/10.1001/jamapediatrics.2017.1488.

Statistics Canada. (2021, March 23). *Canadian income survey, 2019.* https://www150.statcan.gc.ca/n1/en/daily-quotidien/210323/dq210323a-eng.pdf?st=hIqX44FN.

Statistics Canada. (2022a). *Canadian income survey, 2020.* The Daily. https://www150.statcan.gc.ca/n1/daily-quotidien/220323/dq220323a-eng.htm.

Statistics Canada. (2022b). *Labour force survey, January 2022.* The Daily. https://www150.statcan.gc.ca/n1/daily-quotidien/220204/dq220204a-eng.htm.

Statistics Canada. (2022c). *Discrimination before and since the start of the pandemic.* https://www150.statcan.gc.ca/n1/en/pub/11-627-m/11-627-m2022021-eng.pdf?st=fCMCwWN0.

Thompson, N. (2022, June 10). *Canada poised to become first country to add warnings on individual cigarettes.* Global News. https://globalnews.ca/news/8911887/canada-cigarette-warning/

To Do Canada. (2022, April 20). *Rent prices in March 2022 rise at an average of 6.6% from last year across Canada.* https://www.todocanada.ca/rent-prices-in-march-2022-rise-at-an-average-of-6-6-across-canada-from-last-year/#:~:text=Year%20Across%20Canada-,Rent%20Prices%20in%20March%202022%20Rise%20at%20an%20Average%20of,From%20Last%20Year%20Across%20Canada&text=Rentals.ca%20has%20released%20its,of%206.6%25%20from%20March%202021.

Treasury Board of Canada Secretariat. (2019, April 8). *Modernizing the Government of Canada's sex and gender information practices: Summary report.* https://www.canada.ca/en/treasury-board-secretariat/corporate/reports/summary-modernizing-info-sex-gender.html.

Turcotte, M. (2014). *Persons with disabilities and employment.* Statistics Canada. https://www150.statcan.gc.ca/n1/en/pub/75-006-x/2014001/article/14115-eng.pdf?st=Q_tYkPCC.

Women and Gender Equality Canada. (2022). *2SLGBTQI terminology—Glossary and common acronyms.* https://women-gender-equality.canada.ca/en/free-to-be-me/2slgbtqi-plus-glossary.html.

World Health Organization. (1986). *The 1st international conference on health promotion, Ottawa, 1986.* https://www.who.int/teams/health-promotion/enhanced-wellbeing/first-global-conference.

# Health and the Individual

## LEARNING OUTCOMES

7.1 Discuss the key concepts of health, wellness, illness, disease, and disability.
7.2 Explain the main health belief models.
7.3 Discuss changing perceptions of health.
7.4 Examine the psychology of health behaviour.
7.5 Understand the health/wellness—illness continuum.
7.6 Describe four categories of responses to illness and the concept of risk behaviours.
7.7 Review the leading causes of morbidity and mortality in Canada.

## KEY TERMS

| | | |
|---|---|---|
| Cardiovascular disease | Health model | Sick role behaviour |
| Cerebrovascular disease | Holistic | Signs |
| Compensation | Infant mortality | Syndrome |
| Culture | Life expectancy | Symptoms |
| Disability | Morbidity | Wellness |
| Disease | Mortality | Wellness—illness |
| Etiology | Remission | continuum |
| Exacerbation | Self-imposed risk | |
| Health behaviour | behaviours | |
| Health beliefs | | |

Anyone entering a health care profession, either as a hands-on health care provider or as a contributor of administrative or technical expertise, will find it helpful to understand the concepts of health and wellness. It is also important to know what makes Canadians ill. How preventable is poor health? What entities shape a person's outlook on health, wellness, and illness? How has the pandemic affected the health of Canadians? Do circumstances play a role in how ill or healthy we are? The answer to most of these questions vary, depending on the person or population group, their life's circumstances, and the determinants of health. Clearly, the determinants of health (in one way or another) all impact the health and wellness of both individuals and population groups, particularly the social determinants of health such as income and social status (see Chapter 6).

There are, however, medical conditions that *are* largely preventable. Health promotion and disease prevention initiatives addressing lifestyle and risk behaviours are the major focus of primary care in Canada. Some people who are in a position to make healthier lifestyle choices choose to engage in health-risk behaviours, those that cause disease and illness or lead to disability. Why do some individuals ignore basic advice regarding health promotion and illness prevention? For one thing, many people take good health for granted until they are faced with illness or another incapacitating event. Some engage in behaviours that adversely affect their health, such as smoking and taking drugs, and find themselves unable to stop (substance use disorder, which is a disease in itself). Others think they are invincible or immune—it won't happen to them. Some Canadians find themselves in troubling circumstances which, for reasons beyond their immediate control, prevent them from actively engaging in health promotion and disease prevention activities. These circumstances include poverty, racism, marginalization, and mental health issues, and they all increase the risk of poor health from a number of perspectives (see Chapter 6).

Health, wellness, and illness mean different things to different people. Some people will consider themselves well despite the presence of significant health challenges, seeking help when absolutely necessary, and minimizing their health status if asked how they are by family and friends. Others readily succumb to even minor alterations in their health state and require more intervention, understanding, and support. Understanding patients' perceptions of health, their health beliefs, and health behaviours, as well as their corresponding response to diagnosis and treatment, enables health professionals to maximize patients' health outcomes.

Definitions of *health*, *wellness*, *illness*, *disease*, and *disability* evolve constantly, along with social consciousness, the delivery of health care, the affordability of health care services, and advances in medical science.

It is important to recognize the impact of a global society on the health of Canadians as well as people around the world. Diseases formerly considered isolated to certain parts of the world are no longer isolated to specific geographic areas (most recently, COVID-19), the spread of which is enhanced by increased international travel and changing immigration policies. There was a decrease in immigration to Canada 2020 and 2021 because of public health and government restrictions related to the COVID-19 pandemic. However, Immigration Refugees and Citizenship Canada plans to welcome just under a half a million immigrants each year between 2023 and 2025 (Canada Visa, 2022). The goals of this aggressive plan are to strengthen the economy as well as to reunite families and refugees.

Despite experience with previous outbreaks such as Severe Acute Respiratory Syndrome (SARS) in 2002–2003, Canada (as well as most countries around the world) was ill prepared to respond to the COVID-19 pandemic, given how rapidly it spread across the country. As of November 2022 (just as the seventh wave of the pandemic was declared), there were approximately 4,392,747 confirmed cases and 47,468 deaths related to COVID-19 in Canada.

Canada is seeing a resurgence of diseases that were considered all but eradicated, for example, measles and tuberculosis (TB). Measles is appearing again among children who are not immunized. The incidence of TB is 300 times higher among the Inuit population compared to the non-Indigenous population in Canada. The disease spreads easily, especially where there are overcrowded living conditions, poverty, and food insecurity—all relate to inequalities evidenced by the socioeconomic determinants of health (see Chapter 6). For example, Jennifer, who is Inuit, lives in Cape Dorset in crowded conditions. When she was expecting her baby, one of her little brothers was diagnosed as having "sleeping" TB. She was told simply to get as much fresh air as possible and to stay active. Sleeping TB means that her brother had the TB bacillus in his body, but it was latent or inactive. However, the bacillus could become active at any time, risking exposure to everyone in the household. Jennifer lives with her father, mother, seven little brothers and two foster children, in a four-bedroom housing unit.

When considering the health of the individual, the cultural norms and health practices of new Canadians must be considered. There are deficiencies in the provision of care for newcomers settling in the country, from lack of help navigating the system, to not understanding different cultural norms, and language barriers. There are also deficiencies within the system related to the care of Canadians in general, for example, in the area of mental health and medication coverage (see Chapters 3, 4, and 10). Social media has had a profound effect on the health of the individual (e.g., access to health information), including public health campaigns, and how one perceives health and health outcomes (see Chapters 3 and 10 for more detail).

This chapter will explore these issues, provide information on changing trends, and address the leading causes of morbidity and mortality in Canada. We will also discuss the impact of self-imposed risk behaviours on the individual and on the health care system in terms of disease, disability, and cost. The chapter will also reinforce that the health care provider's goal, as part of the health care team, is to help their patients maintain their existing health, assist them in coping with illness, and support them on the road to recovery. Understanding health belief models, the psychology of health behaviour, the ways that individuals respond to illness, and the concept of the health/wellness—illness continuum will assist those pursuing careers in health care how to best support their patients.

## HEALTH, WELLNESS, AND ILLNESS: KEY CONCEPTS

For a long time *healthy* meant "not sick," and *sick* meant "not well." Today the key concepts of health, wellness, and illness are defined in less black-and-white terms. Health care providers should understand the evolution of these definitions—how they have changed to become more multifaceted and inclusive over time.

### Health

What does it mean to be in good health? In the past, the word *health* meant a state of being, of sound mind, and generally suggested a wholeness of the body—that the body was functioning well. Over time, the concept of mental health was integrated into the meaning. Thus, an individual must have both a healthy state of mind and physical well-being to be considered in good health.

In 1948, the World Health Organization (WHO) took the important step of acknowledging that health is multidimensional and not merely the presence or absence of disease. Although a vast improvement over previous definitions, the WHO's definition (Box 7.1) has not formally changed since 1948 and remains largely out of step with current concepts of health and wellness.

### Wellness

Although *wellness* and *health* are often used interchangeably, the two words are not synonymous; however, they share similar concepts. Wellness goes beyond having good health. It considers how a person feels about their health as well as their quality of life.

From a holistic perspective, to achieve wellness, a person must assume responsibility for their own health by leading a balanced lifestyle and avoiding self-imposed risk behaviours. The path toward wellness is not static; it is continuous and must be a lifelong pursuit. Wellness develops from the decisions people make about how to live their lives with quality, good health, and meaning (remember, good health is relative). It is also important to note that wellness for many people depends, to a large degree, on the social determinants of health, where they live, and the inequities they face.

### Dimensions of Wellness

The concept of wellness embraces several categories including, but not limited to, physical, emotional, intellectual, spiritual, and social health. Some wellness models have more recently incorporated environmental and occupational wellness. An even newer and emerging concept is family wellness, which looks at each person in the family unit. If each person is well, the family seems to do well. If a family member considers themselves to be unwell, depending on

## BOX 7.1    Health: An Evolving Definition

In 1948, the World Health Organization (WHO) originally defined *health* as "a state of complete physical, mental, and social well-being and not merely the absence of disease or infirmity."

As perceptions of health evolved, components of this definition have come into question. For instance, some suggested that the word *complete* is unrealistic: How many people can claim to be completely healthy—and what does *completely healthy* mean? The ambiguity of this term is particularly evident today, with individuals living much longer with chronic diseases such as diabetes, cardiovascular disease, and multiple sclerosis as well as those with physical or intellectual disabilities and mental health challenges. Even some forms of cancer are now considered a chronic condition. Accepting such challenges has led individuals to consider themselves healthy within the context of the health issues they are dealing with; their new "normal." This definition also fails to include holistic concepts, such as spiritual wellness and cultural norms. Nurses, for example, must be aware of and respect the spiritual and cultural needs of their patients (e.g., by ensuring patients have access to religious or spiritual resources) when establishing a nursing diagnosis and implementing nursing interventions.

Consequently, the WHO has expanded its concept of health, adding to its definition "the ability to identify and to realize aspirations, to satisfy needs, and to change or cope with environment. Health is therefore a resource for everyday life, not the objective of living. Health is a positive concept emphasizing social and personal resources, as well as physical capabilities" (World Health Organization, 1986).

Sources: World Health Organization. (1948). *Preamble to the constitution of the World Health Organization as adopted by the International Health Conference.* Author; World Health Organization. (1986). *Health promotion: Concepts and principles in action—a policy framework.* WHO Regional Office for Europe.

numerous factors, the family unit, especially relationships, may be adversely affected. A fine line exists between some descriptions of these categories and how they are grouped; various wellness models may divide or label them differently. It is worth noting that some literature refers to the "dimensions of health" rather than the "dimensions of wellness," or the "wellness—illness" continuum rather than the "health—illness" continuum, but these terms are similar in that they consider more than physical and mental health, as well at the fact that health is rarely static (Fig. 7.1).

Some individuals judge themselves to be well despite the presence of disease or infirmity. For example, a patient was diagnosed with amyotrophic lateral sclerosis (ALS, a progressive neurogenic disease for which there is no cure), but he is receiving good medical care and is able to enjoy his family and things that are important to him despite his advancing physical limitations. Therefore, in the present, he considers himself to be well.

Embracing a wellness approach to health for many includes a holistic outlook to health and health practices, which may involve combining traditional (Western) medicine with more nontraditional/unconventional, less invasive treatment modalities. These range from naturopathy, homeopathy, and acupuncture to aromatherapy, therapeutic touch, medication, and yoga. Others may reject Western or traditional medicine altogether in favour of alternative therapies in their quest for wellness and good health (see Chapter 5). Traditional Chinese medicine (TCM), for example, offers a variety of therapies, many that are age-old treatments which many in Canada have embraced.

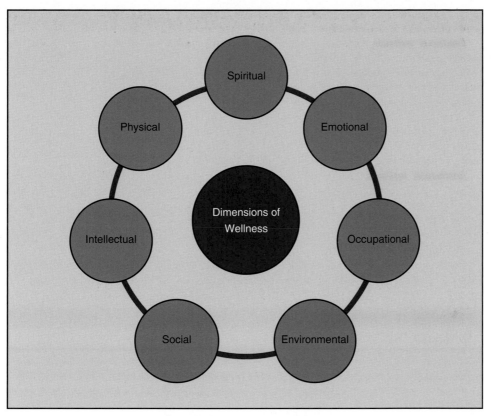

**Fig. 7.1** Dimensions of wellness.

*Physical wellness.* The dimension of physical wellness entails maintaining a healthy body by eating a nutritious, balanced diet; exercising regularly; making informed decisions about one's health; and seeking medical care when necessary. People must understand how lifestyle choices affect physical health to achieve physical wellness. For example, the *Canada Food Guide* recommends avoiding fruit juices and drinking more water instead, as well as moving to a more plant-rich diet, which is also recommended to help address climate change (see Chapter 10).

*Mental wellness.* The WHO defines mental health as "a state of well-being in which every individual realizes his or her own potential, can cope with the normal stresses of life, can work productively and is able to make a contribution to their community." Mental wellness adds a holistic dimension to the definition of mental health. It is being in relative harmony with the dimensions of health and wellness. Mental wellness, like physical wellness, is not static, nor does it mean the absence of mental illness. A person with a diagnosed mental illness under treatment may feel that they are coping well. Consider a person with bipolar disorder. Someone who is bipolar can be well and have their condition controlled for long periods of time with the proper interventions. A person with schizophrenia who responds well to treatment may also consider themselves to be well most of the time. A person may consider it a matter of accepting their diagnosis and all that goes with it—their new "normal." Sometimes just knowing what is wrong and being stabilized with treatment will move the person to the wellness end of the continuum (discussed later in the chapter).

For many Indigenous people, mental wellness along with physical health exists in balance with spirituality and nature (see Chapter 1).

***Emotional wellness.*** Emotional wellness and mental health are often, but not necessarily, interdependent entities. Emotional wellness includes people's ability to understand themselves, to recognize their strengths and limitations, and to accept who they are. The emotionally adapted person effectively handles and controls their emotions, communicates well, and seeks support when needed.

Good mental health allows a person to react proactively when things go wrong—to view adversity as an opportunity to learn and grow. Emotional health very much contributes to this ability. Mental illnesses can affect a person's capacity to deal with stressful situations effectively, especially when a situation poses significant challenges or problems.

***Intellectual wellness.*** Intellectual wellness reflects people's ability to make informed decisions that are appropriate for and beneficial to themselves. From their experiences and learnings, intellectually well people are able to gather information throughout their lifespan and to use that information to make the best of situations. Moreover, these people apply critical thinking skills, prioritize data, and keep informed on current health research, treatments, and health-related issues.

Intellectual wellness may also include occupational health—personal satisfaction from one's career and the ability to balance career with other activities like family and leisure time.

---

### THINKING IT THROUGH

#### *Spirituality and Wellness*

Spirituality has been linked to good health and wellness, with reported benefits ranging from fewer health issues, including anxiety and depression, to a faster recovery. Many people also claim that spirituality provides them with an enhanced ability to deal with stress.

1. What does spirituality mean to you?
2. Why do you think spirituality may contribute to better health?
3. How would you respond to a patient who told you that they wanted to try self-healing through spiritual practice instead of accepting medical intervention for a diagnosed medical condition?

---

***Social wellness.*** Social wellness is about relating effectively to others, including being able to form close, loving relationships, to laugh, to communicate effectively and empathically, to be a good listener, and to respond appropriately. Socially well individuals work agreeably in groups and within the community, are tolerant and accepting of others, and can form friendships and supportive networks. Confident and flexible, socially well people contribute to the welfare of others.

***Spiritual wellness.*** Spiritual wellness is different for most people, and entirely personal. It frequently involves a search for, or achievement of, a sense of purpose or meaning in their lives. It may be based on a faith of some kind, or religion, or encompass a search for harmony and balance with life, themselves, and others. It may encompass a sense of balance—connecting various components of the person's life—achieving a feeling of productiveness and inner peace. Achieving spiritual wellness can involve prayer, meditation, or other spiritual practices. Attaining spiritual wellness may afford a person peace, joy, a purpose in life, and the ability to relate to others in a positive, kind, and meaningful way. Spirituality is an important part of the Indigenous culture and congruent with a holistic approach to personhood, health, and wellness. The spiritually well person often seeks to contribute to society, plays an active role within the community, and displays gratitude and generosity (see Chapter 1, "The Medicine Wheel").

**THINKING IT THROUGH**

*Meditation*

Spiritual wellness is a holistic concept and is often enhanced by meditation—considered a holistic modality. Meditation means to reflect, to concentrate, or to focus on one's breathing or a calming visual image. Individuals who routinely practice meditation claim it provides them with mental, spiritual, emotional, and physical benefits. They claim it connects the body, mind, and spirit, instilling a sense of wellness. Meditation draws one's attention away from whatever is bothersome, calming the mind and spirit. There are several kinds of meditation, such as transcendental and mindfulness. Primary care providers sometimes recommend meditation for conditions such as chronic pain, hypertension (reflection of the body—mind connection, as a calm state of mind has been proven to lower blood pressure), and anxiety disorders. Many therapists will introduce their patients to a variety of meditation techniques or mindfulness (another therapeutic technique) to treat anxiety. Often individuals download meditation apps on their cell phones or "smart" watches and access them as required.

1. Do you believe there is a mind—body connection where meditation can contribute to one's health? Explain your answer
2. Would you or have you tried any meditation techniques? If you have, what benefits have you experienced? If not, why not? Would you be open to trying meditation? Explain your answer.

*Environmental wellness.* Many models of wellness take into account one's relationship with the environment. An environmentally well person is one who engages in a lifestyle that is friendly to the environment and lowering one's carbon footprint. Friendliness to the environment entails consciousness about preserving the external world (climate change), such as walking or biking (instead of driving), recycling, and choosing products that are less harmful to the environment (e.g., less packaging). Families may install alternate heating devices in their homes, such as heat pumps, or using solar panels where possible for heating and cooling homes and running appliances. Environmental wellness also includes strategies to maintain personal health and wellness by, for example, protecting one's eyesight (e.g., using good lighting when reading or working, wearing sunglasses when out in the sung) or limiting exposure to loud noises (e.g., controlling music volume).

Environmental wellness also includes cities, towns, and communities planning for and maintaining outdoor spaces such as parks, walking trails, playgrounds, and recreational activities that promote physical outdoor activity and mental wellness (e.g., interaction with nature) (Box 7.2).

Climate change has become a critical issue that poses an undeniable risk of significant social, economic, and environmental disruption on a global scale. Evidence points to human influences as a direct cause of global warming that is already observable around the world. The changing climate has become a critical issue and poses a serious risk to human health and life. The science says we are beyond reversing the damage to the planet that has already occurred, but with intensive measures, technology, and creative solutions (especially in the energy area) we may be able to mitigate some of the effects of global warming and adapt to a livable future. The problem is, the world (including Canada) is not presently on target to do this. The results of climate change that are already felt around the world (floods, droughts, fires, extreme weather events) will continue to dramatically affect human health and the environment in which we live.

---

### BOX 7.2   Community Structure and Recreation and Wellness Promotion

Public parks and recreational facilities such as playgrounds are essential parts of any community. They play an important role in promoting a healthy physical environment for people of all ages, abilities, and socioeconomic status, encouraging people to embrace the outdoors and active lifestyles. Access to and use of such facilities have been shown to positively impact the health of individuals, from improving the health of those with chronic diseases to encouraging individuals to engage in practices related to preventative and restorative health. Healthy activities related to parks and outdoor space also address cardiovascular disease, diabetes, and cancer by helping to reduce stress, anxiety, and depression. For the most part, there is little or no cost attached to using public facilities.

Source: Based on Park People. (2021). *Accessing the health benefits of parks*. https://ccpr.parkpeople. ca/2021/sections/growth/stories/accessing-the-health-benefits-of-parks

---

***Occupational wellness.*** Occupational wellness occurs when a person feels secure, confident, and valued in their workplace setting. Occupationally well people achieve an adaptive work—life balance, manage work-related stress effectively, and grow professionally. The level of enjoyment people have with their job affects most aspects of their lives—and those of the people around them. Many employers are now offering flexible hours, working at home, especially since the onset of the COVID-19 pandemic. Individuals are also taking a second look at the work they do, the pay scale, hours, and demands, and the impact their work has on their lives and the lives of their families. Many are changing careers, sometimes choosing a better work—life balance and job satisfaction over the amount they are paid.

### Illness

The term *illness*, often used to denote the presence of disease, can also refer to how a person feels about their health, whether or not a disease is present. Despite the absence of pathology or disease, a person may feel ill as a result of tiredness, stress, or both. Although this state differs from feeling healthy and energetic, by definition, it is not a disease.

### Disease

Disease typically refers to a condition in which a person's bodily or mental functions are different from normal. Usually biological in nature, disease may affect various organs of the body and have symptoms that are either observable or difficult to detect. Causes of diseases include the presence of organisms such as bacteria, a virus, or a fungus. Schizophrenia is an example of a disease in which mental functions are affected, resulting in behavioural or psychological alterations, and has a biological or biochemical explanation.

The term *disease* may also be used to describe a group of symptoms (more accurately called a syndrome), which are not related to a clear-cut disease process. *Disease* is often used interchangeably with the vague words *ailment*, *disorder*, *condition*, or *dysfunction*. *Disease* is also sometimes used incorrectly to refer to a disability.

A disease may run a predictable course and subside—with or without treatment (e.g., pneumonia influenza, or COVID-19—in some cases symptoms persist), or it may be chronic and controllable, but not curable (e.g., asthma, diabetes, human immunodeficiency virus [HIV], acquired immune deficiency syndrome [AIDS]). Other diseases are long term and have symptoms that disappear and recur (i.e., go into a period of remission). This reappearance of symptoms and reactivation of the disease is known as an exacerbation of the disease (e.g., as happens with multiple sclerosis and some forms of lymphoma).

Remission of a disease can occur spontaneously or be induced by treatment. In the case of multiple sclerosis, for example, the use of immunosuppressive medications can result in a treatment-related remission. A remission's length varies. The main aim of treatment for leukemia is a complete remission—that is, no signs of the disease from a symptomatic or pathological perspective. If a remission lasts more than 5 years, some consider the person to be cured. In the case of any kind of cancer, however, the word *cure* is used cautiously; some physicians avoid ever saying a person is cured, regardless of the length of time they have been cancer free.

## THINKING IT THROUGH

### Chronic Conditions and Wellness

Suppose you had a chronic condition such as multiple sclerosis (MS) but were managing reasonably well most of the time; for instance, if your MS was in a period of remission. Reflecting on your own definition of *wellness*, answer the following:
1. Do you think you would consider yourself to be well? Explain.
2. Do you think your outlook would be influenced by periods of remission or exacerbation of the condition? Why of why not?
3. Answer the first two questions considering two chronic diseases that people you know may have.

## Disability

A deviation from normal function, a disability can be physical, sensory (e.g., blindness, deafness), cognitive (e.g., Alzheimer's disease), or intellectual (e.g., Down syndrome). A disability can occur in conjunction with, or as a result of, a disease; be caused by an accident; or be present at birth. Invisible disabilities include heart disease and respiratory issues such as chronic obstructive pulmonary disease (COPD). Visual impairment is also a disability and, depending on the degree of visual loss, may or may not be immediately apparent.

The language used to describe people with a disability has changed over the years, moving toward more sensitive, less hurtful terminology. For example, today a person with a cognitive or intellectual disability is most likely to be deemed *intellectually impaired*. Along with improved terminology has come the recognition that people with disabilities deserve the same rights and opportunities as all other members of society (Box 7.3).

Individuals with disabilities still face a degree of ableism and discrimination; others are often impatient with and dismissive of individuals with either cognitive or physical limitations. Invisible disabilities can face similar challenges.

## THINKING IT THROUGH

### Invisible Disability

J.B. has cardiovascular disease and limited ability to walk long distances. J.B. has an accessibility card to put in the window of their car so that they can use a parking space for individuals with a disability. People seeing J.B. park in a spot reserved for individuals with a disability often approach J.B., accusing them of abusing the privilege or using someone else's accessibility designation.
1. Have you ever seen someone seemingly with no physical impairment walking away from their vehicle parked in a spot designated for individuals with a disability and wondered if they are using the spot legitimately? Would you approach the person? Explain.
2. What are your thoughts regarding the concept of disability parking permits?

## BOX 7.3 People With Disabilities: Rights Are Formally Recognized

Historically, people with disabilities have been viewed as individuals who need societal protection, evoking sympathy rather than respect. In an effort to change this perception and to ensure that all people have the opportunity to live life to their fullest potential, December 2021 marked the fifteenth anniversary of the United Nations formally adopting the *Convention on the Rights of Persons With Disabilities*. This was the first such inclusive human rights treaty of this century. The convention covers a number of key areas, including accessibility, personal mobility, health care, education, employment, rehabilitation, participation in political life, equality, and nondiscrimination. All jurisdictions have acts or other pieces of legislation to protect people with disabilities, and almost all are constantly being improved. After consultation with all jurisdictions including Indigenous peoples and individuals with disabilities, Canada ratified this Convention in 2010 and is bound to it by international law.

The UN's initiative Transforming Our World: The 2030 Agenda for Sustainable Development maintained a commitment to ensure that people with disabilities and other vulnerable populations are specifically included in all of the Agenda's goals. These goals are broad and include people, planet, prosperity, peace, and partnership; each has a clearly defined target intended to stimulate defined actions over the next 10 or so years. The statement related to people, for example, states, "we are determined to end poverty and hunger, in all their forms and dimensions, and to ensure that all human beings can fulfil their potential in dignity and equality and in a healthy environment." In 2021, a working group was established to strengthen the rights of women and girls with disabilities and to reduce discrimination.

In Canada, federal legislation protecting people with disabilities includes the *Canadian Charter of Rights and Freedoms, Canadian Human Rights Act*, and the Rights of People with Disabilities. Rights extend to transportation, employment, voting, and rights in criminal procedures.

Sources: Government of Canada. (2018, September 7). *Rights of people with disabilities.* https://www. canada.ca/en/canadian-heritage/services/rights-people-disabilities.html; UN General Assembly. (2015). *Transforming our world: The 2030 agenda for sustainable development, 21 October 2015*, A/RES/70/1. https://www.refworld.org/docid/57b6e3e44.html; United Nations Human Rights Office of the High Commissioner. (n.d.) *Committee on the Rights of Persons with Disabilities.* https://www.ohchr.org/en/treaty-bodies/crpd

## DID YOU KNOW?

### Terry Fox: A Continuing Legacy

Terry Fox, despite his disability, embraced a challenge, leaving a legacy that persists today.

An awareness and fundraising initiative that continues to this day originated with a person by the name of Terry Fox. Terry was born in Winnipeg, Manitoba in 1958. A recognized athlete in high school, at 18 years old Terry was diagnosed with osteosarcoma (bone cancer), which eventually resulted in the need for amputation of his right leg just above the knee. Embracing his physical disability, Terry made the astonishing decision to run across Canada to raise money for cancer research. He began his run—his "Marathon of Hope"—on April 12, 1980, in St. John's, Newfoundland. Terry ended his run near Thunder Bay, Ontario, when, after seeking medical attention for returning symptoms of osteosarcoma (shortness of breath, fatigue, and chest pains), it became apparent that his cancer had returned. Terry died on June 28, 1981, 1 month short of his twenty-third birthday. Every year, Canadians around the world work with communities with support from the Canadian Forces, embassies, and high commissions to organize the Terry Fox Run, raising money for the Terry Fox Foundation. By the end of 2021, an estimated $800 million had been raised worldwide; 78 cents on every dollar raised goes directly to cancer research. Along with the money, the Terry Fox Marathon of Hope continues to raise an awareness of cancer—a disease that touches so many lives.

A bronze statue of Terry Fox was erected in Ottawa in June, 1982, recognizing him as one of Canada's most unique historical figures with his Marathon of Hope and his ability to unite Canadians for his cause. In January 2022, the Terry Fox statue was defaced by protestors opposing vaccination mandates and other public health measures. The condemnation was swift and nationwide, illustrating how highly respected Terry Fox remains among Canadians.

Sources: Terry Fox Foundation. (n.d.). *Terry Fox.* http://www.terryfox.org/TerryFox/T_Fox.html; Terry Fox Foundation. (n.d.). *Facts.* http://www.terryfox.org/TerryFox/Facts.html; The Terry Fox Foundation (2020). *Terry Fox: Impact report 2020/2021.* https://terryfox.org/wp-content/uploads/2021/11/TFF_TFRI_IR_2021_FINAL.pdf

## HEALTH MODELS

A person's health, wellness, illness, disease, or disability—and the resulting interaction with health care providers—usually relates in some capacity to a health model. Defined as a design for delivering health care, a health model can influence both a health care provider's practice and their delivery of health care, which in turn affects treatment, priorities, and outcome measurements. The three most common types of health care models are the medical model, the holistic model, and the wellness model, all of which continue to evolve.

The principles of the wellness model—stressing wellness and illness prevention—are most commonly pursued in our current health care climate. Physicians are embracing evidence-informed decision making and using best practices to deliver patient-focused care in a team-oriented environment.

### Medical Model

The medical model initially focused on the definition that health means the absence of disease. The medical model holds that diseases are identified through a series of predetermined steps such as functional inquiry, objective examination, patient history (subjective information), and diagnostic tests, the results of which lead to a diagnosis and treatment (all scientifically based). More recently, the model has expanded to include the integration of the additional dimensions of health, recognizing, for example, that individuals with chronic diseases can indeed lead healthy lives (even some forms of cancer are now considered chronic diseases that, when controlled, allow a person to live with a reasonable quality of life). The medical model, however, does not typically embrace holistic approaches to caring for patients. The medical model, in general, also does not embrace or collaborate with other approaches to health care, although that practice will vary with individual care providers.

Criticisms of this model include the notion that mental and physical health are more often than not considered as separate entities; the model's focus is more on disease and disability rather than ability and the patient's strengths; and lastly, that the model is paternalistic in the approach to patient care (Swaine, 2011). This approach, however, continues to change, wherein practitioners are involving patients in decision making regarding their own treatment options and plan of care.

## Holistic Model

The holistic approach to health considers all parts of the person. This approach has been used for many years by alternative practitioners, such as naturopaths; only recently has it been integrated into mainstream medicine (see Chapter 5).

Focusing on the positive aspects of health—not on the negatives of illness and disease that inform the medical model—the holistic model strives for a state of health that encompasses the entire person, rather than just aiming for a lack of disease and disability. Although similar to the original WHO definition of health, introduced in 1948 (see Box 7.1), the holistic definition of health goes much further, by recognizing the impact of factors such as lifestyle, spirituality, socioeconomics, and culture on an individual's health.

### THINKING IT THROUGH

#### A Definition of Health

There are many other definitions of health. Consider some of the World Health Organization's (WHO's) international classification systems, such as the International Classification of Functioning, Disability (which measures the relationship between health and disabilities at an individual and population level). These systems are sometimes used in developing current concepts of how health should be defined. The WHO definition does not clearly address individuals with disabilities. Can someone with a spinal cord injury not consider themselves to be healthy? Can individuals who participate in the Paralympics or the Invictus Games not consider themselves healthy? Participants cope with physical as well as mental challenges and show remarkable strength, courage, and perseverance as they achieve their goals.
1. Can anyone really define health in terms that would suit everyone, or is it individual?
2. What would you consider to be a realistic, inclusive definition of health?

## Indigenous Wholistic Theory for Health

With similar concepts to the holistic model above, the *holistic model* is also known as the *Indigenous wholistic theory*. This wholistic approach to health considers mental, physical, cultural, and spiritual well-being, not only of the individual person but of the entire community. The framework incorporates the medicine wheel, which, along with the outlook that Indigenous people have regarding health, is discussed in detail in Chapter 1.

## Wellness Model

The wellness model builds on the medical and holistic models. It considers health to be a process that continues to evolve and to progress toward a future state of improved health. This model requires individuals to practise healthy choices and try to lead a balanced lifestyle. A person's perception of health is based on how they feel about their disease or disability rather than the objective manifestations. The wellness model encompasses an individual's or a group's ability to cope with health-related challenges.

In the wellness model, people assume responsibility for their own health and make informed choices about such things as lifestyle choices that negatively impact all aspects of one's health. The wellness model also considers a person with a disability or illness to be healthy depending on the person's outlook on their life, health, and well-being. This includes whether or not that person can function, meet self-imposed goals, and is not incapacitated by pain.

The common thread linking the holistic and wellness health models is the inclusion of a broad spectrum of factors—physical, spiritual, social, emotional, economic, and cultural.

### International Classification of Functioning Disability and Health

Introduced in the 1980s by the WHO, the International Classification of Functioning Disability and Health (ICF) is both a classification system and a health model. As a classification system, the ICF measures the health of individuals in addition to the health of designated populations. It considers health and health-related issues from the perspectives of the environment, the body's structure and function, and the individual's health-related activities (promoting personal health). As a model, the ICF considers health and disability a little differently. It holds that everyone at some point during their lifespan will experience altered health and may then experience some form of disability. Disabilities are considered common, experienced by many, and not just a few. This model also considers the social components of living with a disability and the effects a disability has on individuals and those around them; it emphasizes the effects of a disability rather than the cause. As a model, the ICF is used clinically by health care providers to assess patients' social and functional challenges and capacities, set realistic goals, formulate treatment plans, and measure outcomes.

## CHANGING PERCEPTIONS OF HEALTH AND WELLNESS

How a person views or perceives health and wellness will affect how that person responds to alterations in health. A person who is feeling happy and optimistic may pass off a minor illness as trivial or as something they can cope with. However, if that same person is feeling down, stressed, or otherwise vulnerable, the same illness may seem more significant. Circumstance and time of day or night can profoundly affect how a person views their health. For example, people sometimes feel more vulnerable at night or in the early hours of the morning. They may wake up in the night and start thinking about things and magnify those things in their mind. A minor illness or concern may seem more profound, or a minor irritation may produce great stress. Individuals who are experiencing serious illnesses, anxiety, and stress over significant events going on in their lives likewise often find their coping mechanisms are diminished during the night. Conversely, when people get up in the morning, interact with others, and start focusing on daily activities, they feel more positive, and things that alarmed them in the night may seem less onerous. Consequently, a positive frame of mind can help a person deal more effectively with stress and fight disease.

### Past Approaches

Until the early-to-mid 1960s, most Canadians held the attitude that if they were sick they would seek medical care, and the doctor would make them better. (People took little responsibility for their own health and rarely participated in decisions related to their treatment.) They did what the doctor told them to do, and most doctors did not expect to be questioned. Doctors and patients functioned very much within the realm of a paternalistic medical model. Few people recognized the impact of lifestyle on their health and safety. Such entities as a sedentary lifestyle, poor nutritional habits, smoking, and alcohol use were rarely directly linked to changes in health status. Within the medical community there was limited education related to promoting a healthy lifestyle. This approach began to change in the 1960s and 1970s. With the help of government initiatives and the establishment of a population health approach to health care (see Chapter 6), Canadians started to see the value of prevention and to consider what they could do on a personal level to stay healthy—that is, they began to take more responsibility for their own well-being. Slowly, community and group involvement in health promotion and disease prevention emerged.

The 1980s and 1990s saw the beginning of changes in the structure and function of how primary care was delivered, further encouraging individuals to not only take responsibility for their own health but also to participate in making decisions about their treatment, which is the norm today. Canadians are now more informed, sometimes looking up pertinent information on the Internet and bringing it in to their health care provider.

Although some information is accurate, some is not; this can have harmful consequences promoting anxiety and stress. Sometimes providers are overwhelmed with the amount of information presented to them by their patients. On the whole, people have become self-advocates, seeking answers if they are not satisfied with what they have been told, perhaps asking for a second opinion. The interprofessional teams that are part of many primary care groups offer more choice of providers to patients. Moreover, individuals are more likely to seek out alternative modalities for treating ailments—anxiety, stress, various diseases, and physical problems. Physicians who are willing to work with alternative practitioners offer their patients the best of both worlds.

Public education regarding lifestyle changes continues to have at least a moderate effect. A federal public initiative, aptly called ParticipACTION, launched in 1971, still promotes a healthy lifestyle through increased physical activity. ParticipACTION has evolved into a network of both public sector and nongovernment organizations (NGOs) whose goals are to promote physical activity, including participation in sports activities. Other organizations do their bit to encourage a healthy lifestyle. The Heart and Stroke Association, for example, sponsors riveting commercials on lifestyle choices (e.g., smoking, inactivity) and related risks. Antismoking campaigns have been launched along with related legislation (including laws governing electronic cigarettes [vaping], see Chapter 8). Similarly, ongoing campaigns (such as Mothers Against Drunk Drivers [MADD]) and laws against drinking and driving continue to reinforce the risks and push for the reduction of alcohol consumption. Now, with implementation of the legalization of marijuana, new challenges are posed in terms of health and safety (see Chapter 8). Canadians, on the whole, pay attention to information being offered and are supportive of related legislation, recognizing that prevention goes a long way. Today, Canadians have a much broader-based understanding of the link between lifestyle and health. Most people recognize that smoking causes lung cancer and respiratory disease. And many know that being active can lower their chances of developing high blood pressure, osteoporosis, cardiovascular disease, and even some types of cancer. People are more aware than ever before that there is a link between obesity, inactivity, and diabetes. Obviously, how individuals respond to this knowledge depends on how they view health, wellness, their own circumstances related to the determinants of health, and their own vulnerability.

## THE PSYCHOLOGY OF HEALTH BEHAVIOUR

Demonstrated by a person's response or reaction to altered health, health behaviour has a significant impact on what a person does to maintain good physical and psychological health. Many factors, including what a person believes to be true about health, prevention, treatment, and vulnerability, influence how people act when they are ill or perceive they are ill. Health behaviour also depends on a person's level of health knowledge, personal motivation, cognitive processes, and perceived risk factors. One's culture and ethnicity will invariably affect all of these areas.

To explain human health behaviour, several models have been developed, including the transtheoretical model, the social–ecological model, the protection motivation theory, and the health belief model (developed in the 1950s by the United States Public Health Service). Elements of the health belief model are relevant in one way or another to all of the other models, so it is described in detail below.

## Health Belief Model

People's health beliefs affect their health behaviour. Health beliefs are things people believe to be true about their personal health and susceptibility to and about illness, prevention, and treatment in general. Beliefs are acquired largely through social interaction and experience. For over six decades, the concept that health beliefs affect health behaviour has been widely accepted and is based on a number of assumptions—for example, if people feel that by taking a certain action they can avoid a negative outcome, they will take that action.

---

### THINKING IT THROUGH

#### *M.M. and Contraception*

M.M. is 17 years old and sexually active. A number of her friends are sexually active as well. J.L., age 16, one of her best friends, became pregnant, claiming that she and her boyfriend were using condoms. J.L. plans to have an abortion and was not particularly upset about the fact that she is pregnant. M.M. has been relying on the rhythm method to avoid pregnancy, not wanting to take the pill for religious reasons. M.M. also felt that becoming pregnant is something that could not happen to her. However, M.M. is now considering an oral contraceptive.

1. Why do you think M.M. thought that becoming pregnant could not happen to her?
2. What difference did the fact that J.L. became pregnant make to M.M.'s way of thinking?
3. What issues might M.M. be struggling with, considering the choice between the risk of becoming pregnant and taking an oral contraceptive?
4. Why do you think she is not considering condoms?
5. What other choice does M.M. have?

---

Another factor that influences people's choices and level of concern is the perceived seriousness of the condition or illness if acquired. M.M. may think that a pregnancy would be devastating, or she may believe that she and her boyfriend will get married and live happily ever after. M.M. may also think that an abortion is a viable option if pregnancy were to occur.

Culture, religion, and spiritual beliefs also influence health beliefs and value systems. As a multicultural country, Canada requires health care providers to pay close attention to and respect cultural and religious traditions and practices. The respect, or lack thereof, shown for such beliefs can affect how the patient feels about seeking health care (e.g., at what point and from whom) and following treatment plans (adherence).

Culture, spirituality and religion may affect a patient's outlook on mental and physical health, wellness, disease, and disability. These beliefs often include the etiology or origin of the infirmity and how it should be treated. Western medicine is largely scientifically based—holding, for example, that an acute infection is caused by a pathogen—whereas some other cultures may believe that spirits, the supernatural, or disharmony with nature may be the cause. Specific beliefs as to the origin of an illness will likely dictate what type of treatment the person will accept and adhere to. One cannot assume that every person from a specific culture will have the same beliefs or practices, as there are other variables involved, such as the person's personal outlook, their upbringing, and experiences. It is best to identify cultural beliefs, preferences, and practices firsthand; if language is a barrier, arrange for someone to act as a translator, or ask that the individual bring a friend or family member to translate for them (although this is not always recommended, especially if privacy of personal information is an issue, or if the person translating assumes a dominant role, interfering with the patient's autonomy).

In Canada, the patient's right to participate in their own health care is valued. Over the past decade, primary care providers have placed great emphasis on involving the patient as a partner in the decision-making process: giving the patient the required information, treatment options, and letting the patient (perhaps with advice from their family) make the final decision. In other cultures, however, the patient's autonomy to make personal health-related decisions is not considered necessary or important; instead, a family member may assume this responsibility. Often in these cultures (e.g., Asian and some Indigenous cultures), the welfare of the whole family is considered in making decisions, possibly without even consulting the patient. Some cultures view doctors and other health care providers as figures of authority, so patients may find discussing their treatment options difficult because they are accustomed to doing as they are told. People within some cultures may not report cognitive problems or mental illness because of perceptions that such illnesses are spiritually induced (i.e., possession by demons), reveal a lack of self-control, or are a source of shame.

Religion, cultural customs, education, and language barriers also influence health behaviours and beliefs and decisions around death and dying. For example, people of Chinese or South Asian descent, Muslims, and Orthodox Jews may question requests for organ donation or the withdrawal of life support, even if the patient is deemed brain dead; the belief that life is sacred dominates. Knowledge concerning the patient's and family's cultural beliefs and traditions is essential if a nurse, for example, is to meet the family's wishes regarding the death of a loved one. Such considerations include how long the family wants to stay with their loved one after death, whether or not it is appropriate to approach the family about organ donation, and if there are special ways in which to prepare the body after death.

It may be that second- and third-generation Canadians do not hold the same beliefs—or do, but not to the same degree—as their parents. Sometimes, within a family, generational differences of opinion may cause conflict when it comes to treatment plans (Euromed Info, n.d.).

### Transtheoretical Model

The transtheoretical model (TTM) of health behaviour is a framework for promoting adaptive changes in a person's health behaviour. The concept proposes that people must progress through the following series of steps before their health behaviour completely changes (i.e., improves): precontemplation, contemplation, preparation, action, maintenance, and termination (Fig. 7.2). Integrated into these steps are 10 cognitive and behavioural activities that further facilitate change. For example, during the *precontemplation stage*, although aware that a behaviour modification may improve their health, the person may initially have no desire or motivation to make a change. During the *contemplation stage, the* person is ready to seriously think about making changes and may consider the risks and benefits of a behaviour change. The *preparation stage* occurs when the person starts planning for the behaviour change (e.g., finds a gym they like, gets more information about joining). The *action phase* is when the person implements their plan, like going to the gym—perhaps engaging a personal trainer, or preparing and eating a healthy meal. The ongoing support of others is important during this phase. If the person is able to adhere to their plan for at least 6 months, they are ready to move into the *maintenance phase,* which must continue for 2 years—continuing with an exercise program and eating a balanced diet. Once achieved, the individual enters into the *termination phase.* At this point, the person's behavioural changes are integrated into their lifestyle and considered permanent.

### Social—Ecological Model

The social—ecological model (SEM) maintains that many levels of influence shape health behaviour, with a focus on health promotion for individuals as well as groups of people within

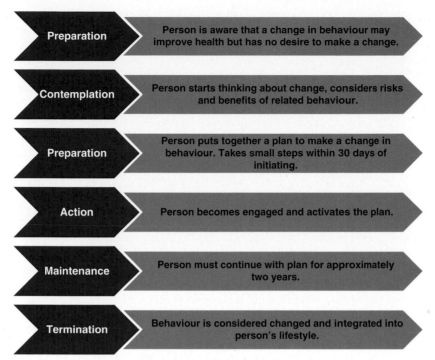

**Preparation** — Person is aware that a change in behaviour may improve health but has no desire to make a change.

**Contemplation** — Person starts thinking about change, considers risks and benefits of related behaviour.

**Preparation** — Person puts together a plan to make a change in behaviour. Takes small steps within 30 days of initiating.

**Action** — Person becomes engaged and activates the plan.

**Maintenance** — Person must continue with plan for approximately two years.

**Termination** — Behaviour is considered changed and integrated into person's lifestyle.

**Fig. 7.2** Transtheoretical model.

organizations. Such influences include a person's education, occupation, or profession; the type of social support (personal, community) they have; their environment (e.g., workplace, availability of health care); and the public policies of various levels of government. The SEM takes into account how various entities put people at risk for developing health, behavioural, and socioeconomic problems, citing individual, relationship, community, and societal factors. Recognizing that there is an interplay between multiple factors promotes an understanding that one affects another.

The ideal situation is one wherein the determinants of health are the foundation for policy development collectively promoting good health, health education, and a healthy workplace.

## Protection Motivation Theory

Building on the health belief model (discussed below), the protection motivation theory asserts that self-preservation is what motivates a person to change their health behaviour. The fear of illness, physical decline, physical disability, mental health problems, or even death can encourage adaptive (or maladaptive) health behaviours. The person's actions depend on how severe they perceive the severity of the threat (e.g., cancer); how likely one is to succumb to the threat (e.g., actually get lung cancer from smoking, or contract a sexually transmitted infection [STI] from having numerous sexual partners); and how likely the preventative action(s) is (are) to be successful. For example, if a person fears that they will develop lung cancer, their health behaviours will be altered by how vulnerable they think they are (i.e., their likelihood of actually getting lung cancer), what they have to do to avoid this threat (e.g., quit smoking), and their ability (or motivation) to take action. See Case Example 7.1.

## Social Model of Disability

The social model of disability recognizes disability as resulting from the interaction between individuals with impairments and the environment around them that consists of physical,

CASE EXAMPLE 7.1   **L.S. and Managing Health Risks**

L.S.'s doctor tells them at a recent visit that their blood pressure, which has been creeping up, is now a concern. L.S.'s last blood panel also reveals a rather alarming rise in cholesterol levels. The doctor tells L.S. that given the fact that they are also overweight, they are at serious risk for a cardiovascular event. L.S. enjoys fast food and is inactive and feels that their lifestyle to date has not contributed to any serious health problems. L.S. has tried losing weight in the past by changing their diet and exercising but has never been very successful in these attempts. L.S. knows people in their 70's who have similar lifestyles and are doing well. Some of them are on antihypertensive and lipid lowering medication, which more or less normalizes their clinical signs. How do you think L.S. perceives the threat of a heart attack or stroke? Do you think L.S. feels they are at risk? Does it appear that L.S. is motivated to engage in lifestyle changes given the information they receive from the doctor? What do you think could change L.S.'s way of thinking? Why?

attitudinal, communication, and social barriers (Inclusion London, n.d.; People with Disability Australia, n.d.). This model holds that the environment must change to accommodate individuals with disabilities, rather than that the individual with a disability must change in order to interact successfully with the environment. For example, instead of a person unable to climb stairs to get to their doctor's office having to figure out how to navigate the stairs, the onus is on the doctor's office to ensure that there is a ramp or an elevator to accommodate the individual. In that context, the social model of disability states that external barriers must accommodate individuals with disabilities, regarding such persons as having the same rights and privileges as someone without a disability (Fig. 7.3).

## THE HEALTH/WELLNESS—ILLNESS CONTINUUM

No matter what health beliefs and religious or cultural background a person has, everyone measures their health (or wellness) and illness in some manner. A *continuum* is a method of measurement usually represented by a straight line with an opposing state at each end. The health—illness continuum (or wellness—illness continuum) measures one's perception of their state of health or level of wellness between "optimum health" and "poor health" or "death." In the middle is a neutral section sometimes referred to as compensation (Fig. 7.4). The wellness—illness continuum includes all of the dimensions of health and wellness, from physical, mental, and emotional health to social, spiritual, and environmental, similar to Health Canada's determinants of health (see Chapter 2).

Movement on the continuum is constant. An individual may wake up feeling good and then develop a headache 2 hours later, altering their perceived placement on the continuum. Also, one person may have a bad cold but not feel particularly ill, therefore may place themselves on the "good health" part of the continuum. Someone else with a similar cold may feel unable to function and place themselves in compensation on the continuum. For example, A.G. is experiencing some epigastric pain—with the diagnosis of a gastric ulcer; to some this is more serious than a cold, but she also considers herself to be in the compensation zone (Case Example 7.2).

People with disabilities also place themselves on different places on the continuum. Consider Dr. Stephen Hawking (who passed away in March of 2018), who was a world-famous physicist and had ALS for many years, and despite his impairments pursued life with a vengeance. Likely he would have placed himself in the compensation range of the continuum.

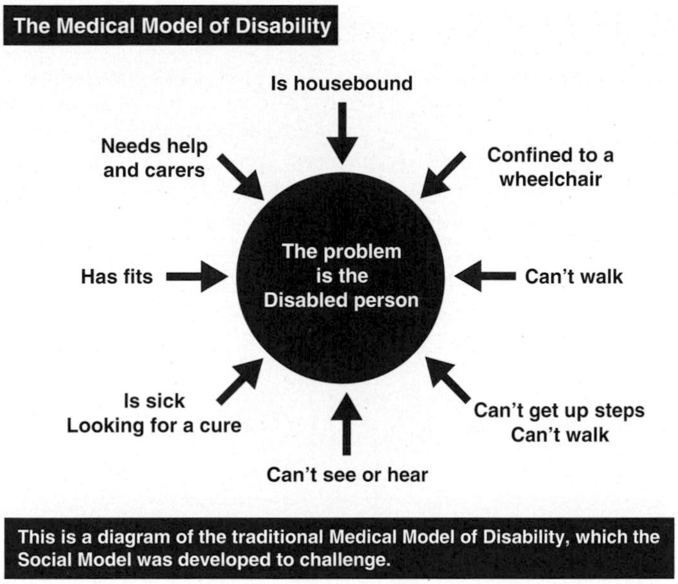

**The Medical Model of Disability**

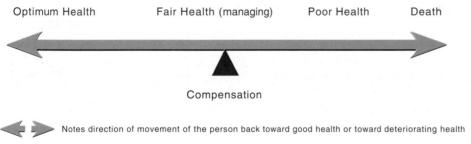

Is housebound

Needs help and carers

Confined to a wheelchair

Has fits

The problem is the Disabled person

Can't walk

Is sick Looking for a cure

Can't get up steps Can't walk

Can't see or hear

This is a diagram of the traditional Medical Model of Disability, which the Social Model was developed to challenge.

**Fig. 7.3** The social model or disability in contrast to the medical model of disability. In the social model or disability, the individual with a disability is at the center. Society is challenged to accommodate the person with a disability rather than expecting the person to adapt to an unfriendly environment (which is congruent with the medical model, wherein persons with a disability are expected to adapt to the environmental challenges they face.) (Source: Inclusion London. (n.d.). *The social model of disability*. https://www.inclusionlondon.org.uk/disability-in-london/social-model/the-social-model-of-disability-and-the-cultural-model-of-deafness/)

Optimum Health        Fair Health (managing)        Poor Health        Death

Compensation

Notes direction of movement of the person back toward good health or toward deteriorating health

**Fig. 7.4** The health continuum (also called the wellness–illness continuum).

He might even have considered himself to be closer to the wellness end of the continuum, accepting his limitations to be within normal limits for him. Consider also Rick Hanson and Ryan Straschnitzki (survivor of the Humboldt bus crash that killed 16 young hockey players). Both men are paraplegics, but with the proper support and an positive outlook went on to achieve numerous goals.

Rick Hanson, known as the "Man in Motion," was, after his accident, dedicated to making the world aware of the potential that people with physical limitations had. His 26-month trip around the world in his wheelchair did just that. The Rick Hanson Foundation remains dedicated to removing barriers for people with disabilities.

CASE EXAMPLE 7.2    **Movement on the Health/Wellness—Illness Continuum**

A.G. has always enjoyed good health and, for the most part, eats sensibly and exercises regularly. Recently, however, she began to have some epigastric discomfort. She was diagnosed with an ulcer and treated accordingly. Symptoms began to improve within a couple of days. On the health—illness continuum, A.G. considers herself to be in compensation but moving toward good health or the wellness end of the continuum. For A.G., the direction of movement would be noted by an arrow moving toward optimum wellness. Fig. 7.5 shows A.G. on the continuum near "fair health" and moving toward "optimum health." What factors might cause Angela to move toward the illness end of the continuum?

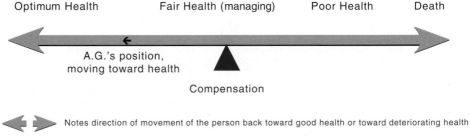

Fig. 7.5 Health/wellness—illness continuum for patient A.G.

Ryan Straschnitzki was to get back on the ice, playing sledge hockey. In 2021, he made Alberta's sledge hockey team, with his next goal being to win the national championship. Both men may have put themselves on the continuum more toward ill health initially, but now more toward the wellness end of the continuum.

Others who, despite trying, cannot accept or cope with a progressive disability or terminal illness may consider their health to be closer to the illness end of the spectrum and find themselves making some difficult choices, including medical assistance in dying (see Chapters 8 and 9).

## SICK ROLE BEHAVIOUR

It is widely accepted that when people are ill, their behaviours, roles, and attitudes change. This response to illness is sometimes referred to as sick role behaviour or behavioural illness response to disease or illness (Thompson, 2022). The stress of being ill can alter people's perceptions and the way they interact with others, from those who are close to them to the health professionals they deal with. Illness can also influence the behaviour of those associating with the unwell person, in large part because these people often have a burden placed on them. They may be required to provide extra support to the ill person or to assume their responsibilities, which may result in a change in their daily routine and increased stress.

To better understand sick role behaviour, consider the fact that we all behave differently at different times, with different people, and in different situations. These varying behaviours affect, among other things, the diverse roles and responsibilities we assume throughout our lifetime. Persons who are ill are often relieved from the roles and responsibilities they have in society—which ones and to what extent depend on the nature and severity of their illness.

---

**CASE EXAMPLE 7.3  A Young Mother's Placement on Wellness —Illness Continuum**

A student nurse was looking after a young mother who was in labour and delivery. Because there were serious signs of fetal distress, after discussing options with the mother and her husband, the decision was made to do a Caesarean birth. The mother became uncommunicative, answering with one word or not at all, making it impossible for the student nurse to assess her needs accurately. The next day, when the student nurse went to see the mother on the postpartum unit, they were greeted by a big smile and an outgoing, chatty, and cheery demeanor. The student nurse could not believe this was the same person. When asked how she felt, the mother responded "good and my baby boy is fine, but that's it. I will never have another child. I have never felt so helpless and afraid in my life. I thought my baby was going to die." The anxiety and fear of the unknown, and worry about the outcomes for her baby, had greatly affected the mother's normal behaviour and her outlook in terms of wanting to go through a pregnancy again. Where do you think the mother would place herself on the continuum when the decision to have a Caesarean birth was made? What about afterward?

---

The majority of people respond to their illness in an adaptive manner. Others will respond by being "more of what they are." For example, sometimes people who consistently complain about their health, call their provider frequently, and rely heavily on health care providers will likely become more extreme in these behaviours when faced with an illness, even a minor one. Alternatively, components of a person's character not usually seen can emerge. A normally easy-going person considered an extrovert may, when ill, become inwardly focused and quiet, or uncommunicative for several reasons, including fear (Case Example 7.3).

Although pronounced changes in attitude are more apt to be evident when a person suffers a serious illness, the stress of a relatively minor illness or accident (for example, a broken leg or pneumonia) can also be problematic—especially if the illness limits or alters the patient's activities, role functions, or ability to work, even for a short period of time. Such limitations will invariably affect the person's attitude and outlook, as well as the attitudes of those close to the person. As noted at the beginning of this chapter, culture may also affect a person's response to illness.

Health care providers can do their part by maintaining their professional role and respecting the fact that patients will present moods and attitudes that differ from those they display in good health (influenced also by the health belief model they affiliate with, and if their locus of control is internal or external). Family members may also become upset, short-tempered, and demanding. It is important to remember that they are also coping with the stress of altered roles and functions and are probably frightened and concerned about their loved one who is ill. Managing patients and family members in such situations requires the ability to remain calm, listen to their concerns, answer questions simply and honestly, and connect them to the appropriate resources as required. A calm, caring, and supportive demeanor most often brings about the most positive responses.

Sick role behaviour may be affected by the setting, such as if a person is hospitalized or treated in the community setting (e.g., at home with home care), or, despite their health problem, if they are still able to carry on with their usual routines of work and looking after a family. Hospitalization is most likely to affect how someone responds to an illness, because they are removed from their home and community and their activities are highly

---

**CASE EXAMPLE 7.4    N.P. and Culturally Safe Care**

N.P., a 65-year-old woman from India, refused to let a male registered nurse assist her with her bed bath. N.P. drew the covers up under her chin and waved the nurse away. Confused, the nurse reported that N.P. had refused care. In N.P.'s culture, modesty is very important, and female caregivers are preferred. What would you do if you were in the nurse's position?

It is important to note that health care providers must avoid stereotyping or generalizing behaviour based on the patient's cultural background. For example, N.P.'s daughter was born in Canada and may not share the same level of modesty.

---

restricted—from the time they get up to the time they are expected to go to bed and the time that meals are served. Patients more or less lose their sense of autonomy.

Health care providers must also take into account the fact that language barriers or cultural or religious beliefs are likely to affect how a patient responds to hospitalization and medical care. It is important to read the patient's body language and responses. When culture is an important component of providing care to a patient, one must find out more about the patient's culture and health care beliefs and practices. Family members can be a resource, as can other health care providers who may be familiar with the patient's needs and expectations.

Health care providers influenced by Western medicine are taught that touch (even a hand on the arm or shoulder) can be comforting to a patient, no matter the setting, and that eye contact is important. Eye contact for the most part is a behaviour influenced by culture. Some Canadians are taught that establishing eye contact engages another person, demonstrating interest and warmth, especially if accompanied with a smile. Eye contact on the other hand, particularly if sustained, is perceived by some as a sign of disrespect or even aggression. Although this is a generalization and varies with individuals, in many cultures, such as Hispanic, Asian, Middle Eastern, and Indigenous, low eye contact is preferred (Raeburn, 2021; Willingham, 2012). Direct eye contact may be perceived as disrespectful and impolite. In some cultures, a woman may interpret direct eye contact from a male health care provider as an unprofessional interest in her. In fact, avoiding eye contact, especially with someone deemed to be in authority, is considered by some people to be a sign of respect and politeness. Modesty is also a concern for people from some cultures (Case Example 7.4) (Chin, 1996; Nursing, 2005; Schwartz, 1991; Thompson, 2022).

Sometimes it is necessary for health care providers to seek the help of other team members to ensure optimal care and treatment. Personal space is another variable that health providers must be aware of. Although personal to some degree, there are cultures that are comfortable with someone moving close to them, and others that are not. Touch, even just putting a hand on a patient's arm, can be perceived as invasive by some, and not by others.

## Sick Role Theory

The sick role theory is based on the assumption that individuals who are ill have certain inherent rights and responsibilities, recognizing the fact that ill persons may be unable to carry out some, if not all, of their normal activities and responsibilities. Society, as such, is expected to understand this, giving leniency to the ill person where they would not for someone who was in good health. For an individual to be accommodated because of their illness, the person must be able to prove that they are ill (e.g., seeing a doctor or other health care provider, be diagnosed, and present proof or illness, for example, at work). Two rights and responsibilities are described in this theory: the right not to be blamed for being ill, and the right to expect others to be tolerant of the fact that the person is unable to carry out certain duties while they are ill. The two responsibilities on the part of the ill person are to seek the proper treatment promptly, and to make seeking treatment a priority. Problems with this theory include the fact that it does not accommodate individuals with chronic illnesses. The person's rights are only active while the person is ill and are thus temporary. How, then, would someone with a medical condition that is going to improve and, in fact, progress, be accommodated?

## Stages of Illness: Influence on Patient Behaviour

A patient's acceptance of a diagnosis and treatment plan normally follows a relatively predictable path through the stages of illness. But a person's response and choice of course of action depend on their health beliefs, health behaviours, and other variables (e.g., the seriousness of the health issue) discussed in this chapter. A person may have an illness "brewing" for some time before symptoms appear. How long the illness has been present will affect the nature and severity of the signs or symptoms of the illness once they do become apparent, as well as the outcome of the illness. The stages of illness and probable responses are summarized in Box 7.4.

---

### BOX 7.4   Stages of Illness

**Preliminary Phase: Suspecting Symptoms**
- Symptoms, possibly subtle, appear; they may progress or abate.
- Person either acknowledges or ignores symptoms.
- Person may seek immediate medical advice or look for information elsewhere (e.g., on the Internet).

**Acknowledgement Phase: Sustained Clinical Signs**
- Person decides symptoms cannot be ignored.
- Person seeks advice from family or friends, self-treats, or considers making an appointment with the doctor.

**Action Phase: Seeking Treatment**
- Symptoms become problematic and concerning.
- Person seeks medical advice.

**Transitional Phase: Diagnosis and Treatment**
- Person receives a diagnosis, a treatment plan, or both.
- Person may seek a second opinion if the diagnosis is serious.
- Person may accept treatment, becoming involved in the treatment plan, or may refuse treatment or even deny the diagnosis (e.g., in the case of a terminal disease).

**Resolution Phase: Recovery and Rehabilitation**
- Person may recover completely with minimal intervention or may require surgery, ongoing care, or rehabilitation.
- Person may or may not embrace and adhere to the rehabilitation plan; if the illness becomes chronic, the person will reposition themselves on the health–illness continuum.

**THINKING IT THROUGH**

### Regulating J.W.'s Blood Sugar

Twelve-year-old J.W. is a diabetic who has their diabetes well under control and has been monitoring their own blood glucose levels and adjusting their own insulin according to their doctor's orders. J.W. has a smartphone app (as do J.W.'s parents) that allows them to check their blood glucose levels regularly (J.W. wears a skin patch allowing for wireless monitoring). Prior to J.W.'s first-semester examinations, the parents noticed that for several days J.W.'s blood glucose levels were much higher than they should be. J.W.'s parents also noticed that J.W. was not eating well and hiding chocolate bars in their room. The parents tried talking to J.W. about it, but J.W. refused to discuss the problem and told the parents they are overreacting. J.W.'s parents make an appointment for J.W. to see their diabetic counsellor. As a dietary assistant, you have been asked to review J.W.'s diet and dietary habits with them. J.W. grumbles about the fuss everyone is making and does not understand the need for any changes to their diet or lifestyle.

1. What do you think is the problem?
2. What approach would you take with J.W.?

## Self-Imposed Risk Behaviours

Examples of self-imposed risk behaviours include not wearing a seatbelt or bicycle helmet, diving into unknown waters, smoking, unhealthy eating habits, and sexual promiscuity. People engage in risk behaviours for a number of reasons, including simple enjoyment, habit, and thrill-seeking. Recall that certain risk behaviours may be considered cultural norms. Also, individuals who have addictions to substances, for example, are not considered to be willingly engaging in risk behaviours. In this example, alcohol and drug use are addictions and not a clear choice that a person makes. To overcome substance use disorders, most people require intervention and treatment.

A common initiator of risk behaviour (that a person willingly engages in) among young people is peer pressure. For example, if a teen's friends smoke or take drugs, the teen may try it rather than risk not fitting in. Risk behaviour in one person often will affect another person. For instance, people who choose not to smoke may nevertheless find themselves in danger of inhaling second-hand smoke (they may not realize the implications, or find it difficult to remove themselves from the situation), or they may drive sensibly but voluntarily ride in a car with an impaired driver. Risk behaviour is dangerous for the individual, and when it results in injury that requires medical or surgical intervention, it places the burden of cost on the health care system.

Some risk behaviours are less obvious, especially in terms of accepting responsibility for one's own health, including awareness of one's own health risks as dictated by family history (genetics), lifestyle, and current health issues. Most primary care providers follow provincial and territorial "best practices" guidelines with respect to preventive medicine. Preventive screening tests such as Pap smears, breast screening, and, when medical history dictates, colonoscopy are examples. Health care providers will sometimes notify their patients when they should be considering medical screening. However, the onus is on the individual to have the screening done. The COVID-19 pandemic has added a complication to this situation as "elective" procedures, including diagnostic tests, were put on hold numerous times, particularly over the first 2 years of the pandemic (and in the fall and winter of 2022 and 2023 numerous surgeries were cancelled to accommodate the rise in pediatric admissions to hospitals and Intensive/Critical Care Units across the country). Cancelling surgeries and procedures has resulted in a backlog of procedures, sometimes with serious consequences. A patient, for example, found a breast lump early in 2021. Because elective procedures had been put on hold, the patient could not have the necessary mammogram for 3 months; after a diagnosis of breast cancer was made, it was another 6 months before the patient had surgery (well outside best practices guidelines), as the surgical dates were pushed back two times. By the time the patient was seen, the tumour had tripled in size, spreading to surrounding lymph nodes. The patient's prognosis now was guarded at best.

Health promotion and disease prevention initiatives undertaken by all levels of government aim to promote healthy lifestyles and avoid activities and behaviours that negatively impact the health of a person or a population group. These initiatives are taken for three reasons: to promote the health and longevity of Canadians, to ease the financial burden on our health care system, and to ease the burden on health human resources.

## THINKING IT THROUGH

### Smoking as a Risk Behaviour

As a nurse in a family health team, you are responsible for counselling patients who want to stop smoking. A friend of yours asks you to see their cousin V.K., who recently immigrated to Canada and is a heavy smoker. Your friend says their cousin has refused all suggestions to try to quit smoking. Your friend is worried and thinks that smoking has compromised V.K.'s health. When interviewing V.K., you find out that prior to coming to Canada they spent 2 years in a refugee camp where stress was high and smoking was common.

1. Is it reasonable to assume that V.K. was willfully engaging in what is termed a self-imposed risk behaviour?
2. What cultural or situational circumstances are likely contributing to V.K.'s smoking?
3. What do you think is the best approach to encouraging V.K. to reduce or quit smoking?

## THE HEALTH OF CANADIANS TODAY

Life expectancy for Canadians is increasing for both men and women. Life expectancy is derived from statistical data of how long populations are expected to live. Based on the latest data available, the Canadian life expectancy at birth is 81.97 years for both males and females (Statistics Canada, 2022a). For males, it is 79.82 years, and for women, 84.1 years (Statistics Canada, 2022a). For individuals at the lower end of the socioeconomic gradient the life expectancy for men is 4 years shorter than those living in higher socioeconomic communities, and 2 years shorter for women.

On a global perspective, men have the longest life expectancy in Iceland, Switzerland, and Australia, whereas women's longest expectancy is found to occur in Japan, Spain, and Switzerland.

## DID YOU KNOW?

### *Life Expectancy in Canada*

Life expectancy in Canada declined by 0.6 years in 2020 compared to the previous year, because of the high COVID-19-related mortality rates. This decline represents the largest annual decrease in life expectancy since 1921, when the vital statistics system was introduced. This decrease was greater for males (0.7 years) than for females (0.4 years). Québec had the largest decline, followed by Ontario, Manitoba, Saskatchewan, and British Columbia.

Life expectancy for Indigenous people in Canada is significantly lower than for non-Indigenous Canadians. This discrepancy relates to the gaps in the delivery of quality health care, socioeconomic inequities compounded by the impact of colonialism, and intergenerational trauma (Tjepkema et al., 2019). Recommendation #19 of the Truth and Reconciliation Commission outlines actions the federal government could take to address glaring inequities related to the social determinants of health and to begin closing this gap:

"We call upon the federal government, in consultation with Aboriginal peoples, to establish measurable goals to identify and close the gaps in health outcomes between Aboriginal and non-Aboriginal communities, and to publish annual progress reports and assess long term trends. Such efforts would focus on indicators such as: infant mortality, maternal health, suicide, mental health, addictions, life expectancy, birth rates, infant and child health issues, chronic diseases, illness and injury incidence, and the availability of appropriate health services" (Truth and Reconciliation Commission of Canada, 2015).

In Canada, among the Indigenous population, the Inuit community has the lowest projected life expectancy. Reported in 2017 (the latest available statistics), the average life expectancy for Inuit was 64 years for men and 73 years for women. First Nations life expectancy was 73 years for men and 78 years for women. The life expectancy for Métis was 74 years for men and 80 years for women (Tjepkema et al., 2019). It is estimated that the life expectancy for Canada's Indigenous population has increased by about 2 years since the early 2000s. In 2017, Indigenous people made up an estimated 4.1% of the Canadian population (Statistics Canada, 2017). For more information on life expectancy for Indigenous people in Canada see Table 7.1. For more information on life expectancy at birth across Canada, see Table 7.2.

### TABLE 7.1   Life Expectancy for Indigenous People in Canada

|  | Men | Women | % of Indigenous Population* |
|---|---|---|---|
| Inuit | 64 | 73 | 4% |
| First Nations | 73 | 78 | 60% |
| Métis | 74 | 80 | 36 |

*The Indigenous population in Canada is estimated to be 1 670 000. The percentage of that population group is shown in the last column.

**Source:** OECD Library. (n.d.) Chapter 1. Profile of Indigenous Canada: Trends and data needs. In *Linking Indigenous communities with regional development in Canada.* https://www.oecd-ilibrary.org/sites/e6cc8722-en/index.html?itemId=/content/component/e6cc8722-en

| TABLE 7.2 Life Expectancy at Birth, 2018–2020 | | | |
| --- | --- | --- | --- |
| | **Both Sexes (Years)** | **Males (Years)** | **Females (Years)** |
| Canada | 81.97 | 79.82 | 84.11 |
| Newfoundland and Labrador | 79.89 | 77.9 | 81.7 |
| Prince Edward Island | 81.9 | 79.7 | 83.8 |
| Nova Scotia | 80.46 | 78.37 | 82.55 |
| New Brunswick | 80.84 | 78.70 | 82.91 |
| Québec | 82.57 | 80.77 | 84.31 |
| Ontario | 82.34 | 80.16 | 84.47 |
| Manitoba | 79.81 | 77.73 | 82.12 |
| Saskatchewan | 80.06 | 77.69 | 82.56 |
| Alberta | 81.46 | 79.15 | 83.85 |
| British Columbia | 82.39 | 79.93 | 84.93 |
| Yukon | 79.0 | 76.0 | 82.1 |
| Northwest Territories | 77.5 | 75.2 | 79.8 |
| Nunavut | 71.8 | 70.3 | 73.1 |

Note: Life expectancies are calculated with a method that uses 3 years of data.
**Source:** Based on Statistics Canada. (2022). Life expectancy and other elements of the complete life table, three-year estimates, Canada, all provinces except Prince Edward Island. Table 13-10-0114-01. https://www150.statcan.gc.ca/t1/tbl1/en/tv.action?pid=1310011401

The infant mortality rate (for infants under the age of 1 year) is often used as a measure of the effectiveness of a country's health care system. Canada's infant mortality rate has declined over the last several decades, but not as fast as the rate in other developed nations. In Canada the infant mortality rate in 2021 was 4.055 deaths per 1,000 live births, representing a 2.71% decline from 2020 (World Population Review, 2022). By contrast, the infant mortality in the United States was 5.8%. On an international level, the country with the lowest infant mortality rate was Morocco, at 1.8%, followed by Japan, Iceland, and Finland. Of interest is that how infant mortality rates are defined differs among countries, making statistics somewhat variable. Some countries, for example, do not include stillborn babies when gathering statistics, whereas others do. The infant mortality rates in percentages for infants aged under a year in 2020 are summarized in Table 7.3.

## THINKING IT THROUGH

### Life Expectancy Calculator

Life expectancy has gradually increased over the past decades, from 60 years in 1920 to more than 80 today. The decline in the mortality rate since 1951 was largely a reduction in deaths from diseases of the circulatory system. A decline in infectious and parasitic diseases and diseases of the respiratory system also contributed significantly to increased life expectancy. This trend can be attributed to numerous variables, from advances in medical technology facilitating earlier diagnosis of diseases to improved treatments, as well as placing more emphasis on health promotion and disease prevention.

The life expectancy calculator (see link on the Evolve site) predicts how long you will live, based on information you enter regarding your current lifestyle and health status to date. If

you are comfortable doing so, complete the questionnaire to determine your own life expectancy.
1. Were you surprised at the results?
2. Would you make any changes in your health-related lifestyle choices, based on your results? If so, what would they be?

Sources: Decady, Y., & Greenberg, L. (2014, July). *Ninety years of change in life expectancy.* Catalogue no. 82-624-X. ISSN 1925-6493. https://www150.statcan.gc.ca/n1/pub/82-624-x/2014001/article/14009-eng.htm; Employment and Social Development Canada. (2021). *Building understanding: The first report of the National Advisory Council on Poverty.* Cat. No: EM12-74/2021E-PDF. https://www.canada.ca/content/dam/esdc-edsc/documents/programs/poverty-reduction/national-advisory-council/reports/2020-annual/Building_understanding_FINAL_Jan_15.pdf

## Leading Causes of Death in Canada

The three leading causes of death in Canada in 2020 were malignant neoplasms (cancer, 26.4% of all deaths), followed by heart disease (17.5%), and COVID-19, accounting for 5.3% of all deaths (Statistics Canada, 2022b). Following these were accidents, cerebrovascular disease, diseases of the lower respiratory tract (COPD, asthma, and pulmonary hypertension), diabetes, influenza and pneumonia, Alzheimer's disease, suicide, and kidney disease. The four leading causes of death for men were cancer, heart disease, accidents, and lower respiratory disease, whereas the four leading causes of death for women were cancer, heart disease, cerebrovascular disease, and chronic lower respiratory disease. It is interesting to note that the mortality rate from influenza and pneumonia dropped to its lowest point in 20 years. Among the theories as to why is the fact that, because of COVID-19 public health recommendations, more people

**TABLE 7.3   Infant Mortality Rates for Infants Aged Under a Year, by Jurisdiction, 2020**

| Province | Infant Mortality Rate |
| --- | --- |
| British Columbia | 3.7% |
| Alberta | 5.3% |
| Saskatchewan | 6.7% |
| Manitoba | 6.7% |
| Ontario | 4.2% |
| Québec | 4.1% |
| New Brunswick | 4.7% |
| Nova Scotia | 3.7% |
| Prince Edward Island | 4.6% |
| Newfoundland and Labrador | 5.0% |
| Nunavut | 14.3% |
| Yukon | Unavailable |
| Northwest Territories | 9.0% |

**Source:** Based on Statistics Canada. (2022, January 24). *Infant deaths and mortality rates, by age group.* Table 13-10-0713-01. https://www150.statcan.gc.ca/t1/tbl1/en/tv.action?pid=1310071301&pickMembers%5B0%5D=1.14&cubeTimeFrame.startYear=2019&cubeTimeFrame.endYear=2020&referencePeriods=20190101%2C20200101

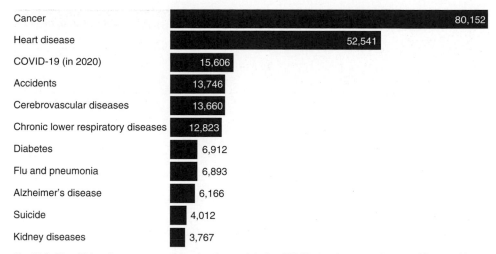

**Fig. 7.6** The 10 leading causes of death, along with the COVID death rate in Canada. (Source: Hurst, C. (2021, September 28). *What are the leading causes of death in Canada?* https://www.finder.com/ca/what-are-the-top-10-causes-of-death-in-canada)

were wearing masks and practising physical distancing, which would also reduce the spread of the influenza and related viruses (Statistics Canada, 2022b).

The following is a brief discussion on the three leading causes of death in Canada (excluding COVID-19): cancer, cardiovascular disease, and cerebrovascular disease (Fig. 7.6).

### Cancer

The incidence of cancer in Canada is alarming, with cancer rates having only slightly decreased over the past decade (1.2%) despite newer treatments and screening initiatives. That said, two in five Canadians will develop cancer in their lifetime. One in four will die from the disease. Men have slightly higher rates of being diagnosed with cancer as well as dying from the disease than women. Lung cancer is the most common type of cancer, followed by colorectal, breast, and prostate cancer making up 44% of all new cancers in the country (Canadian Cancer Society, 2022). See Table 7.4 for statistical details.

The incidence of different types of cancer is influenced by such factors as lifestyle and health habits, environmental factors (pollution), socioeconomic factors (poverty), lack of education, and lack of opportunities for or access to disease prevention and health promotion initiatives (Elflein, 2021). Prompt access to cancer medical services such as cancer screening is another important factor. These factors affect the number of cases and types of cancer seen in regions across the country (e.g., which cancers are seen more frequently in some regions).

The province of Newfoundland and Labrador has the highest cancer incidence rate of any province in Canada (55.8 cases/100,000), followed by Ontario (54.9 cases/100,000) and Nova Scotia (53.9 cases/100,000). New Brunswick's cancer incidence is 50.8/100,000, followed closely by Prince Edward Island at 49.8/100,000 (Elflein, 2021). The incidence rates of cancer are very similar in Manitoba, Alberta, and Saskatchewan (around 48 cases/100,000) (Elflein, 2021). Interestingly, British Columbia and the Northwest Territories have the same incidence of cancer at 48.9 cases/100,000, and the Yukon is lower at 41.5/100,000 (Elflein, 2021). Considering the remote geography of the two territories and their health inequities, why do you think their rates are lower? The highest mortality rate from cancer is in Nunavut.

**TABLE 7.4   Types of Cancer and Percentage of Individuals Affected**

| Type of Cancer | Statistical Information |
| --- | --- |
| Lung | Accounts for 13% of all new cancers |
| Breast | Accounts for 25% of all cancers in women |
| Prostate | Accounts for 20% of all cancers for men |
| Colorectal | Accounts for 11% of all new cancers |

Note: The number of estimated new cases excludes non-melanoma skin cancer cases.
**Source:** Based on Canadian Cancer Society. (2022). *Cancer statistics at a glance*. https://cancer.ca/en/research/cancer-statistics/cancer-statistics-at-a-glance#:~:text=2%20in%205%20Canadians%20(44,expected%20to%20die%20from%20cancer

The cancers with the highest mortality rates are lung, cancer of the bronchus, and breast cancer. In contrast, mortality rates for prostate cancer are relatively low because of early diagnosis, treatment when indicated, 'prostate cancers are slow growing. Because of the low mortality rates, there is controversy over how aggressively to screen for and treat diagnosed cases of prostate cancer. The age of the individual is a factor in treatment (the younger the person, the more aggressive treatment might be). Monitoring the progress of prostate cancer is achieved through periodic assessment (a blood test) that monitors the person's prostate-specific antigen (PSA) levels. Most jurisdictions will cover the cost of a PSA test if recommended by a health care provider for monitoring purposes. The cost is not covered for routine screening in most jurisdictions—a person can request the test but will have to pay out-of-pocket. The average cost of the PSA test in Canada is $40.00.

### Cardiovascular diseases

Heart disease is the second leading cause of death in Canada; cerebrovascular disease is (excluding COVID-19 in 2020) is the fourth leading cause of disease (Statistics Canada, 2022b). Together, these diseases are referred to as *cardiovascular disease* and are frequently grouped as such. Cardiovascular diseases include coronary artery disease (CAD), heart failure, arrhythmia (abnormal heartbeat), and peripheral vascular disease (problems with circulation, primarily in the legs). Of these, CAD is the most common.

Hypertension is the most significant risk factor to developing heart disease. Approximately 25% of men and 23% of women have high blood pressure, with 64% being unaware that they have it.

Other risk factors include smoking, high cholesterol, inactivity, and obesity. Genetics are also a contributing factor. The incidence of heart disease has decreased slightly over the past few years, likely because of improved screening (and treatment) for risk factors, education related to health promotion and disease prevention (risk reduction), and lifestyle changes.

An estimated 1 in 12 Canadians over the age of 20 years is living with some form of heart disease. Mortality rates increase with age. Men are more than twice as likely to develop heart disease, even though men are typically diagnosed on average 10 years younger than women. Indigenous people in Canada are approximately twice as likely to develop heart disease, particularly those who live on-reserve and are subject to a wide range of cardiovascular risk factors, including food insecurity, obesity, and inactivity (inequities related to the social determinates of health).

Generally, population health initiatives implemented by both federal and provincial/territorial governments have contributed to lower mortality rates from heart disease and a healthier lifestyle. Other organizations such as Heart and Stroke Canada and the Canadian Society for Exercise Physiology also encourage an active lifestyle. ParticipACTION initiatives also address the importance of adequate rest (balanced with activity). With heart health in mind, the organization has recently introduced regulations forcing manufacturers to lower the amount of trans fats in prepared foods, launched public campaigns to encourage manufacturers to lower sodium content in foods, and made efforts to reduce the sale of unhealthy foods in schools.

### Cerebrovascular disease

Cerebrovascular disease includes a number of conditions that affect the flow of blood to the brain, the most serious of which is stroke. Stroke occurs when there is a blockage of oxygen to part of the brain, caused by an interruption in the blood flow, most commonly a blood clot. Stroke is the tenth cause of disability-adjusted life years; stroke (excluding COVID-19 related deaths) was the fourth leading cause of death in 2020 (Statistics Canada, 2022b). The Canadian Heart and Stroke Foundation estimates that in the next two decades, the number of individuals living with long-term stroke-related disability will increase by 80% (Heart and Stroke Foundation, 2018).

Nine in ten Canadians have at least one risk factor for stroke (which are almost identical to those for heart disease). Hypertension, as with heart disease, is the most significant risk factor. Additional risk factors for women include pregnancy, menopause, and age. Approximately 10% of Canadians over the age of 65 will experience a stroke (Public Health Agency of Canada [PHAC], 2019). The incidence of stroke is higher in women, and they appear to experience worse outcomes. Of all deaths from stroke in Canada, 59% are women and 41% are men.

Heart disease and stroke together are also one of the leading causes of hospitalization in Canada. Nunavut (which is puzzling given the risk factors in that jurisdiction) and Québec have the lowest mortality rates from heart disease and stroke, while Labrador and Newfoundland and the Northwest Territories have the highest (Conference Board of Canada, 2018). One can only assume from these facts that the message that Canadians can do much to reduce risk factors for acquiring a variety of infirmities, including stroke and heart disease, is somehow not getting through, even though access to health information and teaching materials has been greatly enhanced by the Internet and by the focus on health education in the country. More work is clearly needed to teach Canadians at large that adopting a healthy lifestyle at an early age will increase the chances of enjoying better health in their later years.

## THE IMPACT OF COVID-19 ON THE HEALTH OF CANADIANS

To say the effects of the COVID-19 pandemic and resulting socioeconomic outcomes have had a significant impact on the mental, physical, and emotional health of Canadians is probably an understatement. Canadians of all ages have been affected either directly or indirectly. Without question, those who are considered marginalized and in lower socioeconomic brackets endured more severe health outcomes than did others (Centre for Addiction and Mental Health [CAMH], 2020).

### Long-Term Care Facilities

Older persons in long-term care facilities and retirement homes were disproportionately affected by COVID-19 (Canadian Institute for Health Information, 2021). Individuals in these facilities were more vulnerable because of their age and the presence of comorbidities, resulting in higher morbidity and mortality rates than experienced by the general population. In many facilities residents typically share a room with another person, sometimes two or three others, which contributes to the spread of infection. Infection prevention and control measures were deemed inadequate, as was the supply of personal protective equipment in many facilities. In addition, there was inadequate staffing, so the amount of even the most basic care that residents received was reduced. As well, in many facilities, physician visits decreased, and residents were not sent to the hospital as readily as in the pre-pandemic period. Because of tightened visiting restrictions, residents suffered from isolation and loneliness, which adversely affected their health.

### Mental Health

Canada's existing mental health crisis only intensified as a result of the pandemic. A recent poll revealed that 50% of Canadians reported an increase in mental health issues since the beginning of the pandemic, particularly heightened anxiety and stress, struggling with such entities as uncertainty about their employment and income, housing, and food insecurity. In addition, individuals of all ages have experienced depression, and, for many, an inability to cope effectively with daily life. A January 2023 report released by the federal government stated that young people have been disproportionately impacted by the COVID-19 pandemic, with social isolation, virtual learning challenges, job insecurity, and financial hardship worsening their mental health and well-being.

### Substance Use

The pandemic has intensified another pre-existing public health crisis, substance use—more profoundly, the use of opioids and related drugs. The use of opioids (opioid harms) has increased dramatically, as have the number of opioid-related deaths between 2020 and 2022 (Government of Canada, 2022a). Reasons for this increase include a reduction in addiction supports and services (many of them closed because of public health restrictions). There has also been a decrease in the illegal supply of opioids and other drugs because of travel restrictions and border closures, resulting in increased availability of contaminated, more lethal drugs. There were an estimated 2,772 opioid-related deaths between January and March of 2021 alone (Statistics Canada, 2021). This represents a 65% increase in opioid-related deaths compared to the same time frame a year earlier (PHAC, 2022). Most opioid-related deaths occurred in adults between the ages of 20 and 40, 75% of whom were males. A significant number of these deaths occurred in younger Canadians who lived in Ontario, Alberta, and British Columbia. Modelling by the PHAC indicates that up to 2,000 individuals could die from opioid toxicity in each quarter of 2022 (see Chapter 10).

### Long-COVID

The majority of Canadians who were infected with the SARS-CoV-2 (COVID-19) virus or its variants have recovered. However, a number of individuals have experienced ongoing symptoms, now referred to as *long-COVID*. Although more older Canadians experience long-COVID, younger adults and children may be affected as well. Symptoms include overwhelming fatigue, respiratory symptoms such as shortness of breath and cough, joint and chest paint, and what many describe as "mental fog," or "brain fog," anxiety, and depression (over 100 symptoms have been reported). About 80% of adults reported one or more symptoms in the short term (4 to 12 weeks after being infected), and 60% reported some of these symptoms more than 12 weeks after their initial COVID-19 infection (Government of Canada, 2022b).

Approximately 10% reported that they were unable to return to work in the long term. Just under 60% of children reported symptoms 4 weeks after their infection. Symptoms that children reported include fatigue, headache, stuffy nose, muscle pain, and sleep disturbances. Sometimes these symptoms abate and reappear. There is no single treatment for this syndrome; most treatment is based on symptoms. Individuals who experience long-COVID are often referred to as "long-haulers." Fortunately, research on this syndrome is ongoing, with a better understanding of how to treat it changing frequently (see Chapter 10).

## SUMMARY

7.1 Today, the key concepts of health, wellness, and illness are defined in less black-and-white terms. Definitions of health relate to such things as an individual's own culture, background, and experiences. Wellness goes beyond having good physical and mental health and considers how a person feels about their health and quality of life. The many dimensions of wellness include physical, emotional, intellectual, spiritual, social, environmental, and occupational health. *Disease* refers to a condition in which a person's mental or bodily functions are different from normal. The term *illness*, often used to denote the presence of disease, can also refer to how a person feels about their health, whether or not a disease is present. A *disability* can be physical, sensory, cognitive, or intellectual and can occur in conjunction with or as a result of a disease, or it can be caused by an accident.

7.2 How health care is delivered is reflected in a design, a philosophy, and an approach. Three approaches, or models, are most frequently used: the medical, holistic, and wellness models. The wholistic framework is an approach to health used by many Indigenous people. Some people prefer a natural approach to health care—noninvasive, leaning away from mainstream diagnosis and intervention. Others have more faith in proven treatments. Still others will blend philosophies.

7.3 Several factors influence how people respond when their health is compromised. These include past experiences and one's outlook on life (e.g., optimistic, pessimistic). Over the past several years, Canadians, for the most part, have assumed more responsibility for their own health, assessing their own risk behaviours and focusing on health promotion and disease prevention. Risk behaviours are those activities a person willfully engages in knowing that the activity can negatively affect their health. It is important to note that engaging in such activities or behaviours is not always "willful" per se but be mitigated by the individual's circumstances (e.g., smoking as a coping mechanism for stress).

7.4 Health behaviour is how a person responds to all aspects of altered health. How they react affects their relationship with health care providers, family members, and others close to them. A person's response to an altered health situation is unique to each person and influenced by their background, social and cultural beliefs, and past experiences with the health care system. Understanding that deviations from a person's normal behaviour are just that—and supporting the person appropriately—will go a long way toward helping a patient recover.

7.5 By some standards, such as the health—illness continuum, a person's health is measurable. How a person feels about their health changes frequently and is influenced by the type and severity of an infirmity, personal health beliefs, and the health model the person most closely relates to.

7.6 It is widely accepted that when people are ill, their behaviours, roles, and attitudes change. This response to illness is sometimes referred to as sick role behaviours. This response involves those they are close to (family, friends) and those with whom they work. Although most people respond in an adaptive manner, others become more dependent and sometimes require increased support and understanding. Health beliefs, culture, traditions, and previous experience with the health care system also play a role in an individual's response to illness. Hospitalization may have a greater effect on how a person responds. These responses are referred to as the stages of illness.

7.7    Overall, the health of Canadians has improved over the past decade, yet challenges remain in providing prompt and effective care, particularly for those with cancer and diseases of the respiratory system—the leading causes of morbidity and mortality in the country. In 2020, COVID-19 was the third leading cause of death in the country. Indigenous people are particularly at risk, for socioeconomic reasons and because of geographic isolation, the intergenerational trauma of colonialism and residential schools, and, for many, because of the lack of proximity to larger treatment centres.

The COVID-19 pandemic continues to have a significant impact on the physical, emotional, and mental health of Canadians as well as on the country's economy. Canadians of all ages have experienced increased levels of stress, anxiety, and depression resulting from such variables as social distancing, isolation, and worries related to loss (or potential loss) of income. For many, issues such as precarious housing and food insecurity compound their stress. During the pandemic the use of opioids and the number of opioid-related deaths rose significantly, impacting what was already a national crisis. Most Canadians who contracted the virus recovered, although the mortality rate remains high, particularly among older Canadians with comorbidities living in long-term care and residential facilities. Long-COVID is experienced by a number of Canadians, some who have appeared to recover, with a variety of symptoms reappearing after 12 or more weeks.

## REVIEW QUESTIONS

1. Describe the dimensions of wellness, and explain how wellness goes beyond having good health.
2. Differentiate between a disease and a disability and provide examples of both.
3. Compare and contrast the medical, holistic, Indigenous wholistic, and wellness models or theories of health, identifying the key points of each.
4. What challenges face individuals with physical and mental impairments?
5. Explain how Canadians' attitudes toward their health and well-being have changed over the past several decades.
6. Differentiate between health beliefs and health behaviours.
7. Briefly describe how a person's health behaviour can affect how you as a health care provider treat that person.
8. How can you best provide culturally sensitive health services to a new Canadian?
9. Explain how sick role behaviour may affect where someone places themselves on the health—illness continuum.
10. Describe how the different stages of illness may influence patient behaviour.
11. How and why have the leading causes of death in Canada changed over the past 10 years?
12. What effect has the COVID-19 pandemic had on the misuse of opioids in Canada?
13. Because Canada is a culturally diverse country, it is inevitable that in most health care settings the need to be culturally knowledgeable and culturally sensitive is an essential component of rendering appropriate, unbiased health care. Research the cultural demographic makeup within your community. Choose one culture and familiarize yourself with related health care practices, traditions, and expectations. Construct a short information sheet outlining points that would be useful for a health care provider to have when interacting with a person with that cultural background.

# REFERENCES

Canada, S. (2017). *Projections of the Aboriginal populations, Canada, provinces and territories, 2001 to 2017. Catalogue number 91-547-XIE.* https://www150.statcan.gc.ca/n1/pub/91-547-x/2005001/4072106-eng.htm.

Canadian Cancer Society. (2022). *Canadian cancer statistics.* https://cancer.ca/en/research/cancer-statistics/canadian-cancer-statistics.

Canadian Institute for Health Information. (2021, December 9). *COVID-19's impact on long-term care.* https://www.cihi.ca/en/covid-19-resources/impact-of-covid-19-on-canadas-health-care-systems/long-term-care.

Centre for Addiction and Mental Health (CAMH). (2020, July). Mental health in Canada: Covid-19 and beyond. *CAMH policy advice.* https://www.camh.ca/-/media/files/pdfs—-public-policy-submissions/covid-and-mh-policy-paper-pdf.pdf.

Chin, P. (1996). Chinese Americans. In J. G. Lipson, S. L. Dibble, & P. A. Minarik (Eds.), *Culture and nursing care: A pocket guide* (pp. 74—81). University of California San Francisco Nursing Press.

Conference Board of Canada. (2018). *Mortality due to heart disease and stroke.* https://www.conferenceboard.ca/hcp/provincial/health/heart.aspx.

Elflein, J. (2021 November 18). *Estimated cancer rates in Canada by province, 2021.* https://www.statista.com/statistics/438129/estimated-incidence-rates-of-all-cancers-in-canada-by-province/#:~:text=Rate%20of%20Canadian%20new%20cancer%20cases%20by%20province%202021&text=In%20Nunavut%20there%20are%20around,100%2C000%20in%20Newfoundland%20and%20Labrador.&text=As%20of%202021%2C%20there%20were,in%20Canada%20per%20100%2C000%20population.

Euromed Info. (n.d.). *How culture influences health beliefs.* http://www.euromedinfo.eu/how-culture-influences-health-beliefs.html/.

Government of Canada. (2022a). *Modelling opioid-related deaths during the COVID-19 outbreak.* https://www.canada.ca/en/health-canada/services/opioids/data-surveillance-research/modelling-opioid-overdose-deaths-covid-19.html.

Government of Canada. (2022b). *Post-COVID-19 condition (long-COVID).* https://www.canada.ca/en/public-health/services/diseases/2019-novel-coronavirus-infection/symptoms/post-covid-19-condition.html.

Heart and Stroke Foundation. (2018). *Lives disrupted: The impact of stroke on women. 2018 Stroke Report.* https://www.heartandstroke.ca/-/media/pdf-files/canada/stroke-report/strokereport2018.ashx#:~:text=TIAs%20are%20an%20important%20warning,stages%20for%20stroke%20in%20women.&text=More%20than%2062%2C000%20strokes%20occur,of%20these%20happen%20to%20women.&text=One%2Dthird%20more%20women%20die,women%2C%2041%25%20are%20men.

Inclusion London. (n.d.). The social model of disability. https://www.inclusionlondon.org.uk/disability-in-london/social-model/the-social-model-of-disability-and-the-cultural-model-of-deafness/.

Nursing. (2005). Understanding transcultural nursing. *Nursing, 18,* 21—23, 35, 14, 16 https://journals.lww.com/nursing/Fulltext/2005/01001/UNDERSTANDING_TRANSCULTURAL_NURSING.3.aspx.

People with Disability Australia. (n.d.). Social model of disability. https://pwd.org.au/resources/disability-info/social-model-of-disability/.

Public Health Agency of Canada (PHAC). (2019, December 9). Stroke in Canada: Highlights from the Canadian chronic disease Surveillance system. Cat. *Number.* HP35 88/2017E-PDF https://www.canada.ca/en/public-health/services/publications/diseases-conditions/stroke-canada-fact-sheet.html.

Public Health Agency of Canada (PHAC). (2022, September). *Opioid- and stimulant-related harms in Canada.* https://health-infobase.canada.ca/substance-related-harms/opioids-stimulants/.

Raeburn, A. (2021 December 20). *10 Places where eye-contact is not recommended (10 places where the locals are friendly). The Travel.* https://www.thetravel.com/10-places-where-eye-contact-is-not-recommended-10-places-where-the-locals-are-friendly/.

Schwartz, E. (1991). Jewish Americans. In J. N. Giger, & R. E. Davidhizar (Eds.), *Transcultural nursing* (pp. 491—520). Mosby.

Statistics Canada. (2021, December 22). *COVID-19 in Canada: Year-end update on social and economic impacts. Catalogue no. 11-631-X.* https://www150.statcan.gc.ca/n1/pub/11-631-x/11-631-x2021003-eng.htm.

Statistics Canada. (2022a). *Life expectancy and other elements of the complete life table, three-year estimates, Canada, all provinces except Prince Edward Island. Table 13-10-0114-01.* https://www150.statcan.gc.ca/t1/tbl1/en/tv.action?pid=1310011401.

Statistics Canada. (2022b). *Deaths, 2020.* The Daily https://www150.statcan.gc.ca/n1/daily-quotidien/220124/dq220124a-eng.htm.

Swaine, Z. (2011). Medical model. In J. S. Kreutzer, J. DeLuca, & B. Caplan (Eds.), *Encyclopedia of clinical neuropsychology.* Springer. https://doi.org/10.1007/978-0-387-79948-3_2131

Thompson, V. (2022). *Administrative and clinical procedures for the Canadian health professional. Pearson education.*

Tjepkema, M., Bushnik, T., & Bougie, E. (2019, December 18). *Life expectancy of first Nations, Metis, and Inuit household populations in Canada.* https://www150.statcan.gc.ca/n1/pub/82-003-x/2019012/article/00001-eng.htm.

Truth and Reconciliation Commission of Canada. (2015). *Calls to Action.* https://www2.gov.bc.ca/assets/gov/british-columbians-our-governments/indigenous-people/aboriginal-peoples-documents/calls_to_action_english2.pdf.

Visa, C. (2022). *Canada immigration levels plan* (pp. 2023–2025). https://www.canadavisa.com/canada-immigration-levels-plans.html#:~:text=Under%20its%20Immigration%20Levels%20Plan,reunite%20families%2C%20and%20help%20refugees.

Willingham, E. (2012, October 16). *Low eye contact is not just an autism thing. Forbes.* https://www.forbes.com/sites/emilywillingham/2012/10/16/low-eye-contact-is-not-just-an-autism-thing/?sh=5b92ee4b7f5c.

World Health Organization. (1986). Health promotion: Concepts and principles in action—a policy framework. *WHO Regional Office for Europe.*

World Population Review. (2022). *Infant mortality rate by country 2022.* https://worldpopulationreview.com/country-rankings/infant-mortality-rate-by-country.

# The Law and Health Care

## LEARNING OUTCOMES

8.1  Summarize five types of law that relate to health care.
8.2  Explain the federal and provincial jurisdictional framework related to health care
8.3  Outline the concerns about and the issues pertaining to health care as a right.
8.4  Discuss the legality of offering private services in Canada.
8.5  Discuss the basic principles of consent to treatment.
8.6  Explain the health record related to privacy legislation.
8.7  Describe the legal role of regulated health professions.
8.8  Summarize four additional legal issues in Canadian health care.

## KEY TERMS

Act
Civil law
Code of ethics
Common law
Confidentiality
Conflict of interest
Constitutional law
Contract law
*Controlled Drugs and Substances Act*
Criminal law
Duty of care
Electronic health record (EHR)

Electronic medical record (EMR)
Fiduciary duty
Good Samaritan law
Implied consent
Incident report
Informed consent
Malpractice
Negligence
Oral consent
*Personal Information Protection and Electronic Documents Act (PIPEDA)*

Power of attorney
Privacy
Professional misconduct
*Quarantine Act*
Regulation
Regulatory law
Statutory law
Tort
Whistleblower
Workplace Hazardous Materials Information System (WHMIS)

This chapter provides a practical but cursory overview of the relationship between the law and some elements of health care in Canada. It concentrates on selected basic elements of health care and the application of related legal issues, rather than on specific laws and legislation. Because laws vary among the provinces and territories, it is more meaningful for students to research those within their own jurisdiction to access specific information.

Most health care providers, health care facilities, regional health and other governing authorities, and regulated professions are governed by legislation, regulations, or guidelines, all of which affect how they function (see Chapter 5). This chapter begins by examining the division of legislative powers between the federal government and the provincial and territorial governments where health care is concerned. It also discusses the legal responsibilities of the federal government with respect to safety legislation and sections within criminal law that affect health care. This chapter also looks at the legal rights of Canadians to health care under the *Canada Health Act* and the law according to the Charter of Rights and Freedoms.

Private enterprise in health care is growing across the country and often clashes with the principles of publicly funded health care, and legislation regarding private enterprise varies among jurisdictions. Many Canadians embrace the opportunity to choose between public and private services, and others do not. This chapter briefly discusses restrictions imposed on Canadians with regard to seeking health care from private clinics and the right of Canadians to purchase private insurance for medically necessary services that the provinces or territories cannot provide within reasonable time frames.

Other topics discussed here include the legal guidelines and responsibilities of health care providers regarding consent to treatment and how to facilitate requests for medical assistance in dying. The effects of the law on health care providers, as well as on their moral and legal obligations to patients, are also highlighted. Finally, this chapter addresses health information management, confidentiality, and current privacy legislation—and the challenges presented by electronic health records.

## LAWS USED IN HEALTH CARE LEGISLATION

Laws in Canada include both statutory law (i.e., derived from acts) and common law (i.e., made by judges in deciding cases). Various levels of government are authorized to create laws. Some laws apply to the health care industry more than others, including constitutional, statutory, regulatory, and common (or case) law, all of which are described in the sections that follow.

### Constitutional Law

Constitutional law addresses the relationship between the people and their government, and establishes, allocates, and limits public power. In Canada, cases challenging a person's right to health care have been based on the *Canadian Charter of Rights and Freedoms*, part of the Canadian Constitution. Under the Constitution, everyone has the following fundamental freedoms (*Canadian Charter of Rights and Freedoms*, 1982):
- Freedom of conscience and religion
- Freedom of thought, belief, opinion, and expression, including freedom of the press and other media of communication
- Freedom of peaceful assembly
- Freedom of association

A Canadian citizen denied any of these rights can challenge the person, persons, or organization denying them such rights, based on the related section of the Charter.

### Statutory Law

A *statute* is a law or an act. Statutory laws are the laws passed in Parliament (i.e., at the federal level) or in the provincial or territorial legislatures. Examples of statutory laws under federal authority include those dealing with immigration, taxation, and divorce. Statutory laws under provincial or territorial jurisdiction include those related to education, family, and health care.

### Regulatory Law

Regulatory law, also referred to as *subordinate legislation*, is a form of law that possesses the legally binding feature of an act, because it is usually made under the authority of an act. Although regulatory law may be left to government departments and agencies to complete, regulatory law is not made by Parliament (i.e., at the federal level) or by provincial or territorial legislatures but rather by delegated persons or organizations, such as an administrative agency or a tribunal. The authority to implement regulations, however, must be specifically outlined in a federal, provincial, or territorial act—for example, in Manitoba, the *Regional Health Authorities Act* gives regional health authorities the power to make, implement, and enforce certain regulations. Federally, the *Food and Drugs Act* has authority over Health Canada's food and drug regulations.

In health care, regulatory law affects hospital boards, health care institutions, and bodies governing health care providers. Under provincial and territorial health care professions acts (e.g., Ontario's *Regulated Health Professions Act*), the Minister of Health oversees the manner in which health care professions operate and govern themselves and also retains the power to request that a council make, amend, or revoke a particular regulation.

## Common (Case) Law and Civil Law in Canada

In Canada, law in all provinces and territories except Québec is based on common law. Québec operates under civil law and statutory law, based on the French *Code Napoléon* or *Civil Code*.

Common law is not established within legislature or formally written like statutory law. Also called *case law*, it results from the decisions of the courts. These decisions are based on a variety of historically established laws, consistent with previous decisions or higher court decisions, interpretations of written laws, and other legal principles not outlined in statutory law. Although Québec's civil law system relies heavily on written laws, judges in Québec courts often seek guidance from previous decisions and must also interpret written laws, as is done in common law systems. In addition, common law may govern litigation conducted before the Federal Court of Canada.

## Classifications of Law: Public and Private Law

Laws are classified as public or private. *Public law* pertains to matters between an individual and society as a whole and therefore includes criminal, tax, constitutional, administrative, and human rights laws. For example, when an individual breaks a criminal law, their breach is considered a wrong against society, not just a wrong against another person or a select group of people. There may be variations in public law among jurisdictions.

*Private law* governs matters concerning relationships between people or legal entities and includes contract and property law, matters relating to inheritance, family law, tort law (e.g., negligence), and corporate law. A person can sue a business, a dentist, a doctor, a hospital, a primary health care organization, or any individual for damages under private law. These suits can include torts of libel and slander, breaches in privacy and confidentiality, and negligence suits.

The following example illustrates the difference between public law and private law. If a nurse, Jenna, believed a patient was better off dead and actively helped that person (who was ineligible for medical assistance in dying) to die, the police, acting on behalf of the state, would arrest the nurse and charge her under the *Criminal Code*, part of public law. If found guilty, Jenna would likely be sentenced to jail or be ordered to pay a fine (i.e., to the state). The victim's family could also launch a civil suit against the nurse under private law. If the family were awarded damages, the nurse would have to pay these directly to the family. All jurisdictions have some type of specialized agency, sometimes called Criminal Injury Compensation Boards or similar. In Newfoundland and Labrador, the Newfoundland Crimes Compensation Board is an example of where a victim (or the family of a victim) can apply for damages, bypassing the necessity of launching a civil suit, once an individual has been convicted in a criminal court. The government assesses the damages, which are awarded from public funds.

## Tort Law

A tort occurs when one person or that person's property is wronged or harmed by another, either intentionally (deliberately) or unintentionally. Tort law cases can be complicated—for example, proving negligence over an intentional act.

### Intentional Tort

An intentional tort occurs when the harmful act is deliberate. In health care, it usually involves physical aggression or forcing unwanted medical treatment on a patient. Two examples of an intentional tort are a health care aide proven to have treated a patient roughly, resulting in injury to that patient, or a health care provider successfully performing cardiopulmonary resuscitation (CPR) on an individual who had a known do-not-resuscitate order.

### Unintentional Tort

An unintentional tort occurs when the act caused physical or emotional injury or property damage but was not deliberate or calculated. Unintentional torts usually result from acts of human error, misjudgement, or negligence. For example, human error might be considered the cause if a nurse gave the wrong medication to an older patient causing harm. A physiotherapist might misjudge a patient's ability to ambulate, resulting in a fall the first time they tried to get up independently. Negligence is one of the most common torts, and cases are often complicated.

*Negligence.* Negligence is a type of tort law. Negligence can be in the form of malpractice or, depending on the case, professional misconduct. Negligence occurs when a health care provider (unintentionally) fails to meet the standards of care required of their profession. Negligence can occur when a duty of care owed a person is not completed. In health care, examples may include forgetting to perform a necessary action, not caring or confirming whether a particular and necessary action is performed, providing improper or substandard care, providing a patient with unclear instructions, or failing to successfully instruct a patient in how to follow a treatment plan (Case Example 8.1).

Health care providers may find themselves accused of a tort if a patient experiences physical or emotional injury resulting from something the health care provider did or did not do and negligence is proven.

Duty plays a significant role in both medical ethics and medical law. Health professionals are often held more accountable in terms of their duty to their patients than people in many other professions. Health care providers can face litigation if it is proven that they failed to fulfill their duty to the patient. Duty becomes part of the patient–health care provider relationship as soon as the professional relationship begins. For example, J.R. has made an appointment with a new doctor. Their professional relationship begins once the doctor has seen J.R., assessed J.R., and recommended a treatment plan. Before the appointment, J.R. could

---

### CASE EXAMPLE 8.1   A Physiotherapy Assistant Ambulates a Patient

A physiotherapy assistant has been asked to get 85-year-old E.P. (who has advanced Alzheimer's disease) up for a short walk and then help them back to bed. After leaving the floor, the physiotherapy assistant remembers that they failed to put up E.P.'s bed side rail. Running late, the physiotherapy assistant leaves the hospital thinking, "Someone will have done it by now." About an hour later, E.P. tries to get out of bed alone and falls and breaks a hip. E.P.'s family sues the hospital and the physiotherapy assistant on the grounds of negligence.

not claim that the doctor was negligent in a health-related matter and bring legal action against them. The doctor is responsible for J.R.'s care until the doctor–patient relationship ends and J.R. has transferred their care to another practitioner. Facilities likewise can be held responsible for incidents when substandard care is proven (e.g., inadequate staffing levels in a long-term care facility resulting in harm to a resident), because the facility itself is responsible for setting and maintaining standards of care.

*Litigation and the duty of care.* Almost all health care providers are bound by a duty of care that is in keeping with their profession's standards of care. Litigation in such cases considers the level of competency that a "reasonable person" possessing the required competencies is expected to meet. This standard set out by any regulated profession (e.g., the Ontario Nurses Association or the Nurse Practitioner's Association of Alberta) must be met by all members of that professional association.

## Contract Law

Contract law involves private agreements that are generally enforceable by the courts like many other laws, provided the agreement does not violate other governing laws or is otherwise illegal in purpose. For example, contracts can exist between an employer and an employee, or a health care provider and a patient. They also may be either expressed (i.e., openly spoken or written) or implied (i.e., unspoken but considered understood).

A breach of contract occurs when one of the parties fails to meet the terms of the agreement. A plastic surgeon, for example, can agree to perform a face lift on a patient for a given price. If, for some reason, the physician fails to complete the procedure, or if the patient refuses to pay the agreed-upon price, one can sue the other for breach of contract. Another example: a private health care organization hires a dentist on a 1-year contract. After 2 months, the dentist finds a higher-paying position and leaves. The health care organization can sue the dentist for breach of contract.

## Criminal Law

In Canada, criminal law, with a few exceptions, is set out in federal legislation. Most laws can be found in the *Criminal Code* of Canada, which details descriptions of crimes and criminal law procedures. It is a category of public law that deals with crimes against people, property, or both and those deemed intolerable by society (e.g., murder, racism, theft). In most cases, to be guilty of a crime a person must perform *a wrongful act—actus reus* (what was done) and a *wrongful intent—mens rea* (a guilty mind)—for example, a health care provider who willfully engages in a harmful act with the intent of harming their patient.

Criminal charges involving health professionals and patients consider the "duty of care," the principle of "do no harm," and a health professional's degree of authority, which would be considered in tort liability and could impact sentencing in criminal cases.

Although an extreme case, consider the nurse Elizabeth Wettlaufer, who pleaded guilty, among other charges, to killing eight older Canadians in long-term care facilities in London and Woodstock, Ontario in 2016. She was in a position of authority and trust. She was sentenced in an Ontario court to life in prison with no chance of parole for 25 years. Box 8.1 suggests ways for those in clinical practice to avoid legal problems in the health care environment.

## THE LAW, THE DIVISION OF POWER, AND THE JURISDICTIONAL FRAMEWORK

The *British North America Act* (now the *Constitution Act*) was passed in 1867, granting jurisdiction over some areas of health care to the federal government and jurisdiction over

## BOX 8.1 Strategies for Avoiding Legal Problems

- Most health care facilities require criminal checks both for potential employees and for students who apply to complete a work or co-op placement. Complete any such criminal checks as requested.
- Work only within your scope of practice and competencies (things you have been taught how and deemed competent to do and that are legally within the scope of your professional practice). If asked to do something outside of your scope of practice or something you are not licensed to do, say no. If you feel unsure about how to perform a specific task within your scope of practice, ask for help. It may be a task or procedure well within your legal boundaries but one which you have not done recently and are not confident you can do properly (e.g., administer an inhalation treatment, start an intravenous [IV] line, or change a complex dressing). It is not a crime to seek assistance; you could harm a patient, be subject to disciplinary action, or face litigation if you do not.
- Complete, concise, and accurate documentation protects everyone—you, the organization you work for, and your patient. Keep required charting current and accurate. Prioritize what you are charting, adhering to the protocol of the organization you work for. In the event of litigation, the medical record may be the most important document in determining the outcome of a case. This may be a challenge with computerized charting and documentation, flow charting, and charting by exception. Always adhere to the rules regarding passwords, logging in and out of a computer system, and *never* allow someone else access to your login or to sign a chart under your name.
- Most facilities maintain a formal process for the reporting of adverse events, including prompt reporting according to facility guidelines and completing a form called an incident report. Information on this form must be concise and accurate. In most cases, if the incident involves a patient in the hospital setting, the information recorded on the incident report appears on the patient's medical chart only if it relates directly to the patient's health. The incident report itself is sent to the risk manager, who uses it to assess the occurrence and to implement measures to prevent similar future occurrences.
- Adhere to privacy and confidentiality laws (both in and away from your place of employment). Think before you speak about work or information relating to work. Never access anyone's files (electronic or written) unless you have a legal right to do so. Being a friend or relative does not give you legal access to another's private health information, even something as innocent as disclosing if a mutual friend has had their baby yet. Remember, good news related to health information also must remain confidential.
- In a health care facility, there may be unrealistic workloads requiring you to prioritize care. Always do your best. Never provide substandard care or treatment. If there are things you cannot do, document what they are. If possible, take the extra time to complete a task properly. An ounce of prevention goes a long way.
- Be an advocate for your patients. If you suspect that something is wrong, use the appropriate chain of command and talk to someone, rather than ignoring the incident. Your patient may be afraid to address the situation personally or may feel that they will simply be ignored.
- Do not ignore unethical or illegal activities. Follow protocol, policies, and procedures.
- Ensure that you have some type of liability insurance through your place of employment or your professional college or organization that will cover you for mishaps or wrongdoing.
- Be mindful of wrongdoing as well as unethical practices of others. If you have strong feelings that something is wrong, seek advice. Do not become involved in something you feel or know is illegal.
- Take care of yourself. If you experience harassment in your workplace, seek out the best possible plan of action. Others may be experiencing the same problem. These situations are tricky and sometimes do not end well if not handled appropriately.

other areas to the provincial and territorial governments. Government jurisdiction means that it has authority over specific designated geographic and legislative areas and also possesses the right to draft, pass, and enact laws within its area of authority.

Initially, the provinces assumed responsibility for "the establishment, maintenance, and management of hospitals, asylums, charities in and for the province, other than for marine hospitals" (*Constitution Act*, 1982). As discussed in Chapter 1, health care is essentially a provincial /territorial power; however, there are some areas where the power is left to the federal government, because select populations are left under federal mandate (e.g., federal inmates, and Indigenous peoples falling under the *Indian Act*).

In addition to enforcing the terms and conditions of the *Canada Health Act* and providing financial support to the provinces and territories (see Chapter 2), the federal government oversees certain components of health care activity covered under the *Criminal Code* of Canada. Some of these components are outlined in the *Federal Food and Drugs Act* in addition to the *Controlled Drugs and Substances Act.* The federal government has the authority to establish prohibitions and penalties when violations of the Act occur.

By virtue of the vague phrase "peace, order, and good government" (*Constitution Act*, 1982) the federal government has the authority to pass legislation on matters that would normally fall under provincial or territorial jurisdiction—in particular, the enactment of emergency powers, which occurred as a result of the convoy and occupation of Ottawa in 2022, and matters of national concern such as an epidemic (COVID-19).

## Workplace Safety

Several Canadian organizations—including the Canadian Centre for Occupational Health and Safety (CCOHS), the Workers Compensation Board (WCB, or equivalent), and systems such as Workplace Hazardous Materials Information System (WHMIS)—strive to maintain the health of working Canadians by ensuring that they have safe and healthy workplaces.

Health care providers may have to interact with the CCOHS and Workers Compensation Board in some manner, possibly by helping a patient regain health and mobility in order to return to their current workplace or to transfer to a new career. The following is a brief overview of these agencies.

### Occupational Health and Safety

Occupational health and safety legislation has 14 jurisdictions in Canada—10 provincial, 3 territorial, and 1 federal. Each jurisdiction enacts its own occupational health and safety legislation related to the rights and responsibilities of the employer, the supervisor (if applicable), and the worker. The federal government manages labour affairs for certain sectors, including employees of the federal government and of federal corporations. The federal government also has jurisdiction over individuals working in occupations that cross provincial and territorial lines (e.g., transportation and communication, pipelines, and some Indigenous activities) and in the federal public service sector.

The *Occupational Health and Safety Act* in each province and territory applies to workplaces within that region (with the exception of those overseen by the federal government) and work done by owners in private residences. Oversight is the responsibility of the Ministry or the Department of Labour in most jurisdictions, or the Workers Compensation Board (or commission).

### Occupational Health and Safety Legislation: Objectives

Aiming to ensure a safe workplace for all Canadians and to support the rights of workers to a safe environment, occupational health and safety legislation sets guidelines, provides for legal enforcement of these guidelines, and outlines the rights of employees, including the following:

- The right to be aware of potential safety and health hazards
- The right to take part in activities (e.g., by serving on committees or acting as a health and safety representative) aimed at preventing occupational accidents and diseases
- The right to refuse to engage in dangerous work without jeopardizing their job

### Occupational Health and Safety and Workers Compensation Boards

Workers Compensation Boards work hand-in-hand with the CCOHS but concentrate specifically on assisting injured employees by providing wage replacement, rehabilitation, and training. Legislation related to these boards or commissions, drafted and administered by each province and territory, is typically named the *Workers Compensation Act*. The Northwest Territories and Nunavut share a Workers Compensation Board.

*Workplace Hazardous Materials Information System.* The CCOHS oversees the Workplace Hazardous Materials Information System (WHMIS) legislation, which became law through complementary federal, provincial, and territorial legislation in October 1988.

The national standards for WHMIS legislation were established by the federal *Hazardous Products Act* and the Controlled Products Regulations. Enforced by the federal, provincial, and territorial governments, this legislation applies to all Canadian workplaces in which identified hazardous materials are used. The national office for WHMIS operates as a division within Health Canada.

Some may think that WHMIS legislation would apply only to industrial settings, but hazardous materials are present in many areas of the health care industry. Hospitals, for example, house hazardous substances used in diagnostic testing (e.g., radioactive products), chemotherapeutic agents, combustible agents (e.g., oxygen), infectious material, and medical waste.

### Drugs and the Law

Canada's drug laws are covered primarily by federal legislation called the *Controlled Drugs and Substances Act*. This Act replaced the *Narcotic Control Act* and parts of the *Food and Drugs Act* (Parts III and IV) in May 1997. The new Act established different categories of drugs, called *schedules*. The classification system addresses the properties of drugs and their potential for harm. Schedule I, for example, includes cocaine, heroin, opium, oxycodone, morphine, and codeine; Schedule II addresses cannabis (*Controlled Drugs and Substances Act*, 2018). Amendments are frequently made to the Act.

### Controlled Drugs and Prescriptions

The *Controlled Drugs and Substances Act* outlines who can prescribe controlled substances, and the conditions and terms of use for prescription narcotics. The prescribing of controlled substances occurs under combined federal, provincial, and territorial legislation.

*Dispensing controlled drugs in facilities.* Most hospitals and other health care facilities maintain a closely monitored supply of restricted drugs (e.g., hydromorphone). These drugs must be prescribed by a qualified prescriber and carefully dispensed by the pharmacy. Most jurisdictions require that health care facilities stocking such drugs keep them under double lock at all times. In almost all acute care facilities even controlled drugs are electronically dispensed (with appropriate protocols), reducing the margin of error and misuse. Each dose is carefully recorded.

In the past, only a registered nurse (RN) or a registered psychiatric nurse was allowed to handle or dispense controlled drugs in acute care settings. Increasingly, however, registered or licensed practical nurses (R/LPNs or LPNs) are also assuming this responsibility. In almost all long-term care facilities, LPNs (RPNs in Ontario) may dispense and sign for narcotics.

***Prescribing controlled drugs.*** Under federal legislation controlled drugs can only be prescribed for legal, therapeutic purposes. The legislation states that prescribing practitioners must remain alert for behaviours that suggest patients are seeking drugs for unlawful purposes.

Among the prescription medications that are commonly abused are tranquillizers or benzodiazepines (e.g., diazepam, lorazepam) and opioids such as oxycodone, hydrocodone, codeine, morphine, and Percocet (a combination of oxycodone and acetaminophen).

Other drugs (most often used illegally) include heroin and synthetic opioids such as fentanyl (Canadian Centre on Substance Abuse and Addiction, 2022). These powerful drugs have addictive properties and are targets for illegal use and trafficking, in particular the opioids. Use of these drugs can be tragic, ranging from addiction to death. Increasingly, illegal drugs obtained on the street are mixed with other dangerous compounds that are responsible for severe adverse reactions and the rise in drug-related death rates.

***The opioid crisis.*** Health Canada has called the continuing number of opioid-related overdoses and deaths a national crisis. It has sanctioned a number of initiatives to address the problem, by working with provincial/territorial governments, organizations, and other stakeholders.

One example is the Joint Statement of Action to Address the Opioid Crisis, which outlines a collaborative commitment of numerous organizations to respond to this crisis (Canadian Centre on Substance Use and Addiction, 2017). The joint goal is to address ways to improve treatment, prevention, and harm reduction strategies at a national level.

Another initiative is the Canadian Drugs and Substance Strategy, which is a comprehensive national approach with the goals, among other things, of curbing the availability, supply, and use of illegal drugs and implementing effective harm reduction methodologies (Government of Canada, 2018a). The *Good Samaritan Drug Overdose Act* compliments this strategy (Government of Canada, 2018a). The Act provides a level of legal protection for people experiencing an overdose as well as those seeking help for the person (instead of charging them with possession of a controlled substance). Exceptions are if the person has an outstanding warrant, is known for trafficking controlled drugs, or is wanted for an unrelated offence.

***Prescription drugs.*** In an effort to curb the use of addictive prescription drugs, in 2017 guidelines were released by the Canadian Medical Association detailing best practices recommendations regarding how to prescribe opioids. These guidelines include using opioids as a last resort for pain control for any patient, in addition to identifying individuals at high risk for addiction who should not be prescribed these drugs. The guidelines also recommend alternative methods of controlling pain, including the use of pain management clinics and non-medication interventions. In addition, the Canadian Medical Association is collaborating with Health Canada in implementing regulatory changes supporting take-back programs (for narcotics) and methods to dispose of these drugs in a safe and appropriate manner (Canadian Medical Association, 2015).

Regardless of the precautions that health care providers (e.g., nurse practitioners and physicians) take to prescribe addictive drugs responsibly, some patients will inevitably obtain prescription drugs for their own use or to sell. If a provider is deemed to prescribe controlled drugs too liberally, their practices may be reviewed by their governing body.

Under federal legislation, prescribing practitioners must keep detailed records of all controlled substances prescribed and provide authorized inspectors access to these records upon request. In order to dispense controlled drugs, pharmacies in most jurisdictions must have an original signed prescription.

Health Canada routinely inspects pharmacies selling prescription medications over the Internet or by mail order to ensure they comply with the *Food and Drugs Act* and *Food and Drug Regulations*. Such pharmacies must maintain an established licence to act as a wholesaler, and under federal legislation, only certain categories of medications may be sold in this manner.

## Legalization of Recreational Cannabis

Because the federal government has authority over criminal law, the creation and enactment of the *Cannabis Act* came under federal jurisdiction. The use of recreational cannabis was legalized in Canada in 2018 and is regulated under the *Cannabis Act*. The Act details the legal framework for the production, distribution, sale, and possession of cannabis for recreational use but does not change the policies and procedures for the use of cannabis for medical purposes, which has been legally available for over two decades and is controlled by the Access to Cannabis for Medical Purposes Regulations (Government of Canada, 2021, 2022a).

The *Cannabis Act* also identifies a range of penalties for anyone breaking the law(s), particularly related to illegal distribution of cannabis to younger people. Constitutional powers involving matters affecting cannabis legislation are shared between the federal government and the provinces/territories (Watts et al., 2017). Provinces, for example, have the legal authority over how to regulate the production, distribution, and retail sales of cannabis within their own borders (Crew, 2018).

## The Role of the Provincial and Territorial Governments

Because matters affecting the legislation of cannabis are split between federal and provincial/ territorial governments, differences in regulation occur among provinces and territories (Government of Canada, 2018b). In compliance with federal policies, provincial and territorial governments can license and regulate the distribution and sale of cannabis (where they are sold and under what terms). The provinces and territories are at liberty to adjust the minimum age for purchasing products (e.g., 18 years of age, although that is the age recommended under the Act) and set limits for personal possession.

## Advertising Prescription Drugs

In Canada, direct-to-consumer advertising of prescription drugs is strictly controlled and must meet certain criteria. Under the *Food and Drugs Act*, advertising a prescription drug is defined as "any representation by any means whatever for the purpose of promoting directly or indirectly the sale or disposal of any food, drug, cosmetic or device" (Government of Canada, 2020). Some drugs can be advertised in Canada under the following two conditions:

1. *Reminder advertisements.* Manufacturers can advertise drugs using their brand names, but cannot directly mention their uses. For example, television ads for erectile dysfunction merely hint at the drug's intended use and end by suggesting that viewers ask their doctor.
2. *Disease-oriented ads.* Rather than mentioning a brand name, these commercials discuss a condition, suggesting that the consumer consult their physician for available medications.

## Health Canada's Emergency Powers

The Constitution states that the federal government has an interest in "peace, order, and good government." As a result, the federal government retains the power to enact laws to manage health-related emergencies of national concern. Lessons learned from the severe acute respiratory syndrome (SARS) pandemic in 2003 prompted the federal government to revise the severely outdated *Quarantine Act* in 2005 (which had remained essentially the same since its inception in 1872).

## The *Quarantine Act*

Administered by the federal Minister of Health, the *Quarantine Act* (2005) complements the International Health Regulations by allowing Canadian authorities to respond more rapidly to health threats at Canadian borders and better preparing authorities to deal with threats and risks to global public health. The Act is also designed to complement existing provincial and territorial public health legislation (Chapter 2).

Provisions under the Act address current concerns and threats in society. The federal government now has the authority to:

- Divert aircraft or cruise ships to alternative landing or docking sites
- Designate quarantine facilities anywhere in Canada
- Restrict or even prohibit travellers who represent a serious public health risk from entering Canada

The Act also created two new occupational categories: environmental health officers and screening officers. These officers have the authority to assess, screen, and detain individuals who pose a health risk at the borders; to investigate and detain ships; and to examine goods and cargo crossing into or out of Canadian borders. It is important to note that this Act does not restrict the movement of Canadians from one province or territory to another. Such restrictions were put in place by some provinces (e.g., Ontario and Québec) during the height of the COVID-19 pandemic.

## COVID-19 and Related Laws

At the beginning of the COVID-19 pandemic, the federal government, under the authority of the *Quarantine Act* (S.C. 2005, c. 20) and the *Aeronautics Act* (RSC, 1985, c A-2), closed Canadian borders to most nonresidents, effectively banning "foreign nationals" (identified as persons who are not Canadian) from entering Canada by air travel from a foreign country, with the exception of those from the United States. Shortly after, however, in consultation with the US government, the border between Canada and the United States was closed (both ways) to nonessential travel. The border closure was reviewed periodically and renegotiated and remained in effect for 19 months.

The *Quarantine Act* (S.C. 2005, c. 20) gives the federal government (usually overseen by the Minister of Health) the authority to screen individuals who are suspected of having a communicable disease from entering the country or, upon entry, order them to isolate themselves at designated locations. For example, travellers returning to Canada during the pandemic were initially required to isolate for a period of 14 days. At times, hotels were used to isolate travelers (under the Act the Minister of Health has the authority to establish quarantine facilities anywhere in the country). Noncompliance with these protocols can result in fines or jail terms. The protocols for quarantining and isolating changed several times during the course of the pandemic. There are some exceptions to quarantine restrictions applied to asymptomatic people or groups of people entering the country—for example, a licensed health professional working in Canada (with some restrictions), the crew of an aircraft, a person invited into the country by the Minister of Health who is involved with assessing COVID-19 restrictions, and a person or groups of people providing an essential service.

## The *Aeronautics Act*

Used along with the *Quarantine Act* (S.C. 2005, c. 20), the *Aeronautics Act* (RSC, 1985, c A-2) comes under the authority of the Minister of Transport. The Act deals with regulations involving aviation security and related concerns. This includes rules regarding screening individuals entering an airport or aircraft and outlining the conditions under which they may travel as applied during the pandemic. In addition, the Act allows the Minister to redirect aircraft to various points in Canada or prevent aircraft from landing in the country. Aircraft from countries experiencing acute COVID-19 outbreaks were prohibited from landing, and others (for a period of time) were redirected to four major Canadian centres (Toronto, Montreal, Calgary, and Vancouver) (Statistics Canada, 2021).

### The Role for Public Health Authorities

During the pandemic, the federal Minister of Health, working with the Public Health Agency of Canada (PHAC) (and at times collaborating with other authorities), provided oversite and guidance to Canadians regarding rules, regulations, and protocols to keep Canadians safe. The PHAC also collaborated with jurisdictional public health agencies that have the authority to enact public health protocols within their jurisdictions. Such protocols included, at various points or waves during the pandemic, ordering businesses to close, placing restrictions on public and private gatherings, wearing masks, closing provincial borders, and enforcing vaccine mandates.

The legality of steps taken to suspend and sometimes terminate employees for noncompliance with vaccination protocols is managed at the provincial/territorial level under labour laws.

### International Health Regulations

The International Health Regulations outline strategies to prevent the global spread of infectious diseases to minimize any resulting disruption to the world economy (World Health Organization, 2008). Since the revision of the International Health Regulations, the World Health Organization (WHO) has declared four public health emergencies of global concern: H1N1 influenza (2009), polio (2014), Ebola (2014), Zika virus (2016), and, most recently, COVID-19 and monkeypox.

International regulations offer many benefits in monitoring and containing risks. Under the WHO's constitution, all signatory states agree to be bound by the terms to adhere to the International Health Regulations, which provide ways to identify a global public health emergency and outline measures for quickly gathering and distributing information and global warnings, including travel warnings. Currently, the US Centres for Disease Control and Prevention (CDC) is working with countries around the world to meet the goals of the International Health Regulations, addressing more than 400 diseases, conditions that are associated with significant morbidity and mortality rates and cause disabilities. Partners involved in related programs include experts in surveillance, epidemiology, informatics and diagnostic systems, health ministries, and public health authorities in WHO member countries.

## HEALTH CARE AS A RIGHT

Whether health care in Canada is a legal right is, at times, subject to interpretation with respect to both the Canadian Constitution and the *Canada Health Act*. For example, although all jurisdictions are expected to abide by the terms and conditions of the *Canada Health Act*, because of the jurisdictional division of powers related to health care, the federal government cannot *legally* force the provinces and territories to do so. The federal government can, however, use its constitutional spending power (contributing financially to health care programs) as leverage to ensure jurisdictional compliance (see Chapter 1). For the most part, all jurisdictions do comply with the terms and conditions of the Act, thus health care is considered to be a legal right. This right to health care remains limited by the principles and conditions of the Act in terms of the subjectivity of interpretation of some components of the Act. Therefore, application of the Act varies among jurisdictions, depending on interpretation, resources, finances, and so on. Rights are discussed from an ethical perspective in Chapter 9.

### The Canadian Charter of Rights and Freedoms

With strained resources, there are long waits for some medical and surgical procedures, at times prompting individuals to turn to the *Charter of Rights and Freedoms* for legal means to gain access to specific health care services. Canadians, for the most part, cannot purchase private insurance for medically necessary procedures, as it is disallowed by the Canadian government in order to avoid creating a two-tiered system that would run counter to the concept of universal health care.

The *Canadian Charter of Rights and Freedoms*, embedded in the Canadian Constitution, guarantees Canadians certain rights and freedoms, but is tempered by the phrase "subject only to such reasonable limits prescribed by law as can be demonstrably justified in a free and democratic society" (*Canadian Charter of Rights and Freedoms*, 1982). The Charter does not specifically identify health care, nor does it guarantee in specific terms that Canadians have a right to health care. The Charter does, however, demand that health care be provided to all persons *equally* and *fairly*.

The following sections within the Charter have met with legal challenges relating to the right of Canadians to health care:

- Section 7—life, liberty, and security of person. This section is sometimes used to challenge the government with respect to access (or lack thereof) to timely and appropriate health care (e.g., joint replacement surgery). To determine whether a person's rights have been violated with respect to health care, the court must consider three things: (1) the medical resources available at the time of the person's illness, (2) the demands made on those resources, and (3) the urgency of the individual's medical needs. Under the law, everyone has the right to fair assessment, but this right does not guarantee access to specific services.
- Section 15—equality. Section 15(1) states, "Every individual is equal before and under the law and has the right to equal protection and equal benefit of the law without discrimination and, in particular, without discrimination based on race, national or ethnic origin, colour, religion, sex, age or mental or physical disability." A defendant must prove discrimination (i.e., that they have been treated unequally) on the basis of one or more of the criteria outlined in this section.

Several notable challenges regarding people's right to health care have been made. One of the first was prompted by long waits for access to surgical services. Probably the most significant is the case of George Zeliotis, who required hip surgery and argued that his long wait time for the surgery caused him immeasurable pain, suffering, and immobility, impacting almost every aspect of his life. He claimed he had the right to make decisions that would preserve his quality of life, including the right to *timely* health care. The Supreme Court of Canada ruled that Québec's ban on private insurance in the face of long wait times violated the *Charter of Human Rights and Freedoms*. The courts held that when the public system is unable to deliver care within a reasonable time frame, alternative actions must be considered. The Supreme Court essentially removed restrictions prohibiting individuals from using private insurance to pay for services offered by the public system. The Court held that removing this restriction would guarantee freedom of choice for individuals and improve accessibility of care. Although viable in Québec (because it was argued under the Québec *Charter of Rights and Freedoms*), this ruling did not lead to significant changes in legislation across the rest of the country. It did, however, prompt provinces and territories to set benchmark time frames wherein certain surgeries should be performed.

## THE LAW, THE CONSTITUTION, AND END-OF-LIFE ISSUES

### Advance Care Directives

Advance care directives (part of the overall process of advance care planning) are instructions prepared by a mentally competent individual, outlining their wishes concerning health care decisions in the event that they can no longer decide for themselves. A person may express in advance their wishes about what intervention, medical treatments, or levels of care they will either consent to or refuse. Physicians and other health care providers must honor the person's decisions, even when the recommended treatment can potentially prolong the person's life or otherwise be beneficial to their health.

Similarly, a physician can refuse a decision by the patient's substitute decision maker (the person assigned the power of attorney for personal care when a patient is no longer capable of doing so) that is contrary to the patient's wishes, if the physician believes the patient has changed their mind or that the substitute decision maker is unfamiliar with the patient's wishes.

### Types of Advance Care Directives

There are two types of advance directives: *instructional* and *proxy*. Instructional directives (sometimes referred to as *living wills,* although living wills termed as such have no legal status in Canada) can be specific or general in nature. Specific instructions are detailed and explicit, outlining the person's wishes clearly, relative to presumed circumstances. For proxy advance care directives, general instructions include principles to be followed but give the decision maker the latitude to make decisions on a situational basis (Health Law Institute, Dalhousie University, n.d.).

Legislation determining the details related to legal policies and procedures for advance care directives are province/territory specific. In addition, each jurisdiction has different versions of forms for advance care planning as well as detailed information regarding completion of forms that can be downloaded from the government website. Some provinces also prescribe substitute decision making when not otherwise stated or legally provided for.

### Medical Assistance in Dying

The following includes highlights of the policies, procedures, and standards relating to medical assistance in dying. Details are available on the Government of Canada website at https://www.canada.ca/en/health-canada/services/medical-assistance-dying.html.

Medical assistance in dying (MAiD) became legal in Canada in 2016 (Bill C-14, which amended the *Criminal Code* and received Royal Assent on June 17, 2016). To make this possible, two sections of the *Criminal Code* were struck down: Section 25 of the *Criminal Code* held that helping an individual to end their life was an indictable offence; Section 14 held that it was unlawful for a person to ask someone to help them end their life. Bill C-14 is binding across Canada (Government of Canada, 2022b; Supreme Court of Canada, 2015).

### Amendments to MAiD Legislation

In October 2020, proposed amendments to the legislation for MAiD was introduced to Parliament (Bill C-7), receiving Royal Ascent on March 17, 2021. Changes came into effect that day. The most significant changes involve eligibility for MAiD, and procedural safeguards for individuals applying for MAiD whose death is not foreseeable.

In March 2021, a Senate Joint Committee on Medical Aid in Dying was appointed to review the provisions of the *Criminal Code* related to MAiD and their application to topics such as mature minors' (and their ability or right to apply for MAiD) advance requests, mental illness (particularly concerning safeguards to be put in place when a person with a mental illness becomes eligible to apply for MAiD), protecting people with disabilities, and the status of palliative care in Canada.

Because health care is the responsibility of provinces and territories, some variations exist regarding how the law is interpreted, applied, or both; related training for physicians and nurse practitioners; the application and approval process; the forms used; and the protocol(s) leading up to and for the actual procedure.

### Eligibility

A person must meet all of the following criteria:

- *Age*: Be over the age of majority (18 or 19 years, depending on the jurisdiction) and mentally competent (to make health-related decisions) to apply for medical assistance in dying
- *Health coverage*: Have a valid health card in the province or territory in which they live, or have health coverage through the federal government. This essentially discourages visitors to Canada from trying to apply for MAiD.
- *Health status:* The person must
  - Have a serious disease, illness, or disability, or other irreversible medical condition.
  - Be in the advanced stages of decline that cannot be reversed.
  - Experience unbearable and irreversible physical or mental suffering that cannot be alleviated as a result of the disease or disability such that the person's quality of life is unbearable and unacceptable to them. (Note that the person does not have to have a terminal illness.)
- Proposed legislation extending eligibility for MAID to persons suffering solely from a mental illness and for whom all related safeguards are met was scheduled to come into effect on March 17, 2023. In February 2023, this legislation was extended allowing more time for consultation and review of eligibility criteria.

### Consent for MAiD

Informed consent, as with any medical procedure that requires the applicant to be competent, must ensure that a patient is made aware of, and understands, all the necessary medical details and options the person may not have tried. This includes pain control and other palliative care measures, such as counselling and support for mental and emotional issues, including related anxiety and depression. It is reasonable to assume that many individuals applying for MAiD are experiencing stress and perhaps are depressed because of their situation, but of sound mind and thus clear and certain about their decision. If the attending practitioner is unsure about the person's mental status (including depression), they can request a psychiatric consult.

All details of the procedure itself must be understood by the applicant. The applicant must sign a consent form at the time of the initial interview when the request is made and again at the time of the procedure. The exception is if advance consent has been authorized and given as noted below.

Amendments to MAiD legislation now allow a person with any condition that will likely affect their decision making capacity in the future to sign a waiver exempting them from signing the final consent otherwise required just prior to the MAiD procedure taking place. Thus, a person with progressive cognitive impairment can choose a time for the MAiD procedure farther into the future than they might otherwise have chosen. They do not have to worry that if their impairment worsens to the point where they are incapable of agreeing to the procedure at the time it is to take place the procedure will be withheld.

The person seeking MAiD can withdraw consent at any time. The physician or nurse practitioner must ask the person, if cognitive, one more time prior to the event if the person wishes to withdraw their request. If a person who has signed a waiver exempting them from giving final consent indicates in any way that they have changed their mind, the physician or nurse practitioner will abandon the procedure. This includes the person indicating that they have changed their mind using words or gestures but excludes involuntary physical responses. This criterion is a new safeguard protecting the person who decides that they have changed their mind about receiving MAiD.

### Health Professionals Involved in MAiD

Physicians and nurse practitioners (except in Québec) are allowed to oversee a request for MAiD as well as facilitate the process. Other health professionals (e.g., nurses) are often present to support the individual and perhaps provide indirect assistance. Usually selected family members, friends, or both are present as arranged by the person receiving MAiD.

Health professionals who are opposed to MAiD do not have to be involved in the process. They are, however, expected to refer the patient to the appropriate resources. Most jurisdictions have a referral centre available that individuals without a primary care provider can access for direction.

### Additional Safeguards

Additional safeguards (other than those discussed earlier) ensure that MAiD is not abused or mishandled. These include stipulating that the applicant must make the initial request in writing or have a competent adult who understands the process, its implications, and outcomes make the request for them with the applicant present. A competent adult independent witness must be present when the request is made. This person must also understand the process and its implications. This person cannot be involved in the applicant's circle of care or benefit in any way from the death of the applicant. In addition, a physician or nurse practitioner must agree that the applicant meets the eligibility criteria applicable in their jurisdiction and have this assessment confirmed by an independent physician or nurse practitioner (Government of Canada, 2022b).

Additional new safeguards implemented in March 2021 concern requests made when "natural" death is not foreseeable. For example, one of the two providers assessing the person's eligibility for MAiD must have expertise in the medical condition that is prompting the person to apply for MAiD.

---

### THINKING IT THROUGH

#### *Dementia and MAiD*

Y.V. is 78 years old and has been diagnosed with Alzheimer's disease. Y.V. is still mentally competent and has decided to apply for MAiD. After the required assessments, Y.V. has been accepted. Y.V. signs a waiver exempting them from having to respond to the final consent at the time of the procedure (which Y.V. has already chosen).

1. How would you feel if Y.V. was your parent and at the time of the procedure you felt they were still enjoying a reasonable quality of life, even if they had lost their decision making capacity?
2. Would you try to overrule your parent's decision?
3. Do you agree with the legislative changes allowing someone with dementia to make the decision to have MAiD in advance? Explain your answer.

---

### Types of Medically Assisted Death

There are two ways in which MAiD may occur. A health provider (physician or nurse practitioner) may administer the lethal medication, or they can prescribe medication that the applicant can self-administer. The choice is made by the applicant and will, to a large degree, depend on the individual's physical ability to take medication, as well as their comfort level with the process.

A person who is very sick, weak, or has trouble swallowing is likely to have the physician or nurse practitioner administer the medications intravenously. The person may then feel more confident that the medication will work more effectively and promptly. Others may simply prefer to have the medication administered intravenously, deeming the process to be more peaceful. Those choosing to self-administer the medication may feel that the process is less invasive, less intrusive, and, for them, more peaceful.

---

**DID YOU KNOW?**

### MAiD in Québec

There are minor differences in the process related to medical assistance in dying in all jurisdictions across Canada, but the major parts of the legislation remain the same. There are two key differences in Québec: only physicians, not nurse practitioners, are allowed to participate in MAiD, and there is no option for self-administered MAiD in Québec; the physician must administer the medication.

---

## THE LEGALITY OF PRIVATE SERVICES IN CANADA

As previously noted, Québec is the only jurisdiction wherein a Canadian can purchase health insurance for private health care for designated medically necessary procedures (discussed later). It is, however, illegal for Canadians under *most* circumstances to have medically necessary procedures (e.g., joint replacements) performed at a private facility. Private health care services come at a price for most people, with the exception of groups of individuals (identified in Chapter 3) who have publicly funded insurance that pays for services at private clinics.

Surprisingly, a person can legally have a medically necessary procedure performed privately in Canada, outside of their province of origin (depending on the services offered). If T.J., for example, from one province goes to another jurisdiction seeking a knee replacement, it is perfectly legal for them to do so. T.J., as a nonresident of that province or territory, is not subject to the rules and regulations governing the private health care services in that jurisdiction. But T.J. would have to pay for that service.

---

**THINKING IT THROUGH**

### Eligibility for Private Services

Two individuals are out mountain biking north of Vancouver. M.K. is from Alberta, and L.Y. is from British Columbia. They both fall; M.K. injures his ankle, L.Y. injures his wrist. They call an ambulance. When assisting M.K. onto the stretcher, the paramedic injures his shoulder. A Royal Canadian Mountain Police (RCMP) officer pulls up to see if they can help, and the RCMP officer injures his shoulder as well. All of these individuals were seen in an emergency department. Treatment recommended for all of these individuals includes physiotherapy and surgery at some point in the near future. Wait lists for these surgeries are long, which is problematic for each person in terms of getting back to work. Are any of these individuals eligible to seek (paid) prompt treatment at a private clinic? If so, why? Who is eligible to have surgery at a private clinic? Why?

---

### Independent Health Care Facilities

Health care providers can become involved in other medical businesses or services in addition to their professional responsibilities. Independent facilities include medical/surgical clinics,

> ### CASE EXAMPLE 8.2   Herbal Supplements
>
> N.P., a sports medicine specialist, owns a private physiotherapy clinic in partnership with his partner, T.P., who sells herbal supplements in the same commercial space. Often N.P. would recommend herbal supplements to his patients to treat various conditions to assist with their physiotherapy. These supplements are sold by his partner.

laboratories, physiotherapy, and diagnostic centres. Patients are often referred to these private facilities by their health care providers. Theoretically speaking, private facilities can compensate the referring health professional for such referrals, causing legal and ethical concerns. Any health care provider who is directly or indirectly part of a private clinic who doesn't disclose their connection and obtains monetary gains from referrals is acting both illegally and unethically (Case Example 8.2).

In Canada, common law governs some conflict of interest concerns. The law binds providers to behave with honesty and integrity (i.e., to act according to a fiduciary duty) with regard to their patients and medical practice (see Chapter 9). This includes the duty of the provider to inform patients of any potential conflicts of interest regarding their practice (Office of the Conflict of Interest and Ethics Commissioner, 2014).

As is the case with most aspects of health care, provincial or territorial legislation directs the operation of private health care facilities in Canada. In Ontario, for example, the Independent Health Facilities Program (implemented under the *Independent Health Facilities Act*) licenses—in some cases, funds and coordinates—quality-assurance assessments for private facilities. Additionally, these facilities are subject to routine inspection, often by the provincial or territorial college of physicians and surgeons. In January 2023 the Ontario government announced plans to expand the number and range of surgeries performed in to private-for-profit facilities (all procedures are covered by OHIP).

In Alberta, the *Health Care Protection Act* oversees surgical services provided outside of hospitals. Private surgical facilities must have the approval of both Alberta Health and Wellness and the College of Physicians and Surgeons of Alberta; must have an approved contract authorizing them to provide insured services; must comply with the principles of the *Canada Health Act*; must be a required service within their geographic location; and must not negatively affect the public health system.

Organizations such as Timely Medical Alternatives (https://www.timelymedical.ca) assist Canadians in accessing any type of health care services—some of which can be obtained within Canada, others being outsourced to the United States. In most cases, patients pay for these services themselves.

Should Canadians have the right to choose between private and public health care services? Is it a constitutional right? See Box 8.2.

## PRIVATE HEALTH CARE IN QUÉBEC*

For years, doctors in Québec were allowed (under specific rules) to opt out of Régie de l'Assurance Maladie du Québec (RAMQ) to privately offer procedures covered by the public system.

Despite the *Chaoulli c. Procureur général du Québec, 2005* conclusion issued by the Supreme Court of Canada that prohibition on private insurance contravened the *Québec Charter*

---

* Based on personal correspondence with Pascal-André Vendittoli, MD, MSc, FRCS, Directeur médical de la Clinique Duval, Clinicen chercheur chevronné FRQS, Professeur Titulaire de chirurgie UdeM; Dr. Nicolas Duval, MD FRCS(C); and Dr. Pauline Lavoie, MD, MSc.

---

**BOX 8.2  A Constitutional Challenge: The Right of Canadians to Private Health Care**

Dr. Brian Day is an orthopedic surgeon and co-owner of the Cambia Surgery in Vancouver (Vancouver Sun, 2016). Opened in 1996, Cambie Surgery remains one of the largest surgical centres in British Columbia. Dr. Day is a long-time proponent of the right of Canadians to access private health care when the services they need are not available to them in a timely fashion within the public system. He holds that it is morally and ethically wrong for the government to force people to wait for unreasonable lengths of time to access health care services. Dr. Day claims Canada is unique among all other countries in that almost all provinces have a health care system in which citizens cannot by law, purchase private health insurance to cover "medically necessary" health care and hospital services. His claim was supported by expert witnesses for both plaintiffs and government in the B.C. constitutional challenge (Personal correspondence with Dr. Brian Day, March 18, 2022).

In June 2009, Dr. Day (along with six patients who joined the action as plaintiffs) launched a constitutional court challenge against the B.C. *Medicare Protection Act* on the basis that it violates the constitutional rights of B.C. residents and that the provincial health care system (as it stands) denies patients the right to timely health care. The court challenge was based on two constitutional rights: (1) violation of a person's right to life, liberty and security of persons and (2) on the basis that there are arbitrarily exempted groups who have access to private health care including (as discussed previously) individuals covered by Workers Compensation and those covered under the Public Service Health Care Plan (Personal Correspondence with Dr. Brian Day, March 18, 2022; Public Service Health Care Plan Administration Authority, n.d.). Section 15 of the charter states "Every individual is equal before and under the law and has the right to the equal protection and equal benefit of the law without discrimination and, in particular, without discrimination based on race, national or ethnic origin, colour, religion, sex, age or mental or physical disability." Dr. Day argued that *all* B.C. residents have the right to access private health care if waits in the public system for services are too long. Lawyers for both the B.C. and federal governments countered arguing that allowing what was essentially a two-tiered system, would erode universal health care in Canada, and, among other things, disadvantage older patients and those with complex chronic health conditions. The hearing did not commence until September 2016.

The B.C. Supreme Court (under Justice Steeves) dismissed the court challenge in 2020. Dr. Day appealed to the B.C. court of appeal, which also rejected the challenge. The case now goes before the Supreme Court of Canada.

The decision (when made) by the Supreme Court of Canada will affect all jurisdictions because the challenge was made under the *Canadian Charter of Rights and Freedoms*. This differs from the Chaoulli v. Québec case discussed earlier as its challenge was under the *Québec Charter of Rights and Freedoms*.

Sources: Vancouver Sun. (2016, September 6). *Dr. Brian Day vs. private medicine foes*. https://www.youtube.com/watch?v=A0-OhCYAZeQ; Public Service Health Care Plan Administration Authority. (n.d.). About the PSHCP. https://www.pshcp.ca/about-the-pshcp/

---

*of Human Rights and Freedoms* and Québec law 33 (Loi modifiant la Loi sur les services de santé et les services sociaux et d'autres positions législatives) allowing Québecers to seek private insurance for three surgical procedures (hip- and knee-replacement surgery and cataract surgery), the insurance companies showed little interest in selling such policies. As a result, the opportunity to have these private services covered by private insurance did not become a viable choice.

In spite of this, private clinics in Québec have grown, making private health care in Québec more available than in any other jurisdiction in Canada. These facilities, essentially private hospitals, are referred to as specialized medical clinics, or Cliniques médicales spécialisées (CMS).

There are two types of CMS in Québec:

1. ***Private–public partnerships (PPP)*** which perform services in partnership with the public system (RAMQ). The RMAQ covers the cost of services the patients receive in addition to remunerating the doctors for their services. These CMS do not have hospital beds for a length of stay extending beyond 24 hours. Performed procedures only include minor outpatient surgeries such as arthroscopy, cataract surgery, or hernia repair. If a patient requires a hospital length of stay greater than 24 hours (e.g., for an unforeseen complication), they are transferred to the "home" public hospital of the patient and surgeon.

   Contracts are negotiated between the CMS and public hospitals to provide designated services to their patients and need final approval by the Health Ministry. The profits made by these CMS are negotiated. Before the COVID-19 pandemic, it was 10% of the expenses claimed for a specific procedure, but since the beginning of the pandemic this has been increased to 15%.

   In these CMS, there are two exceptions worth noting that allow patients to pay for their surgery and jump the queue (then RAMQ is not involved):

   - A "grey zone" in the law allows a third-party payer (WSIB/CNESST, employer, etc.) to pay the cost of private surgery. A private bill is submitted to the third party, including a private fee for the doctors (the doctor should be out of RAMQ in this case).
   - Patients who reside outside of the province of Québec can pay for a private surgery because RAMQ does not insure them. A private bill is submitted to the patient, including a private fee for the doctors (again, they must be out of RAMQ).

2. ***Private CMS:*** Patients must pay the clinic for services and care received either out-of-pocket or through private insurance. Doctors working in these CMS must be opted out of RAMQ to privately perform publicly funded medically necessary procedures. Private CMS can have up to five inpatient beds to accommodate patients requiring a hospital stay longer than 24 hours, which would include postoperative rehabilitation services facilitating hip and knee surgeries. The Duval Clinic in Montreal was the first private clinic licensed by the Québec Health Ministry to operate as a fully equipped private facility. These private facilities cannot refer to themselves as *hospitals.*

## INFORMED CONSENT TO TREATMENT

Throughout Canada, before a health care provider may treat a patient, they require the informed consent of the patient. Consent must be both informed and voluntary:

- *Informed:* Patients must understand the treatment or procedure—the nature and purpose of the proposed treatment, the risks, side effects, benefits, and expected outcomes. Patients must also understand the implications of refusing the recommended treatment and be made aware of alternatives, if any, to the proposed treatment so that they have choices. The health care provider has an obligation to use language that is at an appropriate level for the patient and to discuss the information when the patient is not stressed or unhappy.
- *Voluntary:* Patients must not feel compelled to make a decision for fear of criticism, nor must they feel pressured toward any particular decision by the information provider or anyone else. Sometimes in health care, only a fine line exists between coercing and making a recommendation, especially when the health care provider feels strongly that the patient should consent to a treatment, and the patient is leaning toward refusing it.

See Did You Know? Sterilizing Indigenous Women Without Consent.

The Supreme Court of Canada supports the basic right of every capable person to decide which medical interventions they will accept or refuse. An individual also has the right to withdraw consent at any time, even if a procedure has started (College of Physicians and Surgeons of Ontario, 2020). For example, a patient is undergoing an angiogram (to which they have consented) and experiences pain, dizziness and headache, and flushing in the initial stages of the procedure (effects not explained as being "normal" for the procedure). They have the right to halt the procedure until further investigation reveals the cause of their symptoms, even if the physician feels there is no danger in continuing the procedure. Involving patients in all aspects of their health care is important: not only does it show respect for the patient and their right to autonomy; it also improves patient adherence to treatment regimes.

Each province and territory has enacted its own legislation addressing informed consent. Therefore, policies vary somewhat among the jurisdictions. Relevant legislation may include the *Adult Guardianship Act* (RSBC 1996), the *Mental Health Act* (R.S.O. 1990, c. M7), and the *Health Care Consent Act* (1996, S.O. 1996, c.2, Sched. A). Increasingly, physicians and other health care providers are advised to obtain written consent for even minor medical services such as immunizations instead of relying on implied or verbal consent. Written consent also ensures that the patient has had the necessary information explained to them and protects the patient and health care provider.

All health care providers in a position to provide care to a patient have both legal and ethical obligations regarding their patient's consent to proposed care. The ethical components of consent are discussed in Chapter 9.

## DID YOU KNOW?

### Sterilizing Indigenous Women Without Consent

In 2017, reports of Indigenous women in Canada being forced or coerced into having surgery resulting in sterilization (tubal ligations), a practice spanning decades from the 1920s or 1930s to as recently as 2022, were brought to light, largely as a result of a report made public by the health authorities in Saskatchewan (Standing Senate Committee on Human Rights, 2021). Jurisdictions reporting this abuse include British Columbia, Saskatchewan, Manitoba, Ontario, Québec, the Northwest Territories, and Yukon.

In 2018 a class action lawsuit was launched by a Saskatchewan law firm on behalf of a group of Indigenous women in that province, some claiming they had been sterilized without their permission; others consenting to the procedure, not realizing that they had the legal right to refuse it; and still others claiming that they were bullied (or coerced) into giving consent (Zingel, 2019).

The Standing Senate Committee on Human Rights began investigating this issue in 2019 and released a report entitled "The Scars That We Bear" in 2022 (Zimonjic, 2022). The Committee concluded that, even today, Indigenous women were being either coerced or bullied into being sterilized. In addition, the Committee reviewed reports that other population groups, including Black and racialized women, were also subjected to these procedures. The Committee made 13 recommendations, including that "legislation be introduced to add a specific offence to the *Criminal Code* prohibiting forced and coerced sterilization" (Standing Senate Committee on Human Rights, 2022).

Sources: Standing Senate Committee on Human Rights. (2021, June). *Forced and coerced sterilization of persons in Canada.* https://sencanada.ca/content/sen/committee/432/RIDR/Reports/2021-06-03_ ForcedSterilization_E.pdf; Standing Senate Committee on Human Rights. (2022, July). *The scars that we carry: Forced and coerced sterilization of persons in Canada – Part II.* https://sencanada.ca/content/ sen/committee/441/RIDR/reports/2022-07-14_ForcedSterilization_E.pdf; Zimonjic, P. (2022 July 14). *Senate report calls for law criminalizing forced or coerced sterilization.* CBC News. https://www.cbc.ca/ news/politics/senate-report-forced-coerced-sterilization-1.6520592; Zingel, A. (2019, April 18). *Indigenous women come forward with accounts of forced sterilization, says lawyer.* CBC News. https:// www.cbc.ca/news/canada/north/forced-sterilization-lawsuit-could-expand-1.5102981

## Types of Consent

### Express Consent

Express consent can be written or oral (which may be directed by agency policy) and indicates a clear choice on the part of the patient. Express consent requires that the individual be fully informed as to the benefits, risks, and consequences of any treatment options.

### Written Consent

All major medical interventions require signed, written consent as confirmation that the appropriate process for obtaining consent was followed and that the patient has agreed to the proposed intervention (Office of the Privacy Commissioner of Canada, 2021). Ideally, the person signing the consent form understands what the intervention is, including its risks and benefits. Although written consent provides health care providers with evidence of consent, a signed consent form may be weighed against any conflicting evidence and therefore may not provide a solid defence in the case of legal action.

Most consent forms have to be signed by the patient, dated, and witnessed (Office of the Privacy Commissioner of Canada, 2021). People qualifying as a witness to consent vary among jurisdictions and health care organizations. For medical procedures, including minor or major surgery, a physician or registered nurse will usually witness the consent. The witness should be comfortable that the patient understands what they are signing (e.g., a nurse getting a consent for surgery from a patient and signing as the witness). If any doubt remains, the appropriate person (e.g., usually the physician, nurse, or technologist doing the procedure) should speak to the patient and provide clarification. In some situations (e.g., in the hospital), reviewing the nature of the procedure is important, as medical terms can be confusing or misleading; the witness, if a health professional, should ensure that what the patient has been told agrees with the nature of the procedure the patient is consenting to (Case Example 8.3). Consent forms may be mailed or emailed to patients beforehand to be reviewed and signed—in this case it is incumbent upon the patient to seek further information if required.

Note that a multicultural environment may present challenges surrounding consent because of religious, cultural, gender, or social concerns, as well as language barriers. Most hospitals maintain a list of volunteer interpreters to be used should the need arise; however, interpreters capable of delivering health-related information clearly and accurately are not always available. Often, medical staff must rely on a family member to translate for the patient.

### Oral Consent

Equally binding as written consent, oral consent is given by spoken word over the phone or in person. If someone other than the patient is required to give oral consent for surgery over the phone, depending on the situation, some facilities ask that two health care providers validate a telephone consent. For example, if a person gives telephone consent for a procedure for their spouse (assuming the spouse is unable to give consent and their partner is in a legal position to do so), two health care providers must be on the telephone to validate the partner's consent,

---

### CASE EXAMPLE 8.3   Signing Consent

P.K. is prepared to sign a consent form for a hysterectomy and reads through the form given to her by the nurse. The type of surgery named on the form is a *pan-hysterectomy*, which P.K. may not understand. If she does not ask for clarification, she will sign consent for removal of her uterus, fallopian tubes, and ovaries.

that consent was given, that he has had all of his questions answered, and that he fully understands the circumstances under and for which consent is being provided. Protocol may vary among facilities and jurisdictions.

When a health care provider receives oral consent, they should carefully document it in the patient's chart, describing the intervention discussed, stating that the patient has acknowledged understanding of the intervention, and noting that the patient has agreed to it orally. Written consent remains the preferred alternative, however, especially for complex treatments.

## Implied Consent

Implied consent occurs by virtue of the fact that an individual seeks the care of a physician or other health care provider (Office of the Privacy Commissioner of Canada, 2021). For example, many people have received an immunization or another treatment from a family physician without having signed a consent form; the immunization or treatment has been provided under the umbrella of implied consent. As previously mentioned, however, more health care providers are requesting written consent, even for immunizations.

Upon voluntary admission to a hospital, patients imply their consent to certain interventions (e.g., allowing the nurse to render care or to take their vital signs). This also includes the sharing of medical information among those caring for the patient, but not anyone outside their circle of care. However, it is proper and respectful to ask the patient if they are comfortable with certain interventions (e.g., "I am going to begin your exercises now. Is that okay?"; "I would like to change your dressing in about an hour. Are you okay with that?").

## Consent in an Emergency Situation

Even in emergency situations, health care providers should obtain consent from a patient before providing treatment if at all possible. Under some circumstances (e.g., the individual cannot communicate because of cognitive impairment, a language barrier, or being unconscious), a health care provider can administer emergency treatment without the patient's permission if, in the professional's opinion, a delay will result in serious harm or injury (Canadian Medical Protective Association [CMPA], 2021). In such circumstances, however, the health care provider must provide clear, detailed, and concise written documentation explaining the decision to give treatment in the patient's medical record.

## Who Can Give Consent

A competent person receiving the intervention most often gives consent for the treatment. If the individual proves incapable of providing consent (e.g., is not mentally competent or is unconscious), the person's legal representative or next-of-kin (subject to provincial and territorial law) assumes the responsibility. In most jurisdictions, the person who legally has power of attorney for personal care, the person who is named as substitute decision maker (also called durable power of attorney) for health care decisions for the patient, or a person related to the patient usually takes on this duty. Legal agreements assigning someone to make decisions for an incapable person are called *representation agreements* or *health care proxies*.

In the absence of a legally assigned person, most provinces and territories will allow a spouse (whether legal or common law) or another family member to legally provide consent. Some jurisdictions outline a designated order, depending on the availability of particular relatives—for example, a spouse will have such control before a father or mother, who would have control before a sibling, who would have control before an aunt or uncle, and so on.

## Age of Consent for Minors

The age of majority as the benchmark for giving consent for medical treatment is becoming irrelevant. Instead, the maturity of an individual as a marker for giving consent is the benchmark in all jurisdictions except Québec. In Québec, the age for consent for treatment is 14 years under the *Civil Code*.

As long as the minor fully understands the treatment and its risks and benefits, they can make an informed decision about accepting or rejecting the treatment, and health care providers must respect their wishes. This is also true if the young person refuses a treatment (e.g., chemotherapy). There may be jurisdictional variations.

When required, either parent who has legal custody of the minor (or a legally appointed guardian) can provide consent for treatment. If children are travelling, the legal guardian or parent can provide written permission to another adult travelling with the minor to consent to medical treatment in case of an emergency.

In extraordinary circumstances, a province or territory can seek temporary guardianship and order that treatment be implemented. Although the Charter holds that Canadians have the right to freedom of religion, when children are, in the view of the courts, too young to hold and express beliefs or to understand the consequences of receiving treatment or not receiving treatment, courts usually uphold requests made to intervene on the children's behalf; for example, if a religious belief holds that a specific intervention is against those beliefs (especially if the treatment is potentially life-saving).

### Consent for Deceased Organ Donation

Provincial/territorial legislation determines the terms and conditions under which individuals can give consent for organ donation, although fundamental similarities exist across the country (Canadian Blood Services, 2022). In most jurisdictions, an individual must be 16 years of age or older to consent to be an organ donor, usually by signing a document such as a donor card or a driver's licence. Individuals can provide consent by registering online to be an organ donor in British Columbia, Alberta, Manitoba, and Ontario. Saskatchewan is the only province that does not link an individual's permission to be an organ donor to either their health card or driver's licence. Younger individuals who cannot otherwise give consent for organ donation may make their wishes known to their parents. Should such a tragic event arise, parents may feel more comfortable donating a child's organs knowing that is what they wanted.

Donation of organs must occur without payment or compensation of any kind to remain legal in Canada. It is important that individuals who wish to be organ donors discuss these wishes with their family or a close friend to ensure that if the event arises, their wishes are made known to the medical team, even if they have taken formal steps to give consent. Except for Nova Scotia, Canada does not have presumed consent legislation wherein an individual's organs and tissues are automatically donated (if suitable) after death unless they opt out. In April 2019, Nova Scotia introduced this legislation under the *Human Organ and Tissue Donation Act*.

### DID YOU KNOW?

#### *Signing to be an Organ Donor*

Signing a donor registration form does not mean you will become an organ donor. Statistically few registered donors are actually suitable for organ donation as medical criteria (hospital policies and procedures) impose limitations. For example, the person must die in the hospital, most often in an ICU or CCU or must be surviving on a ventilator (meaning that without a ventilator, death would be imminent). Physicians must determine whether the patient is brain dead (neurologically) or facing cardiocirculatory death if not on life support. Organ donation can only be considered after all efforts have been made to save the patient. Up to eight vital organs are potentially used—heart, lungs (two), pancreas, intestine, kidneys (two), and liver.

British Columbia, Ontario, and Québec are among the jurisdictions with the highest donation rates in Canada. These provinces have "donation after circulatory determination of death" programs, and mandatory referral and reporting of impending cardiocirculatory and neurological deaths, alerting specialized teams, which approach family members with information about organ donation options. Organ donation (from deceased donors) was 19.2% (per million population) in 2020, which was a 12% decrease from the previous year (perhaps because of the pandemic), but an increase of 28% since 2011 (Canadian Institute for Health Information, 2021).

Between 2010 and 2019, the Canadian Institute for Health Information (2021) reported a 59% increase in the deceased organ donor rate in Canada and a 42% increase in transplant procedures.

Provinces and territories continually embark on organ awareness campaigns with variable results. However, since Logan Boulet's death, the 21-year-old Humboldt Broncos player who donated his organs to six patients following the tragic bus collision in April 2018, there has been a surge in the number of individuals registering across the country (Canadian Press, 2018).

## THE HEALTH RECORD

Any person who has received health care in Canada at any time possesses a health record, an accumulation of information relating to their interactions with health care services. People who work in the health care industry and deal directly with patients are often in a position to access and record health information relating to services provided for the patient. A significant portion of health information today is electronically recorded and stored.

Depending on the nature of the facility and those involved in the patient's circle of care, a health record may consist of information gathered from many sources. A health record in the hospital setting will have more components than one in a dentist's office, a chiropractic clinic, or a physiotherapy clinic. In the hospital setting, records (manual or electronic) will contain numerous and varied reports and records.

Clinics or offices may also maintain a variety of reports: diagnostic reports, consultation reports, history sheets (sometimes called a *cumulative profile*), and a record of what happened at each encounter (e.g., details of visits to the family doctor, including the reason for the visit and the treatment plan and treatment received).

### The Importance of Accurate Recording

In most disciplines, health care providers must, by law, record information clearly, concisely, and accurately. Possibly one of the most important tasks in the field of health care, careful recording provides valuable information that can ensure continuity of patient care. All entries must be dated and signed or initialed (according to agency protocol) either manually or electronically.

What is recorded and how an entry is worded are also important. A person not in a position to diagnose must use words such as "appears to have" instead of "has" and must never record suppositions or inadvertently label someone (e.g., "Mr. Smith is a schizophrenic"). Each discipline provides related guidelines for appropriate charting.

Health care providers must regard anything that they enter into a health record as information potentially required in any type of litigation. Health records may prove important in a legal proceeding.

## THINKING IT THROUGH

### *Adding an Incorrect Diagnosis to a Chart*

An administrative assistant in a busy family health team was asked to add the code for a diagnosis made by the physician on M.T.'s electronic chart. M.T. was a nurse at the local hospital, had lost her son, and was grieving. Not sure what the diagnostic code was for grieving, the administrative assistant added the one they knew for "mood disorder." That diagnosis appeared on the M.T.'s chart. Later, during admission to hospital for a diagnostic test, nurses who knew M.T. noted the diagnosis of mood disorder, which surprised them. Although keeping all information confidential, the nurses caring for M.T. now were convinced that she had a mood disorder.

1. If you were in the same situation, would you be disturbed knowing that colleagues thought you had a mood disorder (which includes such diagnosis as obsessive-compulsive disorder and other major mental health conditions)?
2. What should the administrative assistant have done when coding the diagnosis?
3. What, if any steps, could M.T. take to correct this?

## Ownership of Health Information

It is important to note that all jurisdictions have legislation that balances the right of access to personal information with appropriate protection of that information. Privacy legislation is discussed later in this chapter. The health care facility or doctor's office that collects the information and creates the health record owns the patient's physical chart. Physicians, dentists, other health care providers, and health care facilities that maintain such records, act as custodians of that information.

The health information itself, however, belongs to the patient, and patients retain the right to request a *copy* of the information in their charts (manual or electronic). Patients may not remove physical records from a health care facility or alter its data. Copies are always made, and information from an electronic chart are downloaded for the patient.

Information for a third party (e.g., an insurance company) may only be released with the patient's consent, unless otherwise ordered by a court of law.

Often patients who are moving or changing physicians will request a copy of their chart, which may be given to the patient in paper format or (more frequently) sent directly to the new health care provider electronically. If the chart predates an electronic version, then copies of the chart are prepared and given to the patient or sent to the new provider, usually by registered mail or courier. In such cases, the physician may send only those documents considered essential. The patient must be made aware of any charges associated with the cost of transferring health records.

Under some circumstances, usually to avoid serious negative effects on the patient's mental, emotional, or physical health, a physician may deny a person access to components of their health information or may selectively remove information from a patient's chart before providing the patient with a copy of it. Although existing provincial or territorial legislation aimed at safeguarding health information usually supports denying a patient access, the physician must be able to justify any such decision. A patient can usually appeal a denial.

## Storage and Disposal of Health Information

If a physician moves, ceases to practise for some reason, or retires, the medical information they accumulated must be retained and stored in such a manner that patients and other health care providers providing care for that patient can access it (with the patient's permission) as needed. If another health care provider assumes responsibility for the practice at the same location, the patients' charts often remain at that location. Patients must receive notification of the change of provider.

When physicians or other health care providers form a group, they should immediately clarify ownership of the charts—for example, does each own the charts of the patients they regularly see, or do all of the records belong to the organization?

When a health care provider leaves a practice and no one assumes direct responsibility for the records (e.g., no one takes over the practice), a custodian—a person or business legally allowed to store or otherwise keep medical records—may take over the charts. Medical file storage companies can charge patients several hundreds of dollars for photocopies of their files. Provincial and territorial governments and regulatory bodies specify guidelines for the storage of records, including how long they must be maintained.

The Canadian Medical Protective Association (CMPA) advises that physicians retain medical records for at least 10 years from the date of the last entry, or in the case of minors, for at least 10 years from the date when the age of majority is reached. Each jurisdiction sets its own policies on health records retention; for example, in *British Columbia*, physicians are required to keep their records for 16 years from the date of last entry or of a patient's age of majority (CMPA, 2022). *Alberta* physicians are advised to keep records for a minimum of 10 years after the patient was last seen, or in the case of a minor, the greater of 10 years or 2 years beyond the patient's age of majority (CMPA, 2022). In *Saskatchewan* the length of time is 6 years from the date of last entry or 2 years from when the patient reaches the age of majority, whichever is later (CMPA, 2022). In *Ontario* the length of time is 10 years from the date of last entry or 10 years from when the patient reaches the age of majority or until the physician ceases to practise if some conditions are met. However, Ontario physicians are advised to keep charts for a minimum of 15 years (CMPA, 2022). In *Québec* the length of time certain physicians must keep medical records is only 5 years (CMPA, 2022). For the *eastern provinces* and the *territories* the length of time is 10 years, with the exception of *Yukon* which, like Saskatchewan, is 6 years (CMPA, 2022).

### Destruction of Medical Records

The ultimate destruction of medical records must be accomplished in a manner that will ensure the information can never again be accessed. For example, a health care provider cannot just delete medical information from their computer; rather, the hard drive on which the information is stored must be professionally wiped clean. Paper records must likewise be shredded and disposed of in accordance to provincial/territorial policies.

### Federal Legislation and Privacy Laws

There are several laws governing privacy legislation in Canada. Two federal privacy laws, enforced by the office of the Privacy Commissioner of Canada, are the *Privacy* Act (1983) and the *Personal Information Protection and Electronic Documents Act* (2004), known as PIPEDA, contribute to this protection (Office of the Privacy Commissioner of Canada, 2018).

Each of Canada's provinces and territories implements its own privacy legislation. Some provinces, including Alberta, Manitoba, Saskatchewan, and Ontario, have privacy legislation specific to health care service providers. (See Web Resources on Evolve for a link to privacy legislation for each of the provinces and territories.)

### Privacy Act

The *Privacy Act* applies to federal government institutions involving any and all information the government collects, uses, and discloses about a person. It requires federal government departments and agencies to limit the private information they collect from individuals (*Privacy Act* (R.S.C., 1985, c. P-21)). The Act restricts the use and sharing of any personal information collected, which usually relates to old age security, employment insurance, Revenue Canada (tax collection and refunds), and for other security issues. Additionally, the *Privacy Act* allows individuals to access and correct any information federal government organizations have about them (Office of the Privacy Commissioner of Canada, 2018).

### Personal Information Protection and Electronic Documents Act (PIPEDA)

*PIPEDA* protects personal information collected that relates to the private sector. The Act supports and promotes both online and traditional commercial activities by protecting personal information that is collected, used, or disclosed under certain circumstances. It defines personal information as "information about an identifiable individual" and includes any factual or subjective information, recorded or not, in any form. For example, the following would be considered personal information:

- Name, address, telephone number, gender
- Identification numbers, income, or blood type
- Credit records, loan records, existence of a dispute between a consumer and a merchant, and intentions to acquire goods or services

Known as consent-based legislation, *PIPEDA* requires any organization collecting and using personal information to present patients with consent forms that fully disclose how their personal information will be collected and managed, and to have these forms signed. For example, a dentist's office collecting information for research purposes for commercial gain must reveal to the patient all personal information gathered and seek permission before using it.

For a number of years now, all Canadian businesses have had to comply with the privacy principles set out by *PIPEDA*, except those businesses in provinces with privacy legislation similar to *PIPEDA* (e.g., British Columbia, Alberta, and Québec). *PIPEDA* protects information throughout Nunavut, the Northwest Territories, and Yukon because most organizations, other than hospitals and schools, remain under federal jurisdiction there.

*PIPEDA* does not usually affect hospitals and other health care facilities since most are not overtly involved with commercial activities. Some commercial endeavours in hospitals, such as third-party enterprises operating within the facility (e.g., commercial food businesses, paid parking) must comply with PIPEDA unless there was similar provincial/territorial legislation that would override it.

Any health care providers with private practices and involved in any type of commercial activity (e.g., dentists, chiropractors, and optometrists) are subject to PIPEDA unless similar public (provincial/territorial) legislation applies (Office of the Privacy Commissioner of Canada, 2015).

The legality of exempting some publicly funded organizations from *PIPEDA* legislation has been questioned, because some functions within health care facilities (e.g., a privately owned diagnostic clinic operating within the hospital) mimic those of a private organization.

In most jurisdictions, personal information collected by health care facilities remains under the protection of province- or territory-generated, public-sector legislation (e.g., in Ontario, the *Personal Health Information Protection Act [PHIPA]*; in British Columbia, both the *Freedom of Information and Protection of Privacy Act [FIPPA]* and *Personal Information Protection Act [PIPA]*). FIPPA, for example, gives individuals the right to access their own records as well as the right to insist that any errors found are corrected. At the same time, the Act outlines limited exceptions to the right to access.

While other provinces and territories have also passed their own health privacy laws, these have not been declared substantially similar to PIPEDA. In some of those cases, PIPEDA may still apply.

Newfoundland and Labrador, New Brunswick, Nova Scotia, and Ontario have health-related privacy legislation deemed "substantially similar" to PIPEDA with respect to health information (Office of the Privacy Commissioner of Canada, 2020).

## Confidentiality

All health care providers must legally and ethically keep all health information confidential. The concept of confidentiality refers to the health care provider's moral and legal obligation to keep a patient's health information private. Conversely, the concept of privacy refers to the patient's right for their health information to remain confidential and to be released only with their consent.

Any health care provider involved directly in a patient's case—the circle of care—can legally access relevant portions of the patient information for legitimate reasons while providing care. Depending on the circumstances, administrative personnel also have access to a person's health information and likewise must keep it confidential. Almost all places of employment—particularly in the health care sector—require employees to sign a confidentiality agreement (see Web Resources on Evolve for a link to a sample agreement) and to adhere to the principles and policies within the document. Every facility is expected to have policies and procedures for protecting patient confidentiality, including the fact that they are seeking care, to any and all health information in all forms, including oral exchanges between or among health care providers. As a rule, health care providers should never discuss health information with anyone other than members of the health care team responsible for the patient's care. For example, it is unacceptable to mention to a friend that S.O. just had a baby boy or that P.D. broke his leg and has a cast (Box 8.3).

Under some circumstances, health care providers (e.g., physicians) may have a moral and legal responsibility to *release* confidential health information (e.g., when an individual has harmed or is in danger of harming themselves or others). Also, some health conditions, such as communicable diseases, must be reported to the local public health authority (CMPA, 2015).

A patient who discovers a breach of confidentiality can bring a lawsuit against the individual, organization, or both that are responsible for the breach, whether the breach was intentional or not (Case Example 8.4).

## Security

Health records of any type must be kept in a manner that is both safe and secure, meaning they should be protected from fire and damage from environmental disasters such as flooding,

---

### BOX 8.3 Confidentiality: An Age-Old Concept

The concept of confidentiality was outlined in the Hippocratic Oath 2,500 years ago as follows:

Whatever, in connection with my professional practice, or not in connection with it, I see or hear, in the life of men, which ought not to be spoken of abroad, I will not divulge, as reckoning that all such should be kept secret. While I continue to keep this Oath unviolated, may it be granted to me to enjoy life and the practice of the art, respected by all men, in all times. But should I trespass and violate this Oath, may the reverse be my lot.

Source: The Internet Classics Archive. (n.d.) *The oath, by Hippocrates.* http://classics.mit.edu/Hippocrates/hippooath.html

---

### CASE EXAMPLE 8.4    Breach of Confidentiality

While at a party, a student nurse was conversing with a classmate, who commented on how fast their mutual friend delivered her baby boy last week. "Imagine," said the classmate, "her delivery lasted only 3 hours. That's really fast for her first baby." The student nurse responded, "But that wasn't her first delivery, and second babies usually come much faster."

The minute she uttered the words the student nurse knew they had broken a confidence, but the damage was done. Their mutual friend had had a baby 4 years prior, as a teenager. She'd given the baby up for adoption and told no one. Now the secret was out, causing hurtful and damaging information to circulate among their friends. Think of the possible implications if their mutual friend's husband did not know her history!

1. As a member of a health care team, what reminders can you put in place to ensure that you guard the confidentiality of your patients?
2. What, if any, steps could the student nurse take now?
3. Would your trust in a friend, let alone a health provider, change if you knew they had broken a confidence?

---

among other possible scenarios. In the case of electronic records, the use of encrypted software and passwords is essential. All health information must be stored in such a manner that access is restricted to authorized persons. Hard copies of electronic information and copies of paper-based information must be carefully tracked. Anyone who has access to health information must be bound by confidentiality agreements (from physicians to administrators to nonregulated health care providers). Every functioning electronic system should have a functioning audit trail. Any health care worker who suspects an unauthorized person of trying to access health information, whether within a clinic or a hospital unit, should question the person's identity and intent. Most health care providers and health facilities have protocols for both storing and allowing access to health information they are responsible for.

### Electronic Health Information Requirements

Both electronic and hard-copy records are subject to the principles of confidentiality and the protection of health information. However, the electronic environment poses unique challenges to maintaining confidentiality and privacy standards.

Electronic health records and electronic medical records are essentially separate collections of elements of the same material. Whereas electronic medical records (EMRs) are housed in one facility and pertain only to care received at that facility, electronic health records (EHRs) provide the "bigger picture." Compiled in a central database accessible to authorized persons for the purpose of providing care, electronic health records contain information from several different sources (e.g., a hospital, pharmacy, doctor's office).

Since an electronic health record contains information from various sources, several people will have access to the information. The more people involved, the more likely it is that a breach of confidentiality can result. As with all electronic information, the potential exists for information theft by hackers or by individuals who gain unauthorized access to information because of carelessness with passwords. It is much easier for a person who illegally accesses hundreds of medical files on a hospital computer system to remove or copy those compared to someone trying to walk off with thousands of files in hard-copy format.

There are times when medical records stored in offices, clinics, or in other secure facilities go missing. Although electronic records are deemed more secure than paper records, neither is foolproof.

The consent rules that apply to information stored in hard-copy format also apply to information managed electronically, according to *PIPEDA* and territorial and provincial health privacy legislation. The information custodian must disclose to the patient who will have access to the information and any auxiliary purposes for which the information may be used. The patient also has a right to know what safeguards the facility has in place to protect the information. Some information custodians believe that once people give consent to have their information stored on an electronic health record, implied consent allows for other uses of that information.

Many health care facilities use patient information for research purposes. Strictly speaking, the health care facility should obtain the patient's consent and additionally provide clear and accurate information about the research.

## HEALTH CARE PROFESSIONS AND THE LAW

The regulation of health care providers is discussed in detail in Chapter 5. This section briefly looks at the significant legal responsibilities of regulated health professions.

### Regulated Health Care Providers

Most health care providers who hold a professional designation in Canada are members of a regulating body that assumes a high level of responsibility for the ethical, moral, and legal conduct of its members. Most regulated professions have a system in place for handling complaints against their members and for dealing with members charged with an offence (e.g., a physician who has been disciplined by the provincial regulating body or who has been charged with a criminal offence may be suspended or they may lose their licence). Likewise, regulating bodies will support members when claims prove unfounded. That said, the emphasis of regulated professions is to provide protection for the public, ensuring that care rendered by its members is professional, competent, and culturally safe.

Although litigation against health care providers happens far less often in Canada than in the United States, it is becoming increasingly common here; therefore, all health care providers should purchase some type of liability insurance. Most regulated health care providers obtain malpractice or liability insurance through their professional college or the organization they work for.

### Unions, Health Care, and Legal Implications

Many health sector employees are involved with one or more organizations (e.g., a regulatory body, professional organization, or union). Each organization has its own mandate, structure, and purpose, although there is some overlap. Unions advocate for the well-being of the employee and share concern for the public in terms of having access to safe, high-quality health care.

A *union* is an organization that represents and advocates for its members, usually regarding employee–employer issues. A union, like other organizations, has rules, regulations, policies, and protocols. Unions represent groups of workers within a facility and advocate for and protect the social and economic rights of its members, often in the form of collective bargaining. Issues may relate to human rights, improving employees' wages, hours worked, working conditions, and benefits. They also provide member support in the face of complaints.

Unions are not legally obliged to represent members in anything other than labor relations. Some unions will have insurance, which all members have access to for legal representation and advice in other forums as required (which may include such things as human rights complaints, testifying in coroner's cases, and other litigation). When criminal charges are filed, the support offered may range from none at all to allowing reimbursement if a not guilty verdict is returned.

For discipline hearings and terminations, a union provides a representative to be present at all meetings between members and the employer. The union representative ensures that procedures are followed correctly, that members are made aware of their rights, and that support is provided for members as required (e.g., challenging a termination or disciplinary action, perhaps in the form of a grievance, or going to arbitration).

In many cases, a union will also protect an individual's job. For example, if someone outside of the hospital applied for a clinical secretary's position as well as someone deemed equally qualified from within the facility, the existing collective agreement would ensure that, if proper protocols are followed, the individual already employed within the hospital generally gets the job. Depending on the terms of the collective agreement, it could be that the person employed by the hospital was working in housekeeping, but either trained on the job or took relevant courses, and the individual applying externally was a graduate from a 2-year health office administration program and had an undergraduate degree in health sciences. If it can be proven that the hospital employee can meet job qualifications, that person will likely get the job.

The number of unions representing individuals in a facility can depend on the size of the organization and the number of employees. The Labor Board may stipulate that the union must represent all employees, although there may be some exceptions.

Relative to the number of employees, if several professions are represented, unions may choose to create separate bargaining units for each. In such cases it would be unlikely for more than one category of worker to legally be in a strike position at the same time. In larger organizations, such as hospitals, different categories or professions may be represented by different unions, such as the provincial/territorial Nurses Association for Registered Nurses and the Canadian Union of Public Employees (CUPE for L/RPNs). Such situations may well be dependent on or influenced by the unions involved and workforce actions. What a union environment looks like in any particular workplace is usually influenced by the collective will of those who work there and who are eligible to organize as a union.

### "Sorry, I Made a Mistake"

Although apology legislation is not limited to the health profession, the focus here is on health provider–patient incidents. When an adverse event occurs because of human error, the health professional has the legal and moral obligation to inform the patient of all relevant facts. Examples include a medication error, negligence contributing to a patient falling, misinterpretation of a diagnostic test, or an incorrect diagnosis. Historically, apologizing for the mistake has been seen as opening the door to impending litigation. One of the objectives of apology legislation is to reduce concerns regarding liability in a variety of situations.

Currently in Canada, only Québec does not have apology legislation. British Columbia was the first province to do so, and New Brunswick, the Northwest Territories, and Yukon the latest. The principles of the Canadian legislation are similar in all jurisdictions in terms of protection under the various acts and those outlined by the CMPA. Most pieces of legislation hold that an apology does not constitute an admission of fault or liability, must not be taken into consideration in determining fault or liability, and is not admissible as evidence of fault or liability. Protection offered by this legislation is effective in tribunals, college disciplinary committees, and coroner's inquests and before the courts.

The offer of an apology reduces the tendency of patients to resort instantly to litigation and allows health care providers to deal with their patients in a compassionate manner by recognizing the importance that an apology can play in settling disputes. Apologizing can reduce anger and hostility, showing that the health care provider is caring and acknowledges regret.

### Ending a Physician–Patient Relationship

A primary care provider (usually a physician or a nurse practitioner) becomes legally responsible for the care of a person when active treatment begins. If a physician or other health care provider refuses or ceases to care for a patient without due process (e.g., notifying the patient), they can be charged with abandonment. A variety of situations may cause a patient and a provider to part ways, such as personality conflicts that interfere with effective patient–provider interactions or that restrict necessary communication to ensure best care, including significant disagreement between the patient's expectations and the provider's ability to meet those expectations, or aggressive or unacceptable behaviour on the part of the patient. De-rostering a patient is not the same as firing a patient (see Chapters 3 and 5).

In most jurisdictions, the provider must address the termination of a patient–provider relationship after documented written and verbal warnings, and, finally, in writing in the form of a letter (often called a *Dear John letter*). The administrative assistant working for the physician or nurse practitioner usually bears the responsibility of handling this correspondence, which is most often sent by registered mail or courier to gain proof that the letter was received. Physicians must continue to provide care for any such patients until the patient has found another doctor—which is a challenge, given the current shortage of doctors in Canada.

Conversely, patients can simply walk away from their provider—with no formal separation process—never to return. If they return, even after a protracted time frame, they are entitled to treatment unless the practitioner or group has terms addressing such situations that are made known to the patient.

### Physician Authority: Involuntary Confinement

In all jurisdictions, under a provincial or territorial *Mental Health Act*, doctors have the power to temporarily commit a patient to a mental health facility under certain circumstances, whether acting either independently or in conjunction with the patient's family. In some jurisdictions, patients who pose a danger to themselves or others and who are noncompliant with requests to receive treatment may be subject to a physician's enacting this authority. Some regions require the physician to sign a form, which designates a time frame (e.g., 72 hours) within which the patient will receive an evaluation. Afterward, the patient can be discharged and, if need be, readmitted on a voluntary or involuntary basis. In the case of the last situation, to protect the rights of the patient, a physician other than the one who signed the original form would have to provide an assessment. In most jurisdictions, the patient and their family must also have access to a trained rights advisor or advocate, who may provide an avenue for appeal of the decision for involuntary commitment.

## OTHER LEGAL ISSUES IN HEALTH CARE

### The Use of Restraints

Restraints are used in a health care facility when all other interventions have failed and a patient's behaviour poses a danger to self or others, and to ensure the safety of the patients and of those caring for them. Restraints can be mechanical, environmental, physical, or chemical (medications). The use of restraints of any kind must be ordered by a physician and, in the best-case scenario, with permission from the patient's family or the person who has the power of attorney for personal care.

Most facilities have a "least restraint policy," which means that health care providers must reserve the use of restraints as a last resort, employing every possible intervention to calm or reason with the patient before restraints are used. The type of restraint should be the least invasive type possible and one that least interferes with freedom of the patient. Chemical restraints are used to sedate an agitated patient and not for direct therapeutic reasons. Chemical restraints, although not visibly restraining a person, come with risks and side effects. Using medications as restraints should also be a last resort.

Injury can result from using restraints, perhaps more easily than when they are not used in some situations. A person may become more agitated and confused, particularly if they are cognitively impaired. If someone were to arbitrarily apply restraints in a health care facility, it is likely they would be in violation of the facility's policies and procedures and could potentially face litigation if the patient was injured.

## Patient Self-Discharge From a Hospital

Unless confined under legislation, any inpatient can leave a hospital at any time without a physician's permission. Typically, a doctor will decide to discharge a patient when they feel that hospital care is no longer required. When a discharge order is written, plans for the patient's discharge are activated, and a discharge time suitable for the patient and in keeping with facility protocol is arranged.

When a patient decides to leave a hospital against a doctor's recommendations, the facility should have the patient sign a form releasing the hospital, the physician, and other members within the patient's circle of care from responsibility for that patient's well-being. Once the patient leaves, they assume all responsibility for any unforeseen effects of their action. If a patient refuses to sign a release form, the person managing the discharge must clearly and concisely document the patient's refusal. Including quotes documenting what the patient has said may helpful in proving an accurate account of the incident.

## Good Samaritan Laws

Good Samaritan laws legally protect anyone who offers to help someone in distress if something goes wrong from litigation—as it did in Thinking It Through: The Help of a Good Samaritan. Most jurisdictions in Canada have some form of Good Samaritan legislation. For example, Manitoba, British Columbia, and Ontario have Good Samaritan acts, and Alberta has its *Emergency Medical Aid Act*. Under Québec's *Civil Code*, every citizen must act as a *bon père de famille*, meaning that every person must act wisely and in a reasonable manner to help someone in distress if it does not pose a serious threat to the person. In other words, any person responding to an urgent situation is expected to do so within their scope of practice, knowledge, and level of expertise. A person with no medical training would be held less accountable than would a nurse or a doctor.

---

### THINKING IT THROUGH

#### *The Help of a Good Samaritan*

A person was having a heart attack and an off-duty ICU nurse found them on the ground with no vital signs. The nurse assessed the person and initiated CPR. The person survived the heart attack but suffered a punctured lung as a result of a rib that was broken when the nurse began cardiac compressions. In provinces with a Good Samaritan law, the nurse who came to the aid of person who had the heart attack would likely be protected if that person tried to sue them for causing the broken rib and collapsed lung. What are the Good Samaritan laws in your jurisdiction? Would you be inclined not to start CPR if you were in a similar situation, for fear of litigation?

## Whistleblowing

A **whistleblower** is a current or past employee or member of an organization who reports another's misconduct to people or entities with the power and presumed willingness to take corrective action. A whistleblower may also be a member of the public with no formal ties to an organization. Unfortunately, even when provincial/territorial legislation is in place, whistleblowers often suffer a backlash, such as demotion, suspension, or termination for their efforts. In addition, exclusive of repercussions in their workplace, the person may experience backlash from friends or colleagues outside of the workplace setting. Reprisals can take a heavy toll on the whistleblower socially, financially, physically, and mentally.

Employees who report wrongdoing within their organization to law enforcement officials have some protection under Section 425.1 of the *Criminal Code of Canada* (Criminal Code, 1985). Under this law, it is an offence for employers to threaten, take any type of disciplinary action, or terminate an employee for whistleblowing. It does not protect employees if they report to other sources, for example, the media, but there are cases where other legislation might.

### DID YOU KNOW?

#### *The Whistleblower*

In 2020 (during the COVID-19 pandemic), Mr. Fories, a migrant worker from Mexico working at Scotlynn Farms in Norfolk, Ontario, was fired after going public and speaking to the media about the crowded living conditions on the farm. The case was eventually brought to the Ontario Labour Relations Board under the *Occupational Health and Safety Act*.

After a lengthy hearing, the Board ruled in Mr. Flores' favour, determining that Scotlynn Farms had breached s.50 of the Act when it fired Mr. Flores for raising concerns about health and safety on the farm, ordering compensation for the plaintiff.

Source: Ontario Labour Relations Board. (2020, November 9). *OLRB Case No: 0987-20-UR Health and Safety Reprisal Luis Gabriel Flores Flores, Applicant v Scotlynn Sweetpac Growers Inc., Responding Party.* https://migrantworkersalliance.org/wp-content/uploads/2020/11/Gabriel-Flores-OLRB-Decision_Migrant-Workers-Alliance.pdf

In addition, the federal government provides legislation to protect public servants. The *Public Servants Disclosure Protection Act (PSDPA)* applies to most of the public sector, including government departments and agencies, parent Crown corporations, and the Royal Canadian Mounted Police. Interestingly, excluded are some organizations, such as the Canadian Armed Forces and federal public sector and Crown corporations (Office of the Public Sector Integrity Commissioner of Canada, 2021). At the federal level, investigations concerning reprisals (against a whistleblower) are investigated by a Public Sector Integrity Commissioner and, if they believe there is a legitimate reprisal, the matter is referred to the Public Servants Disclosure Protection Tribunal. Between 2011 and 2021, the Tribunal heard only eight cases. In its current form, the federal legislation places the onus on the whistleblower to prove that the employer has discriminated or otherwise taken action against them—a provision that has drawn criticism from across Canada. In June 2017, a subcommittee in the House of Commons tabled a report recommending significant changes to the Act, providing more protection for whistleblowers.

At the provincial and territorial level, a whistleblower in the public sector in all jurisdictions except the Northwest Territories and Prince Edward Island (legislation in Prince Edward Island was introduced in 2017 but has not been enacted) is protected against retaliation by legislation very similar to the PSDPA. One difference is that statutes at the provincial/territorial level do not provide protection for a whistleblower reporting misconduct by someone employed in the public sector (Del Riccio, 2021).

In general, whistleblowing legislation among jurisdictions in Canada differs depending on the jurisdiction itself as well as the nature and conditions under which the disclosure occurs. A whistleblower program was implemented in Ontario in 2016 (the first of its kind by a Canadian securities regulator), based on a "bounty for tips" initiative, which offers financial rewards (of up to $5 million) to individuals who report corporate wrongdoing.

Along with provincial legislation, individuals may have protection under their provincial or territorial *Occupational Health and Safety Act* regarding violations to enforcement of the rules, regulations, and policies of the organization (SARS Commission, 2005).

Common law also affects whistleblowers in terms of how and what they report and potential reprisals. Under common law, an employee owes their employer the general duties of loyalty, good faith, and, in appropriate circumstances, confidentiality (Public Service Whistleblowing Act, 2002). When an employee breaches these duties by revealing a confidence or some information, believing it is in the public interest, the employer usually takes disciplinary action, which may include dismissal. In the face of such punishment, employees may seek protection from the courts, or if they are governed by a collective agreement, through a grievance procedure.

It is important for a person to be aware that most public organizations have a protocol for someone to follow if they feel they must reveal information they believe to be problematic for those within the organization or to the public. A person must seriously consider all options before blowing the whistle on a person or organization, be sure that they have all the facts, be aware of the protocols they must follow, and, importantly, be prepared for any retaliation or reprisals as a result of their actions.

Because whistleblowing protection varies across the country, many, including those working in health care, may hesitate to report wrongdoing unless they are confident that they will be protected from reprisals. Health care workers, for example, should feel free to alert the proper authorities to such incidents as breaches in infection prevention and control protocols in health care facilities (an ongoing concern during the COVID-19 pandemic), mistreatment of residents or patients in hospitals or long term care facilities, and other information important to protect the health and well-being of others. It has not been uncommon during the pandemic for nurses and other health care workers to blow the whistle on their workplace, speaking anonymously to the media (with their name protected) out of fear of reprisals. In 2020, a personal support worker in Ontario reported that the staff in a long-term care facility were being denied proper personal protective equipment because the facility's administration wanted to stockpile the products in case of a serious outbreak. She claimed that she was not even allowed to use a mask when tending to a patient with a cough (Haines, 2020).

## DID YOU KNOW?

### *Whistleblowing and Canada's Rating*

In March 2021, the Government of Accountability Project (GAP) and the International Bar Association reported the results of a study involving national whistleblowing laws involving 37 countries (Devine, 2016; Nieweler, 2021). Scoring was based out of 20, with each country assigned a score based on international best practices for whistleblower policies established by GAP. Out of the 37 countries, Canada had the lowest score, along with Norway and Lebanon. The highest scores were achieved by the European Union, Australia, and the United States.

Sources: Devine, T. (2016, July 22). *Government Accountability Project.* https://whistleblower.org/international-best-practices-for-whistleblower-policies/; Nieweler, A. (2021, March 29). *Canada's whistleblower law falls last in international rankings.* Whistleblower Security. https://blog.whistleblowersecurity.com/blog/canadas-whistleblower-law-falls-last-in-international-rankings https://blog.whistleblowersecurity.com/blog/canadas-whistleblower-law-falls-last-in-international-rankings

# SUMMARY

8.1  In Canada, various levels of government are authorized to create laws, including constitutional, statutory, regulatory, common, and civil law. Most of these apply to health care in varying degrees. Constitutional law, for example, involves challenges to a person's right to health care that have been based on the *Canadian Charter of Rights and Freedoms*. Tort law is commonly applied when negligent acts on the part of health care workers are proven to occur or because of a compromised standard of care within a health care facility. Criminal law, with a few exceptions, is legislated by the federal government.

8.2  Under the Constitution, jurisdictional authority over some areas of health care is primarily the responsibility of the provincial governments. The federal government provides funding and ensures that the provinces and territories are compliant with the principles and conditions of the *Canada Health Act*. The federal government also has legal authority over spending, issues related to some areas of workplace safety, criminal law (e.g., the regulation and distribution of controlled drugs), and the right to enact federal powers in the event of a national emergency such as during the COVID-19 pandemic under the *Quarantine Act*. Although there are jurisdictional divisions in law, all levels of government work together to address issues such as the current opioid crisis and to continually improve policies and procedures related to the legalization of cannabis.

8.3  As the Canadian health care landscape changes, so do the expectations for our health care system. Many Canadians regard health care as a moral and legal right, even though it is not specifically identified as such in the *Canadian Charter of Rights and Freedoms*. Under a universal health care system, certain health care services are indirectly guaranteed under the *Canada Health Act*. Access to health care services is not always equal, for example, in remote communities. In addition, what is deemed medically necessary is at times subjective, thus a procedure that is covered in one jurisdiction may not be in another. This can sometimes lead to both inequities in and barriers to the type of care people believe they are entitled to. Challenges relating to the right to health care, however, often arise under sections 7 (life, liberty, and security of person) and 15 (equality) of the Charter.

8.4  Canada prohibits its citizens from purchasing private insurance for health care services that are publicly funded (e.g., joint replacement or cardiovascular surgery). The fear is that allowing parallel systems of health care, public and private, will lead to inequities in care and a two-tiered system. Canada has always had a mix of private and public health care, with private services regulated by federal, provincial, and territorial governments. With few exceptions, a service considered medically necessary, theoretically, can be privately purchased. Private health care services have flourished more in some provinces than in others, for example, in Québec; whether it is complementary to or in opposition with the concept of universal health care remains a question. Canadians can buy private insurance for dental care, medications, optometric services, as well as anything not considered medically necessary.

8.5  Consent to treatment is a complicated and sometimes controversial subject. Express consent means that a person gives clear written or verbal consent for a procedure; implied consent can be ambiguous. Most providers now ask for consent even for minor procedures, such as giving immunizations. Also contentious is the right for minors to make their own decisions (legal now in most provinces and territories if the individual is deemed to be a mature minor) and situations wherein parents make decisions for children that contravene what a health care provider deems best or essential.

8.6  Confidentiality, the protection of health information, and consent to treatment are issues covered in some cases by both federal and provincial and territorial legislation. The *Personal Information Protection and Electronic Documents Act (PIPEDA)* federally regulates how organizations may collect, store, and use personal information, including medical records, for commercial purposes. Provinces may displace provisions of this federal legislation by implementing their own similar legislation.

8.7   Almost every major health profession has a regulatory body that governs (or controls) such things as educational standards, provincial, territorial, or national registration, and entry-to-practice requirements for that profession. They also maintain standards of practice and will review complaints against a professional member submitted by the public. Title protection ensures that only qualified professionals can use a designated title, for example, that of a registered nurse. Each profession also has a code of ethics, but such codes are not legally binding.

8.8   Some important legal issues in Canadian health care include the use of restraints, self-discharge from a health care facility, and whistleblowing. A whistleblower is a current or past employee or member of an organization who reports another's misconduct to people or entities with the power and presumed willingness to take corrective action. A whistleblower may also be a member of the public with no formal ties to an organization. Most jurisdictions have their own whistleblowing legislation. Anyone who does decide to blow the whistle must carefully consider the backlash from several sources.

## REVIEW QUESTIONS

1. Under what conditions might the federal government enact emergency powers under the *Quarantine Act?* Give examples in your answer.
2. What is the purpose of occupational health and safety legislation?
3. What are some drug-seeking behaviours to watch for in your profession?
4. Why is an individual's right to health care sometimes contentious?
5. What are two controversial components of the legislation limiting an individual's right to apply for medical assistance in dying?
   a. What were the recent changes to the legislation for medical assistance in dying?
6. Under what circumstances would a health practitioner who owns a private health care facility be in conflict of interest?
7. What are the two types of private clinics operating in Québec?
8. What are three essential criteria for a person to be able to give informed consent?
9. What is a mature minor?
   a. Do you think an age limit should be imposed on giving consent? Justify your answer.
10. What is the purpose of a power of attorney for personal care?
11. How long must a health care provider or facility retain medical records?
12. What is meant by chemical restraints?
13. What are some things a person should consider before blowing the whistle?
14. Explain the whistleblowing legislation in your jurisdiction.
15. What protection does a union offer to an employee member?

## REFERENCES

Canadian Blood Services. (2022). *Organ and tissue donation and transplantation—Privacy notices.* https://blood.ca/en/about-us/organ-and-tissue-donation-and-transplantation.

Canadian Centre on Substance Use and Addiction. (2017). *Joint statement of action to address the opioid crisis: A collective response.* https://www.ccsa.ca/sites/default/files/2019-04/CCSA-Joint-Statement-of-Action-Opioid-Crisis-Annual-Report-2017-en.pdf.

Canadian Centre on Substance Abuse and Addiction. (2022). *Prescription drugs.* https://www.ccsa.ca/Eng/topics/Prescription-Drugs/Pages/default.aspx.

Canadian Charter of Rights and Freedoms. (1982). *Part I of the* constitution act. *1982, being Schedule B to the* Canada act 1982 *(UK) c* (p. 11).

Canadian Institute for Health Information (CIHI). (2021, December 16). *Organ replacement in Canada: CORR annual statistics.* www.cihi.ca/en/organ-replacement-in-canada-corr-annual-statistics#:~:text=Canada's%20living%20donor%20rate%20in,performed%20in%20Canada%20in%202020.

Canadian Medical Association (CMA). (2015). *Harms associated with opioids and other psychoactive prescription drugs.* https://policybase.cma.ca/list?ps=20&q=opioids&p=1.

Canadian Medical Protective Association (CMPA). (2015, March). *When to disclose confidential information.* https://www.cmpa-acpm.ca/en/advice-publications/browse-articles/2015/when-to-disclose-confidential-information#:~:text=The%20CMA's%20Code%20of%20Ethics,%2C%20to%20the%20patients%20themselves.%E2%80%9D.

Canadian Medical Protective Association (CMPA). (2021, April). *Consent: A guide for Canadian physicians.* https://www.cmpa-acpm.ca/en/advice-publications/handbooks/consent-a-guide-for-canadian-physicians#:~:text=For%20consent%20to%20treatment%20to,risks%20involved%20and%20alternatives%20available.

Canadian Medical Protective Association (CMPA). (2022, February). *How to manage your medical records: Retention, access, security, storage, disposal, and transfer.* https://www.cmpa-acpm.ca/en/advice-publications/browse-articles/2003/a-matter-of-records-retention-and-transfer-of-clinical-records#:~:text=10%20years%20from%20the%20date,if%20some%20conditions%20are%20met.

Canadian Press. (2018, April 9). *Organ donation by Humboldt Broncos player inspires others.* CBC News. https://www.cbc.ca/news/canada/calgary/humboldt-broncos-organ-donation-increase-1.4612143.

College of Physicians and Surgeons of Ontario (CSPO). (2020, May). *Consent to treatment.* https://www.cpso.on.ca/Physicians/Policies-Guidance/Policies/Consent-to-Treatment.

Constitution Act. (1982). *1982, being schedule B to the* Canada act *1982 (UK).* c. 11, s. 92 http://laws-lois.justice.gc.ca/eng/CONST/INDEX.HTML.

*Controlled Drugs and Substances Act* (S.C. 1996, c.19). Last amended 21 June 2018. https://laws-lois.justice.gc.ca/eng/acts/C-38.8/FullText.html

Crew, I. (2018, June 28). *Federal/provincial power and pot:* How constitutional distribution of power affects deregulation. *Queen's certificate in law. Blog post.* https://certificate.queenslaw.ca/blog/federal-provincial-power-and-pot-how-constitutional-distribution-of-power-affects-deregulation.

Criminal Code. R.S.C. (1985). c. C-46 as amended https://laws-lois.justice.gc.ca/eng/acts/c-46/.

Del Riccio, J. (2021, May 25). *Employee whistleblower protections in the time of COVID-19.* Canadian Bar Association. www.cba.org/Sections/Labour-Employment/Articles/2021/Employee-whistleblower-protections-in-the-time-of#:~:text=Section%2019%20states%20simply%20%E2%80%9Cno,are%20not%20themselves%20public%20servants.

Devine, T. (2016, July 22). *Government accountability project.* https://whistleblower.org/international-best-practices-for-whistleblower-policies/.

Government of Canada. (2018a). *Prevention: Canadian drugs and substances strategy.* https://www.canada.ca/en/health-canada/services/substance-use/canadian-drugs-substances-strategy/prevention.html.

Government of Canada. (2018b). *Legalizing and strictly regulating cannabis: The facts.* https://www.canada.ca/en/services/health/campaigns/legalizing-strictly-regulating-cannabis-facts.html.

Government of Canada. (2020, August 11). *Illegal marketing of prescription drugs.* https://www.canada.ca/en/health-canada/services/drugs-health-products/marketing-drugs-devices/illegal-marketing/prescription-drugs.html.

Government of Canada. (2021, July 7). *Cannabis legalization and regulation.* https://www.justice.gc.ca/eng/cj-jp/cannabis/.

Government of Canada. (2022a). *Cannabis laws and regulations.* https://www.canada.ca/en/health-canada/services/drugs-medication/cannabis/laws-regulations.html.

Government of Canada. (2022b). *Medical assistance in dying.* https://www.canada.ca/en/health-canada/services/medical-assistance-dying.html.

Haines, A. (2020, March 31). *Whistleblower says workers at nursing homes aren't being given protective gear.* CTV News. https://www.ctvnews.ca/health/coronavirus/whistleblower-says-workers-at-nursing-homes-aren-t-being-given-protective-gear-1.4877005.

Health Law Institute, Dalhousie University. (n.d.) *End of life law & policy in Canada: Advance directives.* http://eol.law.dal.ca/?page_id=231.

Nieweler, A. (2021, March 29). *Canada's whistleblower law falls last in international rankings. Whistleblower Security.* https://blog.whistleblowersecurity.com/blog/canadas-whistleblower-law-falls-last-in-international-rankings. https://blog.whistleblowersecurity.com/blog/canadas-whistleblower-law-falls-last-in-international-rankings.

Office of the Conflict of Interest and Ethics Commissioner. (2014, April 1). *Overview of the conflict of interest act.* https://ciec-ccie.parl.gc.ca/en/publications/Pages/CoIA-LCI.aspx.

Office of the Privacy Commissioner of Canada. (2015, December). *The application of PIPEDA to municipalities, universities, schools, and hospitals.* https://priv.gc.ca/en/privacy-topics/privacy-laws-in-canada/the-personal-information-protection-and-electronic-documents-act-pipeda/r_o_p/02_05_d_25/.

Office of the Privacy Commissioner of Canada. (2018, January). *Summary of privacy laws in Canada.* https://www.priv.gc.ca/en/privacy-topics/privacy-laws-in-canada/02_05_d_15/.

Office of the Privacy Commissioner of Canada. (2020, May). *Provincial laws that may apply instead of PIPEDA.* https://www.priv.gc.ca/en/privacy-topics/privacy-laws-in-canada/the-personal-information-protection-and-electronic-documents-act-pipeda/r_o_p/prov-pipeda/.

Office of the Privacy Commissioner of Canada. (2021, August 13). *Guidelines for obtaining meaningful consent.* https://www.priv.gc.ca/en/privacy-topics/collecting-personal-information/consent/gl_omc_201805/.

Office of the Public Sector Integrity Commissioner. (2021, June 30). *The public servants disclosure protection act.* https://psic-ispc.gc.ca/en/public-servants-disclosure-protection-act.

Public Service Health Care Plan Administration Authority. (n.d.). *About the PSHCP.* https://www.pshcp.ca/about-the-pshcp/.

*Quarantine Act* (S.C. 2005, c.20). https://discussions.justice.gc.ca/eng/AnnualStatutes/2005_20/.

SARS Commission. (2005, April 5). *7. Whistleblower protection. The SARS commission second interim report: SARS and public health legislation.* The honorable Mr. Justice Archie Campbell, Commissioner http://www.archives.gov.on.ca/en/e_records/sars/report/v5-pdf/Vol5Chp7.pdf.

Standing Senate Committee on Human Rights. (2021, June). *Forced and coerced sterilization of persons in Canada.* https://sencanada.ca/content/sen/committee/432/RIDR/Reports/2021-06-03_ForcedSterilization_E.pdf.

Standing Senate Committee on Human Rights. (2022, July). *The scars that we carry: Forced and coerced sterilization of persons in Canada — Part II.* https://sencanada.ca/content/sen/committee/441/RIDR/reports/2022-07-14_ForcedSterilization_E.pdf.

Statistics Canada. (2021, January 13). *Leading indicator of international arrivals to Canada by air, fourth quarter 2020. The Daily.* https://www150.statcan.gc.ca/n1/daily-quotidien/210113/dq210113c-eng.htm.

Supreme Court of Canada. (2015). *Judgment in appeal. Carter et al v. Attorney general of Canada,* 2015 SCC 5 https://scc-csc.lexum.com/scc-csc/news/en/item/4815/index.do?r=AAAAAQAjY2FydGVyIHYuIGNhbmFkYSAoYXR0b3JuZXkgZ2VuZXJhbCkB.

Watts, M., Austin, M., & Mack, A. (2017). *Cannabis in 2017: Setting the stage for legalization.* www.mondaq.com/canada/x/659326/food+drugs+law/Cannabis+in+2017+Setting+the+stage+for +legalization.

World Health Organization. (2008, January 1). *International health regulations (2005).* https://www.who.int/publications/i/item/9789241580410.

Zimonjic, P. (2022 July 14). *Senate report calls for law criminalizing forced or coerced sterilization.* CBC News. https://www.cbc.ca/news/politics/senate-report-forced-coerced-sterilization-1.6520592.

Zingel, A. (2019, April 18). *Indigenous women come forward with accounts of forced sterilization, says lawyer.* CBC News. https://www.cbc.ca/news/canada/north/forced-sterilization-lawsuit-could-expand-1.5102981.

# Ethics and Health Care

## LEARNING OUTCOMES

9.1  Define relevant ethical terms.
9.2  Discuss five significant ethical theories that shape health care decisions.
9.3  Explain the ethical principles that are important to the health care provider.
9.4  Summarize the rights that Canadians have with respect to health care.
9.5  Describe ethical behaviour expected of health care providers.
9.6  Explain ethical considerations relating to end-of-life issues.
9.7  Discuss issues relating to the allocation of resources in health care.
9.8  Briefly debate the ethics around abortion, genetic testing, and genome editing technology.

## KEY TERMS

| | | |
|---|---|---|
| Advance directive | Ethical principles | Involuntary euthanasia |
| Autonomy | Ethical theory | Paternalism |
| Beneficence | Ethics | Rights in health care |
| Compassionate | Fidelity | Role fidelity |
| interference | Fiduciary relationship | Self-determination |
| Continuity of care | Medical assistance in | Teleological theory |
| Deontological theory | dying (MAiD) | Values |
| Divine command ethics | Morality | Values history form |
| Double effect | Morals | Virtue ethics |
| Duties | Nonmaleficence | Voluntary euthanasia |

Health care providers are held to a high level of accountability because the personal and sensitive nature of health care demands it. Entering a health care profession means entering into a moral and ethical contract with patients, peers, and other members of the health care team. A person must employ the highest standards of professionalism and ethical behaviour and make a commitment to excellence in practising in one's chosen field. Anyone entering the health care field must respect the rights, thoughts, and actions of patients; advocate for them; put aside biases; and assist patients in their quest to achieve wellness. Finally, health care providers must work collaboratively with all health care team members, respecting their areas of expertise and scopes of practice.

Ethical decisions made in the same or similar situation by different people may vary based on their own moral ethical codes. This chapter briefly outlines four ethical theories that form the basis for most ethical decisions. Recognizing the perspective from which a person makes an ethical decision helps those who disagree with the decision to show tolerance. It is important to realize that understanding and supporting the patient does not require one to compromise one's own beliefs and values.

Health care providers have a duty to adhere to six **ethical principles** that have particular relevance to the health care profession. This chapter addresses these principles from the perspective of clinical and administrative practice, emphasizing the importance of ethical behaviour, professionalism, and patient **autonomy**.

## WHAT IS ETHICS?

Ethics is the study of standards of right and wrong in human behaviour—that is, how people ought to behave, considering rights and obligations, as well as virtues such as fairness, loyalty, and honesty. Various systems, approaches, and conceptual frameworks deal with how human actions are judged. Ethics involves examining the criteria we use to determine which actions are right or wrong.

Ethics also involves values, **duties**, and moral issues. Ethics is neither religion nor determined by religion—if it were, nonreligious persons would be considered unethical. Ethics also remains separate from the law, although ethical and legal issues are at times closely connected. Ethical choices do not always fit with what is legal, and things that may be legal—or legal decisions—are not always ethical. Moreover, being ethical does not mean following social norms; behaviour considered ethical in one society may be deemed unethical in another. For example, homosexuality is not tolerated (considered either unlawful or unethical or both) in countries such as Russia, Iran, Saudi Arabia, Indonesia, Algeria, and Libya, to name only a few. Polygamy is deemed by most people in North America to be immoral, and for the most part it is illegal. Yet in some regions of the world, including regions in the Middle East, Asia, and parts of Africa, it is both legal and morally acceptable. Abortion is legal in Canada, yet many would consider abortion unethical and immoral; it is legal in some parts of the United States and not in others, where it is thought to also be deeply unethical and immoral, even in cases of rape (discussed later in this chapter).

The term *ethics* also refers to a code of behaviour or conduct. Our behaviour reflects our belief system, which is shaped by many factors, including how we are parented, our home environment, and societal factors such as religion, friends, and school. Our ethical viewpoints are continually influenced by events and experiences and change over time. Ethical standards are influenced by **morals**, values, and a sense of duty—all elements critical to ethical practice in health care.

### Morality and Morals

Almost always linked to ethics, **morality** extends from a system of beliefs about what is right and wrong. It encompasses a person's values, beliefs, and sense of duty and responsibility and can extend to those actions a person believes are right or wrong. Morals are what a person believes to be right and wrong regarding how to treat others and how to behave in an organized society. For example, a person may have a moral belief that one must always tell the truth, regardless of the consequences. Someone else might believe that to be untruthful if it spares someone pain and does not hurt anyone is a moral action.

Morals can be said to define a person's character. Ethics can be described as an individual's *collection* of morals. More broadly, ethics is a social system in which a collection of morals from a number of people are applied. As a professional code of conduct, ethics encompasses the morality and moral beliefs of the profession. People bring their own moral code to their profession; it influences how they behave as professionals and the degree to which they honour their profession's code of ethics. That said, there are individuals who have a different code of ethics that applies to their professional life, and one that is different in their personal lives, although inevitably there are basic similarities.

The differences between morals and ethics are subtle and may be best illustrated by an example. Suppose the Taylors' infant son was born with a condition considered incompatible with life. At best he only had a few days to live. He would likely die of respiratory failure or have a cardiac arrest. The Taylors and their physician have agreed to apply a do-not-resuscitate (DNR) order. In addition, the parents declined interventions that might modestly lengthen the baby's life, for example, intravenous hydration and oxygen. Amy, a registered nurse working in the neonatal intensive care unit, does not morally agree with the decision, believing that all attempts to save or just prolong the infant's life should be taken. However, ethically (i.e., out of respect for the parent's choice and their autonomy), Amy must abide by the decision the parents and the doctor have made and refrain from initiating CPR should she be present if the baby has a cardiac arrest or from intervening by hydrating the baby or giving him oxygen. That said, there are times when a care provider might object so strongly to a decision that a patient and the family have made that the provider feels they cannot abide by a decision they disagree with. In such cases, most facilities allow the care provider to remove themselves from that person's circle of care.

Health care providers who understand their own values and moral standards come better prepared to deal with issues that may arise in their professional role. Moreover, they typically possess a better sense of their commitment to practise in an ethical manner.

Many grey areas exist in ethics and in beliefs regarding what is morally right or wrong. Often, no *absolute* right or wrong exists, and the health care provider's personal beliefs may affect how they deal with difficult situations or react to patients. Understanding and feeling comfortable with one's own beliefs in such areas can make accepting the decisions of others easier. Morally charged topics include the right to die, withholding treatment, DNR orders, withholding information from a patient, and interfering with the patient's right to self-determination—the freedom to make their own decisions. However, not all topics are that intense.

Less dramatic moral issues are more common and are as follows: Is it proper to accept a gift from a patient, or will the act bind a health care worker to providing the patient with preferential treatment? Is it morally acceptable to cover up a medication error that did not cause harm to a patient? Is it acceptable for a health care provider to chart care not given because they were so busy that there was time only to do the basics but feared repercussions if their supervisor found out that some components of care were not rendered? Is it OK to take hospital supplies home for personal use as long as there are plenty left for those that need them? Is it morally acceptable to treat a patient disrespectfully or tell a colleague something you were asked to keep in confidence? Is it acceptable to take pencils or pens home from the clinic you work in, or use the photocopier after hours for your son's school project? How one decides what is acceptable and unacceptable behaviour will depend on their moral code and values. The common denominator with respect to some of the previous situations is that there is plenty to go around and no one is disadvantaged. At school, is it OK to copy someone's assignment? Is it OK to get someone else to complete a project for you? Is it OK to cheat on an exam? Is it OK to shun another student because you don't like them on cultural or religious grounds?

## Values

Values, beliefs important to an individual, guide a person's conduct and the decisions they make. People can have personal values, social values, and workplace or professional values. A person who greatly values friendship may consider their relationship with a particular person more important than, for example, a material object. And although a person may value friendship in general, one friend may be more valued than another. Context may also influence values and, therefore, behaviour (Case Example 9.1).

### CASE EXAMPLE 9.1    T.C. and the Value of Work versus School

T.C., an occupational therapy student, has a part-time job as an orderly. T.C. clearly values professional conduct at work more than personal conduct at school. At work, they maintain an excellent attendance record, are never late, and do their job well. However, at school, T.C. talks in class, frequently texts on their cell phone, hands in assignments late, and has poor attendance—especially on Friday afternoons. T.C. also often misses a day of classes prior to an exam or test. T.C. may place more importance on work for several reasons, including earning money for rent and other amenities. T.C. may not (at least not yet) value education or see it as a means to an end—establishing a career and becoming financially secure.

In health care, particular value is placed on certain virtues—truthfulness (*veracity*), respect for others, empathy, compassion, competency, responsibility, and the right to autonomy and to proper medical care. For example, one cannot effectively establish therapeutic relationships with patients or trusting relationships with colleagues without truthfulness (the foundation for trust) and respect for others. A nurse or a dental assistant may not particularly "like" their team leader or supervisor for any given reason as a person, but may value their managerial and organizational skills. Suppose R., a respiratory therapist, had a friend, J., who was also a colleague. If J. broke a confidence by telling R. something another friend had asked them not to disclose, what would R. think? Could R. trust J. either as a friend or at work regarding the disclosure of patient information?

### THINKING IT THROUGH

#### *A.V.'s Vaccination Status*

A.V. was invited to a friend's house for dinner. When asked, A.V. assured these friends that they were fully vaccinated against COVID-19, but A.V. was unvaccinated and went anyway, knowing there was someone who was immunocompromised in the household. The host found out that A.V. was unvaccinated a couple of days later. When confronted, A.V.'s response was that it was "no big deal" and that they had no COVID-related symptoms anyway. Some people might not think this is a problem, depending on their view on the value of vaccinations. Even the fact that A.V. was untruthful might not be considered an issue given the circumstances.

1. What do you think of A.V.'s actions?
2. Which part of this situation is more problematic—the fact that A.V. went to the gathering unvaccinated or that they lied about it? Or both?

### Duty

Duties often arise from others' claims. If a patient depends on you (i.e., has a claim on you) for your professional services, you have a duty, or obligation, to deliver these services. As a member of the health care profession, you also have a duty to behave in an ethical, moral, and competent manner. Alternatively, duties may be self-imposed. For example, a person who values honesty will make it their duty to be truthful.

Health care providers, by the very nature of the field they work in, have a moral and ethical duty to care for their patients in a competent manner, in addition to a legal obligation, called the "duty of care." As discussed in Chapter 8, the legal component of this duty requires health care providers to provide patients with a reasonable standard of care in accordance with their profession's standards of practice. In terms of a moral obligation, health care providers are expected to provide care even in situations that may threaten their own lives or health; however, they may not be legally bound to do so.

---

**THINKING IT THROUGH**

### The Duty of Care

In Canada, the United States, and across Europe there have been numerous incidents recorded of health care providers in long-term care facilities fleeing their workplace amid an outbreak of the coronavirus, leaving the residents all but unattended. In one case, two nurses were left caring for residents in a 150-bed private long-term care facility. Residents were found in deplorable conditions, some of whom had died. These actions clearly are in opposition to the duty of care.

1. Do you think the care providers gave thought to the duty of care before they left?
2. Do you think they were justified? Explain your answer.
3. What problems do you think these care providers were dealing with that may have exacerbated their decisions to leave?
4. What do you think you would do in a similar situation? Justify your answer.

---

## ETHICAL THEORIES: THE BASICS

Health care providers face making ethical decisions that affect them individually, other members of the health care team, as well as their patients. They also face exposure to ethical situations in which decisions made by others may affect them, perhaps not directly, but emotionally.

An ethical theory guides people toward making an ethical decision. The discussion of ethical theories that follows, although not in-depth, will help you see how some individuals make difficult decisions.

### Teleological Theory

Teleological theory, also referred to as *consequence-based theory of the ends theory*, defines an action as right or wrong depending on the results it produces. Theoretically, the "right" action brings about the most benefit for the most people. Consider Case Example 9.2, which, although it seems extreme, is a true story.

In Case Example 9.2, to say nothing becomes the group's ethical decision. The individuals involved determine what they thought would be the best result and made their decision accordingly. Of less importance to them was that by choosing this action, they would conceal the truth (not to mention the legal implications of their decision—by law, a patient must be told when a medical error has occurred). Applying teleological theory, the decision brings about the best outcomes for the most people (sparing the patient and the family pain). However, one could argue that a decision to tell the truth would bring out the best outcome for the most people: telling the truth, preserving trust, and saving those involved in the decision from possible litigation. What would you do?

---

### CASE EXAMPLE 9.2   Making an Ethical Decision

P.K., a 68-year-old patient, had surgery for lung cancer. It was discovered that the cancer had spread to several other organs. The surgeon closed without any intervention. P.K.'s prognosis was limited to a few weeks at best. Post-surgery it was discovered that a small sponge was left inside the patient. The staff members present, along with an operating room technician, decided it was in everyone's best interests to say nothing. Considering the alternatives, the decision was based on the fact that the sponge would not hurt P.K., but opening them up and removing it could hasten their death and cause them more pain. Another consideration was the fact that the family, already trying to cope with P.K.'s impending death, would be distressed over the incident. Also considered: it was a simple mistake—why get the surgeon and nurses in trouble?

---

### Deontological Theory

*Deontology* developed from the word *duty*. In the case of deontological theory, a moral and honest action is taken, regardless of the outcome. If in Case Example 9.2 the team had used a deontological approach and did the "right" thing, they would have removed the sponge, or they would have told the family what had happened, explained the risks, and allowed them to make the decision. In this scenario, one could argue that following "duty" ethics and teleological theory could result in the same conclusion (depending on the choice as to which decision brought about the most good for the most people, using either theory).

In this case, the truth soon became evident, as all members of the operating room team did not feel comfortable with the initial decision to conceal it. They were aware of the legal implications and felt that honesty, despite consequences, was the best policy. The family appreciated the honesty, recognized that a mistake had been made, decided to leave the sponge where it was, and were thankful to the team for coming forward. There was an investigation into the incident by the hospital. No charges or disciplinary action resulted, but steps were taken to put additional safeguards in place to reduce or eliminate the chances of this incident from recurring.

### Virtue Ethics

Virtue ethics looks at the ethical character of the person making the decision, rather than at their reasoning. This theory operates under the belief that a person of moral character will act wisely, fairly, and honestly and will uphold the principles of justice. Therefore, virtue ethics, unlike teleological and deontological theories, does not provide guidelines for decision making.

In Case Example 9.2, several people were present for the post-surgery discovery. Person A may have decided that it would be best not to divulge the incident about the sponge, whereas Person B may have decided that the incident must be exposed. Each person would make an individual decision based on their own set of values and morals. However, a common decision must often be reached. When people disagree about the course of action to take, sometimes the majority will rule; other times, one person may have the authority to make a call. However, each person should still feel comfortable with their own actions, because each person might have to take responsibility for such actions. In the case example, individuals following the principles of virtue ethics may believe that the surgeon has high moral principles and therefore will refrain from questioning the surgeon's decision. In addition, they may believe that loyalty to the surgeon is a virtue. Then again, the act is both illegal and contrary to hospital policy, so these individuals may take a personal risk by complying with the decision not to report the incident. Ultimately, each person must weigh the situation, determine to whom they owe the greater loyalty, and decide according to their own conscience.

## Divine Command

The most rigid ethical theory, divine command ethics, follows philosophies and rules set out by a higher power. For example, Christians must live by the Bible's Ten Commandments, a list of religious-based moral laws. Muslims follow the rules outlined in the Koran, such as maintaining a just society and engaging in "appropriate" human relationships. In Case Example 9.2, followers of divine command ethics would without question decide that the incident should be reported because honesty makes up an essential part of the divine command theory.

---

### THINKING IT THROUGH

#### *Withholding the Truth From a Patient*

Dr. K. decides not to reveal to J.V. (an older patient who lives in a long-term care facility with no relatives or emotional support system) the nature of their illness—amyotrophic lateral sclerosis (ALS)—until they becomes more clinically symptomatic. This is a disease that causes progressive paralysis, eventually leading to the inability to swallow or breathe. Dr. K. believes this course of action will spare J.V. unnecessary grief, at least in the short term.

1. Is Dr. K. justified in not telling J.V. about this condition and the prognosis?
2. Would it make any difference if J.V. had family or friends to support them?
3. What ethical theory do you think Dr. K is following? Explain why.
4. What decision would you have come to? Why? Based on what theory?

---

## ETHICAL PRINCIPLES AND THE HEALTH CARE PROFESSION

Common to all ethical theories, ethical principles—acceptable standards of human behaviour—provide guidance for decision making and therefore form the basis of ethical study. Ethical principles can be personal or professional in nature. In the best-case scenario, individuals practise similar principles in both their personal and professional lives. Personal principles predominantly guide a person's actions and form the foundation from which professional principles evolve. People who believe in showing kindness and helping those in need in their personal life will likely do the same in their professional life. Those with an uncaring, indifferent attitude toward others in their personal life may or may not be able to show genuine caring, support, or respect, be patient, or give adequate care to a patient.

Outlined below are a number of ethical principles that lend themselves particularly well to health care. These important elements of ethical decision making almost always appear in the codes of ethics adopted by health care professions.

### Beneficence and Nonmaleficence

The foundation of health care ethics, beneficence refers to showing kindness to or doing good for others. No matter what ethical theory is used, beneficence guides the process toward a morally right outcome. Often treated as a separate principle from beneficence, nonmaleficence refers specifically to causing no harm, whereas beneficence encompasses the duties to prevent harm and to remove harm when possible. All health care providers have a duty to do good, to prevent harm, and to not cause harm. Criteria related to what causes harm have shifted over the past few years, perhaps more so since the legalization of medical assistance in dying (MAiD). Is assisting a person who has chosen MAiD to die causing harm? Some would say, yes, it is. Others would disagree with that (discussed later).

Similar to beneficence, the principle of double effect requires a person to choose the option that achieves the most favourable outcome or that causes the least harm. When secondary and potentially negative outcomes or side effects can be predicted, these must not be the intended outcome of the action. For example, A.B., who has terminal cancer, takes high doses of morphine sulphate controlled-release (MS Contin), which has proven to be the only means of controlling the pain. However, A.B. now experiences respiratory distress (respiratory depression is a known adverse effect of MS Contin), which could well hasten the patient's death. Despite this, making A.B. comfortable is considered ethically and morally the action of choice. It could well be that the family are in favour of using the medication despite this adverse effect, believing that, at this point, death would be a relief for the patient. If cognizant, the patient might agree as well.

### Respect

Another key ethical principle is respect. All patients have the right to be treated with respect by those who care for them. Health care providers and their colleagues also have the right to be treated with respect by patients as well as by those they work with. Respecting others involves honouring their right to autonomy, being truthful, not withholding information, and honouring their decisions, whether stemming from personal, religious, cultural, or societal influences. All too often, respect is absent when bias and racism enter into a situation. See the cases of Brian Sinclair and Joyce Eschaquan (discussed later) for examples.

### Autonomy

*Autonomy* comes from the Greek *autos*, meaning "self," and *nomos*, meaning "governance." The ethical principle of autonomy underscores a person's right to self-determination. Autonomy recognizes the right of a mentally competent individual, given all of the relevant facts, to make independent decisions without coercion (i.e., pressure or force).

The principle of autonomy serves as the basis for the principles involved in informed consent and self-determination regarding treatment choices. Patients must be mentally capable and fully informed about their situation to be able to make autonomous and knowledgeable decisions about their health care (see Chapter 8). It falls on the health care provider to ensure that patients have the appropriate information, to help patients understand the information, and to answer patients' questions regarding their situation. Patients also have the right to seek a second opinion. Often patients will ask the provider for input, advice, or recommendations regarding what to do when a decision has to be made, even in relatively low-risk situations. For example, J.O.'s doctor explained some treatment options regarding minor surgery. J.O. understood the choices, but asked the doctor, "If it were your partner, what would you do?" How do you think the doctor should answer?

The move to patient-centred care supporting the patient's right to autonomy has resulted in the creation of a contemporary version of the Hippocratic Oath that remains more aligned with modern concepts, philosophies, and practices, including medical aid in dying (Box 9.1). Although this oath is associated with physicians, it reflects values and ethical implications that impact all health care providers.

### Fidelity

The principle of fidelity—faithfulness or loyalty—requires health care providers to adhere to their professional codes of ethics and the principles that define their roles and scopes of practice, and also to fulfill their responsibilities to patients by practising their skills competently. The term *fidelity* comes from a Latin root word meaning "to be faithful." Fidelity, therefore, requires faithfulness and loyalty to patients, colleagues, and employers (Case Example 9.3). Health care providers are also expected to uphold the rules and policies of the organization (or person) for which they work. In the workplace, role fidelity becomes an

## BOX 9.1 A Modern Version of the Hippocratic Oath

I swear to fulfill, to the best of my ability and judgement, this covenant:

I will respect the hard-won scientific gains of those physicians in whose steps I walk, and gladly share such knowledge as is mine with those who are to follow.

I will apply, for the benefit of the sick, all measures [that] are required, avoiding those twin traps of over-treatment and therapeutic nihilism.

I will remember that there is art to medicine as well as science, and that warmth, sympathy, and understanding may outweigh the surgeon's knife or the chemist's drug.

I will not be ashamed to say "I know not," nor will I fail to call in my colleagues when the skills of another are needed for a patient's recovery.

I will respect the privacy of my patients, for their problems are not disclosed to me that the world may know. Most especially must I tread with care in matters of life and death. If it is given me to save a life, all thanks. But it may also be within my power to take a life; this awesome responsibility must be faced with great humbleness and awareness of my own frailty. Above all, I must not play at God.

I will remember that I do not treat a fever chart, a cancerous growth, but a sick human being, whose illness may affect the person's family and economic stability. My responsibility includes these related problems, if I am to care adequately for the sick.

I will prevent disease whenever I can, for prevention is preferable to cure.

I will remember that I remain a member of society, with special obligations to all my fellow human beings, those sound of mind and body, as well as the infirm.

If I do not violate this oath, may I enjoy life and art, and be respected while I live and remembered with affection thereafter. May I always act so as to preserve the finest traditions of my calling and may I long experience the joy of healing those who seek my help.

Written in 1964 by Louis Lasagna, Academic Dean of the School of Medicine at Tufts University. Source: Nova Online. (n.d.). *The Hippocratic Oath: Modern version.* http://www.pbs.org/wgbh/nova/doctors/oath_modern.html

## CASE EXAMPLE 9.3 Fidelity

A manager of a number of urgent care clinics is on a bus and overhears a conversation between two young people in the seat in front of them. "That clinic is the worst," says one. "They expect me to do everything they ask, and they want it done, like, yesterday."

"Yeah," responds the other, "I know what you mean. I bet you hate working there. It sounds like that manager is a real dragon. I'd never go to that clinic—unless I was dying and there was nowhere else to go!"

What do you think the manager should do? Clearly the principle of fidelity was not one that the staff member was adhering to.

important ethical principle for health care providers as they work to honour patients' wishes and to earn the trust essential to the professional–patient relationship. In some settings, health care providers may be asked to assume different responsibilities that they are not happy about. Depending on the situation, they may have to weigh what they want to do with their professional obligations or duties and the concept of fidelity to their employer.

**THINKING IT THROUGH**

*Professional Obligations or Personal Choice?*

You work in a large acute care hospital, in a transplant unit that is fairly far removed from where patients with COVID-19 are admitted, and at the other end of the hospital from the Intensive Care Unit (ICU), which is functioning beyond capacity with COVID-19 patients on ventilators. When you arrive at work one morning, your manager tells you that you have been transferred to the ICU because of staff shortages. Would you carry out your professional responsibilities because it is your duty to do so, or would you refuse go? What factors would you consider when making your decision?

## Justice

The principle of justice applies, in one way or another, to most ethical situations. In health care, for example, it raises questions such as the following: Do all patients get the appropriate (i.e., just) treatment? Are health care resources fairly distributed? Are the patient's rights honoured? The three main types of justice are distributive, compensatory, and procedural. *Distributive justice* deals with the proper and equitable distribution of health care resources (the allocation of resources). Distribution may not be equal, because it is prioritized and based on need. Distribution of resources may also be inequitable because of geography, such as that experienced by Indigenous people in remote communities or for people living in a rural area (e.g., there is a shortage of doctors and other health care services). *Compensatory justice* relates to the paying of compensation for wrongs done. For example, in June 2022, all provinces and territories agreed to a $150 million settlement of a class action lawsuit with Purdue Pharma, the money to be used to recover health care costs related to the sale and marketing of opioid and opioid-related medication such as oxycodone (Charlebois, 2022). *Procedural justice* points to acting in a fair and impartial manner (e.g., seeing patients on a first-come, first-served basis, or seeing patients on the basis of the seriousness of their complaint; not giving preferential treatment to a friend).

The *Canada Health Act* entitles all Canadians to equal access to prepaid health care and physician and hospital services. However, with resources stretched to their limits and long waiting lists for many services, equal access is compromised, along with other principles of the Act. Health care providers must do what they can to provide the best services to their patients with the resources they have (see Chapter 1).

Health care providers must practise within the boundaries of the law and report any actions that break the law or compromise the health or safety of a patient. Most organizations set up a process for reporting unethical or illegal behaviour. It is important to learn this process and to follow it, no matter whom—an employer, a peer, or a superior—one finds acting unethically. By simply having knowledge of an illegal or immoral act and not reporting it, a person may be considered guilty in the matter. Consequences can range from a tarnished professional and personal reputation to legal action and patient harm. In Case Example 9.2, the operating room technician may disagree with the decision not to report the missing sponge, and by not reporting it they could share the guilt in any ensuing legal action.

## Veracity/Truthfulness

The principle of truthfulness impacts all other health care principles. Truthfulness (also referred to as *veracity*), a valued principle that patients should expect of a health care provider, contributes to building a bond of trust vital to any patient—health care provider relationship (called a fiduciary relationship). Without this bond an effective relationship is all but impossible. Withholding or distorting the truth on the part of any member of the health care team is rarely justifiable, shows disrespect, and works against a person's autonomy and rights. This is particularly so in circumstances when the patient feels that the care provider or other members of the health care team retains a position of power over them because they rely on these health professionals for their care. If a patient views their provider as an authority figure, they may not feel free to express concerns about their diagnosis and treatment plan, whether they trust the provider or not. They may relinquish their right to autonomy in being participatory in their own care.

Expecting that others will be truthful and honest is central to trust, even in our daily lives. The patient-focused (not provider-focused) approach to treatment requires providers to keep the patient fully and truthfully informed. Denying information to patients, giving them incomplete information, or deceiving them causes more harm than good in most situations.

Being truthful supports the key ethical principles of respect, autonomy, fidelity, justice, beneficence, and nonmaleficence. Acting with beneficence involves doing only what is proper and right. Refraining from doing harm is nonmaleficence, and autonomy is the right to self-determination. It is necessary to tell the truth to uphold these principles and to adhere to the concept of duty, which is central to health care ethics.

Truthfulness is necessary to build and maintain trust among colleagues and others with whom one works, regardless of the nature of the professional relationship. If a nurse cannot trust other nurses, a respiratory therapist, an administrative assistant, a member of the dietary staff, or the maintenance staff in a hospital (and vice versa), that relationship is compromised. The same holds true for those working in a doctor's office, clinic, or any other workplace setting. There is a certain amount of interdependence among health care workers that depends on honesty and trust that each person will be accountable and responsible and work within their scope of practice, maintaining the ethical code of their profession.

---

### THINKING IT THROUGH

#### M.P. and a Partial Truth

M.P. has a serious illness, but a treatment option that will potentially cure their illness is available. Their doctor tells them about the treatment, but fearing M.P. may decide to refuse the treatment, the doctor does not elaborate, minimizing the seriousness of the adverse effects that M.P. will likely experience.

1. Do you think the physician is showing respect for M.P.? Explain your answer.
2. What ethical principles has the physician breached?
3. How might the doctor have otherwise approached M.P. about the treatment?

---

## RIGHTS IN HEALTH CARE

*Rights* are entitlements or things that can and should be expected of health care providers and the health care system. Rights may be tangible (real, something measurable, physical, e.g., the right to see a specialist covered under the provincial or territorial plan) or intangible (something one cannot see or touch or is not easily measurable, such as treating a patient with respect).

Numerous moral controversies surround rights in health care, such as the right to die, the right to self-determination, the rights of a fetus, the rights of women to abortion (discussed at the end of this chapter), the right to be treated with respect and fairness regardless of one's race, religion, culture, socioeconomic status, or sexual orientation, and the rights of an individual to health care.

Patients' rights in Canada are vaguely addressed in the *Canadian Charter of Rights and Freedoms*. They are also outlined in the *Canada Health Act*, and although theoretically guaranteed equally across the country, variations occur in each province and territory. All Canadians have explicit rights to health care itself and to certain rights within the system, such as care within a reasonable time frame (discussed below). Other rights that are more vague have been challenged under the Charter—for example, the right to medical aid in dying, although legal for those who meet established criteria, is not comprehensive enough for many and too broad for others (see Chapter 8). Rights *within* health care, established in law in most provinces and territories, include patients' right to their own medical records, the right to confidentiality concerning their health affairs, and the right to informed consent. Intangible rights are more vague, such as the right to unbiased, respectful, competent health care. This right has been blatantly disregarded in numerous circumstances, with occurrences within some facilities demonstrating outright racism (Box 9.2 describes the

---

### BOX 9.2   Respect, Rights, and Racism Within the Health Care System

There are numerous incidents of racism involving health care and Indigenous people in Canada, but few as publicized and poignant as the stories of Brian Sinclair and Joyce Echaquan. Both cases clearly demonstrate the presence of systemic racism that many Canadians find hard to accept. As you read these cases, form your own opinion about each. What do you think prompted health care providers to act or respond the way they did? What ethical principles were ignored or violated? What ethical theories do you think came into play? Clearly the rights of both Mr. Sinclair and Mrs. Echaquan were ignored or simply disregarded. In what ways were the health professionals, and perhaps the hospital, in violation of the duty of care? What might the legal implications of abandoning the duty of care be (see Chapter 8)? Was there a duty of care applied in either case? What changes do you think could prevent either of these cases from occurring again?

**Brian Sinclair**

Brian Sinclair was an Indigenous man who fits well in the category of being marginalized. His experiences included intergenerational trauma. He grew up in poverty, compounded by a family history of substance misuse, racism, and alcoholism. As an adult, Brian Sinclair experienced ongoing challenges. He had multiple health problems accentuated by a history of addiction and chronic illness. In addition, he was mentally impaired and a double amputee. In September 2008, Mr. Sinclair was seen in a clinic in Winnipeg, complaining of abdominal pain and no urinary output in the previous 24 hours (he had an in-dwelling urinary catheter). The attending physician referred him to the emergency department (ED) at the Winnipeg Health Sciences Centre, noting in a referral letter that he should be seen immediately. Mr. Sinclair registered in the ED and was told to wait in the waiting area. He did so, for an astonishing 34 hours. Upon the urging of someone in the waiting room who noticed that Mr. Sinclair was not breathing, the professional staff attended to him, but he was pronounced deceased shortly afterward. The official cause of death was peritonitis secondary to an acute urinary tract infection related to a neurogenic bladder.

At an inquest later, investigations revealed evidence that the professional staff ignored Mr. Sinclair, making assumptions that, because of his shabby appearance and being Indigenous, he was in the ED because he was homeless and perhaps "sleeping it off," not in need of medical attention. Ultimately, the judge did not order an inquiry to determine the role of

---

**BOX 9.2 Respect, Rights, and Racism Within the Health Care System—cont'd**

stereotyping or racism as a contributing factor into Mr. Sinclair's death. The inquest did prompt the hospital to admit that it failed Mr. Sinclair and to make appropriate changes to improve the equity of care to patients. Please see the video on Evolve about Brian Sinclair's treatment (or lack thereof) and the recommendations made (following an investigation) to the hospital to avoid such an event from recurring.

**Joyce Echaquan**

Joyce Echaquan, a 37-year-old Indigenous woman and mother of seven children, was admitted by ambulance to a Québec hospital on September 26, 2020. She was complaining of severe abdominal pain. After admission, and in bed, her arms and legs were restrained. On September 28, Mrs. Echaquan live-streamed 7 minutes of her hospital stay, during which time she appeared to be in continued distress and was pleading for help. At least two employees entered the room (later identified as a nurse and an orderly) toward the end of the video and were heard directing cruel and blatantly racist comments at her. Joyce Echaquan died soon after live-streaming this event. The nurses that admitted Mrs. Echaquan incorrectly identified her as a drug abuser in withdrawal, delaying the treatment she required related to her actual medical condition. Her death was attributed to pulmonary edema. The nurse involved was subsequently fired.

Almost a year later, a coroner's report concluded that racism and prejudice contributed to Mrs. Echaquan's death. The report also stressed that the Government of Québec must acknowledge that there is systemic racism in the province's institutions (e.g., health care and education), something denied by the Québec premier. The coroner, Géhane Kamel, told reporters in Trois-Rivières that "we were witnesses to an unacceptable death" and that "we must ensure that it is not in vain." According to a statement of claim filed at the courthouse in Joliette, Québec in the fall of 2022, Joyce Echaquan's family launched a $2.7 million civil lawsuit against the Centre intégré de santé et de services sociaux (CISSS) de Lanaudière, the nurse captured on video insulting Echaquan, and the doctor assigned to provide her care.

Sources: Global News. (2018, September 21). *Ten years since the death of Brian Sinclair*. https://globalnews.ca/video/4473299/ten-years-since-the-death-of-brian-sinclair/; Nerestant, A. (2021, October 1). *Racism, prejudice contributed to Joyce Echaquan's death in hospital, Québec coroner's inquiry concludes*. CBC News. https://www.cbc.ca/news/canada/montreal/joyce-echaquan-systemic-racism-quebec-government-1.6196038; Laframboise, K. (2021, October 5). *Joyce Echaquan's death "unacceptable," Québec coroner says in addressing inquiry findings*. Global News. https://globalnews.ca/news/8243732/quebec-coroner-systemic-racism-joyce-echaquan/; Geary, A. (2017, September 18). *Ignored to death: Brian Sinclair's death caused by racism, inquest inadequate, group says*. CBC News. https://www.cbc.ca/news/canada/manitoba/winnipeg-brian-sinclair-report-1.4295996

cases of Brian Sinclair and Joyce Echaquan, discussed later in the chapter). Every Canadian has the right to be treated with dignity and to have, wherever possible, their traditions and practices acknowledged, including when seeking mental health services and in long-term care facilities. All Canadians also have the right to privacy, and the right to a reasonable quality of care, including continuity of care. Usually contained in the codes of ethics of health care professions, these latter rights tend to be described more as elements that health care providers must deliver, rather than as rights the patient is entitled to. The right to treatment within a reasonable time frame and to quality care has come into question given the stressors experienced within the health care system that appeared to reach a breaking point in some jurisdictions in 2022 and 2023 (e.g., accessibility, with the temporary closure of many emergency departments). Such situations are beyond the control of health care providers and relate, among other things, to a critical shortage of health human resources.

Although difficult to enforce and at times subjective, the principles of the *Canada Health Act* address Canadians' right *to* health care (with limitations). You will recall that services offered within each province and territory vary, with all jurisdictions offering selected services that surpass the requirements of the *Canada Health Act.* Also, some procedures remain fragmented and uncovered by provincial or territorial plans, resulting in those who cannot afford them doing without these procedures, creating the basis for the argument that a person's right to adequate health care has been violated. Such procedures include the full cost of gender-reassignment surgery in a person's own province or territory and in vitro fertilization. Some also question the ethics of eligibility criteria restricting a person's right to certain procedures (usually based on a person's age or health status). For example, there are age limitations on who can be a living organ donor, which makes sense from a medical perspective in terms of maximizing health outcomes for both organ donors and organ recipients.

### DID YOU KNOW?

#### *In Vitro Fertilization*

Most jurisdictions do not cover the full cost of in vitro fertilization (IVF) (implanting a fertilized egg into a person's uterus) but will cover such procedures to rectify some causes of infertility, such as unblocking fallopian tubes. Providing public funding for IVF is provincially regulated, and how this is funded varies. The (medical) cost for just one IVF cycle is between $10,000 and $20,000, with many patients requiring more than one cycle to conceive. This poses a financial barrier for many people, even with limited public funding. Ontario funds one round of IVF, Manitoba offers a tax credit to couples for money spent on IVF, and New Brunswick funds partial costs of IVF treatment through a grant. In Québec, the public system will cover one IVF cycle for people between the age of 18 and 42 (with some restrictions). For same-sex female partners, only one partner is eligible. Single people are also eligible.

In addition to age, there are restrictions in most jurisdictions on the number of embryos that can be transferred into a person's uterus at one time. In Québec, for example, the number of embryos transferred depends on the person's age (up to three if the person is 37 years of age or older). This is because the older a person is, the less chance an embryo transfer will be successful. There is no coverage in the six remaining provinces or in any of the territories for IVF treatments.

Do jurisdictions with eligibility criteria for IVF treatments discriminate against older people? Should there be limits on the number of embryos implanted? Is it ethical for jurisdictions to fund fertility treatments as they see fit, or should the treatments be offered equally across the country? Is the cost of offering these fertility treatments a justifiable burden on an already financially stressed health care system when the money could, for example, go to cancer treatments or increasing the capacity of human health resources in an emergency department?

#### Expanded Employee Benefits

Early in 2022, several large companies, including most of Canada's large banks, expanded their benefits to include surrogacy and fertility treatments as well as costs incurred related to adoption. This move is, at least in part, an attempt to help employers recruit and retain staff during a restricted labour market, as well as a response to demands made by employees in view of varying methods available for family expansion.

Source: MacNaughton, L. (2022, May 15). *Fertility perks are key benefit companies can offer in tight labour market, advocates say.* CBC News. https://www.cbc.ca/news/business/fertility-benefits-tight-labour-market-1.6451824

In terms of timely health care as a right, over the past number of years, a growing number of Canadians have become impatient with long wait times for health care services. Some are also challenging this right under the *Charter of Rights and Freedoms* when what is considered "reasonable" or benchmark wait times are exceeded, for example, for joint surgery. Despite commitments from the federal, provincial, and territorial governments to shorten wait times, waiting lists in most regions are actually getting longer. This has been greatly impacted by the delays incurred for diagnostic procedures and surgeries during the pandemic. To shorten these wait times, some provinces are resorting to having procedures done in private clinics (with public funding). Other Canadians have gone to the United States to have procedures done, paying for them themselves (see Chapter 8).

---

**THINKING IT THROUGH**

*The Right to Prompt Treatment*

During various waves of the COVID-19 pandemic, to accommodate the numbers of hospitalized people with COVID-19 infections, hundreds of surgeries and procedures across the country were postponed. Some individuals whose procedures were postponed argue that their surgeries, although termed "elective," were in fact urgent, as delays could (and did) result in a worsening of their conditions and, in some cases, death.

1. How were the rights of those whose surgeries and procedures were delayed violated?
2. What strategies do you think would be more effective for triaging patients so that everyone had equal access to the care they needed in a timely manner?

---

## A Patient Bill of Rights

Many countries have developed a patient bill of rights—a statement of the rights that patients are entitled to when they receive medical care—that usually include rights to information, fair treatment, and autonomy over medical decisions. Legislation in countries such as Norway, New Zealand, the United States, England, Spain, Sweden, and Italy supports these bills of rights. In some other countries, patient bills of rights exist only as guidelines, not laws. In Canada, provincial and territorial governments have adopted a range of approaches. Canadian patients' bills of rights are listed by jurisdiction at https://canadianhealthadvocatesinc.ca/patient-rights/.

Even some hospitals create their own patient bill of rights. Many include a section outlining the responsibilities of the patient, which include sharing accurate health information with health care providers; taking an active role in their health care; being courteous to health care providers, other patients, and staff members; and respecting hospital property.

## Duties and Rights

If a patient has a right *within* health care or *to* health care, for the most part, the health care provider has the responsibility, or duty, to grant that right (the duty of care) in an ethical, competent, and timely manner. Moreover, at the heart of patients' rights in health care is the previously discussed principle of autonomy, which has prominence over most other things. Thus duties, rights, and autonomy are necessarily joined.

To fulfill one's duty to honour patients' rights, the health care provider must either act to carry out a responsibility or refrain from acting or interfering in a situation. In other words, a patient's right to something may require one to take steps to provide a service (e.g., educate the patient to aid their decision making); alternatively, it may require one to do nothing (e.g., refrain from pointing a patient toward a particular treatment option). Patients' rights include noninterference regarding some aspects of their health care, supporting the patient's right to autonomy.

As a result of this shift toward patients independently determining what is best for themselves, physicians committed to beneficence may face moral dilemmas—for instance, when a patient refuses life-saving treatment. In most cases, however, health care providers both respect and uphold patients' decisions. When, on occasion, they do not, significant stress and sometimes litigation result.

---

**THINKING IT THROUGH**

*Seeking Advice*

Patients frequently ask health care providers for advice based on their specific professional knowledge and expertise. For example, A.T., an asthmatic, may ask a respiratory therapist whether they should use their inhalers as often as prescribed by their medical specialist.
1. Is it acceptable for a health care provider to give treatment advice to a patient based on their own judgement and experience—for example, "If I were you, I would do this?"
2. Where do you draw the line between strongly suggesting the patient follow your advice, the advice of another provider, and allowing the patient to make an independent choice?
3. What alternatives can you think of if you disagree with the medical practitioner's recommendations?

---

## Parental Rights, Ethics, and the Law

When a patient is considered an adult, self-determination takes precedence over paternalistic intervention, even when the patient's life is at stake. However, paternalism and the legal system sometimes join forces when life-saving treatment is thought to be necessary for a minor yet is refused—for example, when parents make decisions for their minor children that the health care provider believes will compromise the health or life of the child, as in the case of Jehovah's Witness parents refusing a blood transfusion that would save their child's life. In these cases, the parent's or guardian's rights are not absolute, and the provincial or territorial courts will almost always obtain legal custody for the child and allow the recommended treatment. Numerous cases have surfaced over the past few years involving children from newborns to teenagers. This is changing with the recognition of a "mature minor" wherein the wishes of the child may be honoured.

All involved parties want what is best for the patient, but what one considers best may differ from what another considers best. Values, cultural and religious beliefs, and ethical codes can conflict. Who is to say which path should be followed? Do parents not have the right to make decisions for their underage children? Do children who clearly have the maturity to make their own decisions not have the right to do so? Do physicians not have a both a moral, ethical, and legal obligation to preserve life? There are times when individuals, parents, guardians, and even persons considered minors make decisions that conflict with the recommendations of the physician—even in the face of serious, deadly outcomes. It comes down to the rights of the person from an ethical and sometimes legal perspective. Decisions can be related to numerous entities, including personal, social, and cultural values.

A very good example is the 2015 case of Makayla Sault, an 11-year-old First Nations (Ojibwe) girl from Ontario who was diagnosed with a form of leukemia; she was given a 75% chance of going into remission with chemotherapy. After experiencing the difficult adverse effects of chemotherapy, Makayla, along with her parents, decided to terminate this treatment plan (based on spiritual and cultural beliefs), exercising her Indigenous rights (and legal rights awarded to her under the *Health Care Consent Act*) to pursue traditional and alternative therapies. This case was at the centre of numerous discussions from a number of perspectives, not the least of which concerned the right of "competent minors" to make life-and-death decisions, as well as the need to both understand and respect Indigenous health traditions and practices, even if one believed that "Western" medicine (e.g., the chemotherapy) offered the highest chances of survival. What do you think?

A person also has the right to make decisions based on religious beliefs. Adult Jehovah's Witnesses are able to make their own decisions in the face of life-threatening situations where the recommended treatment involves a transfusion of blood or blood products. In the case of minor children considered not competent to make their own decisions, the adults make the decision for them. They do not want their children to die, nor do they refuse other medical treatments, including surgery. Their religious beliefs dictate their course of action. Physicians, on the other hand, observe duty ethics; their duty is to treat the patient. Some might argue for a teleological approach—treating the patient saves the patient's life and in the end benefits everyone involved. Could that outcome be argued, however, if the patient is ostracized by their community for having had a blood transfusion, and if the patient feels wronged for having been forced to do something contrary to their religious beliefs? If you were a health care provider and were tasked with trying to convince someone (an adult or an adult making a decision for a child) to accept a blood transfusion, what course of action would you take? Would you be comfortable abiding by the person's decision, or would you do everything you could to persuade them otherwise?

## Rights and Mental Competence

Conflict with a patient's autonomy frequently arises when a question of mental competence exists. Consider a person with anorexia nervosa, a devastating eating disorder that primarily affects young women, although individuals of all ages are vulnerable. It is often caused by another physiological disorder, or vice versa. Conditions associated with anorexia include obsessive-compulsive disorder, borderline personality disorder, bipolar disorder, post-traumatic stress disorder, and depression. The nature of these diseases often hinders the patient's ability to make rational decisions.

Does a person whose illness skews their ability to make rational decisions have the right to self-determination? Concerns over such situations led a psychiatrist, Marian Verkerk, to propose the concept of compassionate interference, wherein physicians could justify treating individuals against their will. Dr. Verkerk argued that treatment restores patients to a sound physical and mental state, allowing them to make informed decisions. This is an ethical concept, not a legal approach to treatment, bearing in mind that all jurisdictions have laws governing the rights of individuals to refuse care, and legal steps that must be taken if care is imposed.

In British Columbia, minors are legally able to refuse treatment for addictions such as opioid addictions. In addition, they have the right to prevent an attending physician from informing the minor's parents that their child has an addiction. In a *Fifth Estate* episode (available on the Evolve site), a mother explains how much she wanted the right to help her daughter, perhaps saving her life.

As discussed, there are numerous cases in which parental authority has been removed when parents or guardians refuse medical treatment deemed necessary to save a child's life. These cases can become even more complex—for example, when the child in question also refuses treatment but is considered mentally unfit to make such a decision.

Another contentious issue is whether or not an individual who is severely mentally or physically disabled should have children if they are considered incapable of raising a child without full-time social assistance. Is it reasonable to have the authority to prevent individuals in such a situation from having children? Would there be a difference if the person was financially able to pay for this assistance instead of being on social assistance? Whose rights does one consider? Is there a duty to consider allocation of resources used for health care and social assistance? Does that take precedence over an individual's right to autonomy? Or the moral and ethical obligation to treat every person with respect and dignity? This obligation was violated when Indigenous women were sterilized, sometimes without their express consent, sometimes bullying them into the procedure, and sometimes carrying out the procedure without the woman's knowledge (see Chapter 8). In addition, duty of care, along with almost every other ethical principle, was abandoned by health care providers within the circle of care of these individuals.

## ETHICS AT WORK

All regulated health care professions have codes of ethics, as do many places of employment. Review the one belonging to your profession or organization. If none exists, you should consider recommending that one be created and implemented. Many ethical situations arise in the health care industry, and codes of ethics significantly help professionals make appropriate decisions.

### The Code of Ethics

A formal statement of an organization's or profession's values regarding professional behaviour, a code of ethics provides guidance for ethical decision making, self-evaluation, and best practices policies. Most codes cover expectations related to professional conduct that, if violated, can result in loss of the person's professional license, dismissal from employment, or legal action. All ethical codes stress the importance of treating all people equally, with respect and dignity, and without bias. The Canadian Association of Social Workers' Code of Ethics, for example, states, "Social workers respect the unique worth and inherent dignity of all people and uphold human rights"(Canadian Association of Social Workers, n.d.). The Code of Conduct for the Registered Nurses Association of Ontario states, "Nurses respect the dignity of patients and treat them as individuals" (College of Nurses of Ontario, 2019). Unfortunately, these principles are not always upheld, as in the true events recounted in Box 9.2.

### Boundaries and Relationships

#### Relationships With Patients

Personal relationships between patients and health care providers in any discipline are, for the most part, prohibited while the formal relationship remains, and sometimes even for a period of time after the professional relationship ends. Codes of ethics for physicians clearly outline these boundaries. Doctors may not ethically establish personal relationships with patients under their care. In most circumstances, it is recommended that a physician not date a former patient for 1 year after the termination of the patient–physician relationship. Most other health care professions take a similar, though often not as strict, stand on developing personal relationships with patients. For example, no formal objection exists to a physiotherapist starting a relationship with a former patient after their professional relationship has ended.

Often, especially in small towns, a patient admitted to hospital knows many of the staff members. Depending on the nature of the relationship, this may or may not cause concern. If the health care provider feels uncomfortable caring for a particular patient, or the other way around, it would be in the best interests of both to have someone else assume that patient's care.

### Relationships and Friendships With Colleagues

Inevitably, you will develop friendships in the workplace. Unless these friendships interfere with how you do your job, doing so is not considered unethical. However, you must remain impartial and not choose favourites among the staff. Developing alliances by forming cliques at the expense of others is both unprofessional and destructive. Tight-knit groups in the workplace make it difficult for new staff members to integrate and feel welcome. Starting a new job is difficult enough. A warm and inviting environment goes a long way toward helping new employees fit in and begin to function competently as a member of the health care team. Tight-knit groups in the workplace can also alienate current employees, making them uncomfortable, and result in a toxic work environment.

Personal business has no role in the workplace, either. Discussing last night's party, tomorrow's trip, or someone's recent breakup remains inappropriate in any work environment. This extends to the use of one's cell phone during work hours—save texting and calling for breaks.

### In the Hospital Setting

Health care providers employed in a hospital setting are expected to carry out their duties in a professional, legal, and ethical manner. All health care facilities have procedures, policies, and guidelines governing ethical conduct. Employers also expect health care providers to uphold the ethical codes of their individual professions. Although members of the health care team should support each other, overstepping certain boundaries can breach ethical conduct (e.g., moving a colleague's family member up a wait list).

Health care providers also have an obligation to report a fellow health care provider's misconduct or incompetence, whether regarding their job performance or a violation of the principles of confidentiality. Most health care environments develop procedures outlining what to report and whom to report it to. Ethical issues unresolved at a lower level, in most facilities, will be reported to an ethics committee.

---

**THINKING IT THROUGH**

*Establishing a Friendship With a Patient*

In the workplace setting, you will meet a wide range of people, some of whom you are drawn to and feel a natural desire to want to develop a friendship with.
1. Is it ever ethical for a health care provider to exchange phone numbers with a patient with the intent of dating after the patient is discharged?
2. Does it make a difference if the exchange of phone numbers is for the purpose of developing a platonic friendship?
3. What moral or ethical problems could arise from either scenario?

---

### Rationale for Boundaries

#### Trust

A health care worker providing medical services for a patient does so within a therapeutic relationship. Patients trust the health care provider to perform their professional services impartially and competently, without bias or discrimination. Not only is changing the nature of that relationship ethically and morally wrong; it can also interfere with the care and compromise the ability of the health care provider to fulfill their professional duties. The higher the professional's level of responsibility (e.g., a physician versus a physiotherapist, respiratory therapist, or medical administrative assistant), the more damaging such a change can be.

### Balance of Power and Transference

In a physician–patient relationship, decisions made by the physician can have a significant impact on the patient's health and recovery. Along with feeling vulnerable, the patient may be in awe of the physician and misread feelings for the patient. Patients somewhat commonly feel a sense of "falling in love" with physicians or other health care providers. The health care provider has a responsibility to recognize the relevant signs and to ensure the relationship remains formal. In some cases, physicians have to stop providing care for the patient.

All health care providers dealing with patients should be aware of the possibility of such situations. Patients have a right to equitable and fair care—and to trust that they receive it. Therefore, any personal ties with a patient have the potential to interfere with the care of that patient or others, to interfere with a trusting relationship, and to put the patient in a vulnerable position. Nonadherence to maintaining a professional relationship with a patient for a health provider can result in litigation—even a comment can have negative professional consequences. For example, a surgeon made a comment to a 17-year-old female patient that she had a nice "backside" and nice legs (he was known for inappropriate comments to nurses and patients but had never been challenged). The patient and her parents complained to the provincial College of Physicians and Surgeons. After an investigation, the surgeon was suspended for a period of time.

### Accepting Gifts

Patients often give gifts to health care providers who have cared for them, usually as an expression of gratitude. Little literature is available about the ethics of accepting gifts. A box of chocolates for the nursing station when a patient leaves the hospital, some flowers sent to the office, or a card with a small ornament are examples of acceptable gifts. Accepting anything more is inappropriate and may place the health care provider in a difficult position because the patient may expect favouritism, such as access to special treatment or an appointment whenever they want it. Some health care providers make it a policy not to accept anything—ever. If an employer or regulatory college has guidelines about accepting gifts, these must be followed.

Seasonal gifts may be an exception. During the holidays, especially Christmas, patients often give health care providers and their office staff gifts, such as home baking, wine, or other tokens of appreciation—usually with no strings attached. Some people get a true sense of satisfaction from the opportunity to express gratitude. Common sense and familiarity with the patient are the best guidelines when accepting seasonal gifts if the workplace or regulatory college does not address the issue.

### The Ethics Committee

An ethics committee consists of a group of people—often volunteers—who listen to, evaluate, and make recommendations about acts perceived as unethical. Members of such committees usually come from a variety of backgrounds and may include doctors, nurses, social workers, physiotherapists, lawyers, ethicists, and members of the public. Public members do not require special qualifications other than the ability to listen and assist with making fair and unbiased decisions. Members remain on the committee for designated time frames.

Aside from evaluating unethical acts, ethics committees may supply health care providers with guidance in making controversial medical decisions and compile research for policy development within the facility. In the health care profession, decisions are often neither unanimous nor easy. All matters discussed and reviewed by an ethics committee remain strictly confidential.

## END-OF-LIFE ISSUES

End-of-life issues that raise ethical concerns range from establishing do not resuscitate (DNR) protocols, a patient wishing to withdraw life-saving measures and requesting supportive or palliative care, to requesting medical assistance in dying (MAiD).

DNR orders are seen frequently both in hospital and in long-term care facilities, usually requested by individuals who are gravely ill (regardless of their age) and feel that extending their lives would leave them with a life devoid of quality. The phrase *allow natural death* (AND) is sometimes used as an alternative to DNR and is deemed less harsh and more appropriate to some, allowing nature to take its course. This includes withdrawing or not initially implementing life-saving or life-prolonging measures. Comfort measures remain in place. Palliative care is also supportive in nature, avoiding active treatment but ensuring the patient is comfortable and, for the most part, pain free. Palliative care rarely raises ethical issues among patients, their families, and health professionals.

### DID YOU KNOW?

#### *Suicide versus Euthanasia*

The term *suicide* is applied widely to the intentional action of taking one's own life for any reason and is one of the major causes of premature and preventable deaths globally. In 2021, Statistics Canada reported that there are 10 deaths attributed to suicide each day in Canada (Government of Canada, 2022). Suicide is often committed out of despair, depression, and other forms of mental illness. The term *euthanasia* is more frequently associated with the taking of life to alleviate pain and suffering, either with or without the request of the person—for example, voluntary euthanasia (the patient asks someone to end their life, also called *assisted suicide*) or involuntary euthanasia (someone deliberately ends the patient's life without their express consent, which likely ends in a charge of murder).

The term *euthanasia* is used less frequently now that medical aid in dying is legal in Canada, but that is not to say that use of the term does not still occur.

Source: World Health Organization. (2018). *Suicide data.* http://www.who.int/mental_health/prevention/suicide/suicideprevent/en/

### Ethics and Medical Assistance in Dying

MAiD will always be controversial, with some Canadians quite happy to be able to make the choice, and others who disagree with the concept for a variety of reasons. There are also those who remain ambivalent. The concept raises a number of concerns, including fears of misuse of the process for disabled and otherwise vulnerable people—for example, ending Aunt Sally's life to inherit her money, or trying to arrange for the death of a person (adult or child) who is disabled to the point where they cannot make their own decisions, but for whom some see death as a relief and a kindness, or for whom the caregiver feels they cannot attend to the person's needs any longer. This may be for financial reasons or because the demands of the care that the person needs is too difficult for a family to cope with. There are also concerns that a person may choose MAiD for socioeconomic reasons (e.g.; living in poverty, homelessness), feeling that there is no way forward or adequate support.

Recall the changes made to MAiD eligibility criteria discussed in Chapter 8. These changes, although welcomed by many, have raised concerns among others, based on legal, ethical, and moral standards. These concerns include the rights of a person with dementia to have MAiD if they are unable to give consent at the time of the procedure, as well as the concept of being eligible for MAiD based on the grounds of a mental health diagnosis. In addition, the concept of advance requests has come into question.

---

**THINKING IT THROUGH**

### Advance Requests for MAiD

As of September 2022, an advance request for MAiD for a person with dementia (exclusive of physical health) is illegal in Canada, but there are growing demands to increase eligibility to allow a person to make an advance request for this purpose. For example, H.W. has been diagnosed with Alzheimer's disease. Although in the very early stages of the disease, H.W. wants the right to be accepted for the MAiD procedure but have the procedure activated sometime in the future. H.W. will describe the conditions under which they feel that life would be intolerable as a result of dementia (e.g., losing the ability to recognize loved ones and being dependent on others for all aspects of H.W.'s care).

1. What objections do you see that some individuals might have with legalizing MAiD under these conditions?
2. What ethical principles are involved?
3. What impact might allowing this eligibility criteria have on the person's family and loved ones?

When answering Question 3, consider who might have to make the final decision as to when the procedure should actually take place, how they would make that decision, moral and ethical issues the decision maker might struggle with, and the potential influence of other family members on the situation.

---

## Ethical Principles and Medical Aid in Dying

### Rights

A person's right to self-determination is central when it comes to medical ethics. This includes, but is not limited to, the right to equitable health care, the right to accept or refuse treatment, and with respect to this discussion, the right to die with dignity in accordance with the MAiD legislation. The principles involved in legalizing MAiD include the right of a person to autonomy and dignity. Opposing values concerning the sanctity of life were considered when MAiD was legalized, but the rights of a person to end their life to prevent intolerable pain and suffering took precedent. The rights of physicians and nurse practitioners who facilitate the process of MAiD must also be considered. In Canada, health care providers are not obligated to actively participate in the process on the basis of conscientious objection, which may be for religious, spiritual, social, professional, personal, or institutional reasons (Case Example 9.4). At present, physicians are required to refer patients to a physician or nurse practitioner (except in Québec) who will navigate them through the process of seeking MAiD, as health care providers have a duty of care to their patients and should not abandon them. Institutions that refuse to actively participate in MAiD (particularly those with religious affiliations) do so because of religious beliefs and principles but will refer and transfer a patient to another location or facility that does participate in MAiD. This protocol is a discussion all on its own and brings into question the right of a hospital (e.g., a Catholic hospital) to refuse this type of care if it is publicly funded.

---

### CASE EXAMPLE 9.4 B.T. and Conscientious Objection

B.T. is a nurse who is opposed to MAiD for religious as well as moral and ethical reasons. B.T. is one of several registered nurses providing home care for a patient who has end-stage liver disease. The patient has arranged for a MAiD procedure. B.T. was scheduled to provide care for the patient on the day of the procedure but felt they could not do so. Another nurse changed shifts with B.T. If B.T. was in a similar position working in the hospital, they would also be able to remove themselves from caring for the patient. It is important to stress that when a MAiD procedure takes place in the home or the hospital setting, the nurses have no part in carrying out the procedure; their only obligation is to provide general care for the patient.

---

#### Autonomy

Proponents of MAiD claim that the legislation supports the rights of the individual to autonomy, self-determination, and to choose their destiny when faced with an illness or disability causing intractable, intolerable pain and suffering. The principle of self-determination is often central in medical decisions. The key is that the person is mentally competent to make their own decision.

#### Values

When weighing the ethical rightness or wrongness of seeking MAiD, a person's values must be considered. For example, most people value their personal dignity. Personal dignity may include a person's self-worth and sense of pride—for example, in being able to look after themselves as a result of a chronic illness (not necessarily if death is inevitable) or in the final stages of an illness. The person may fear a loss of dignity if they cannot render self-care or depend on others for meeting such needs as feeding and elimination, entities the person associates with quality of life (or lack thereof). Loss of dignity is almost always associated with cognitive impairment and feared as an illness progresses (consider the patient in their quest for advance requests for MAiD).

#### Trust

Primary care providers almost always have a mandate to preserve life, to do no harm, and to bring about good (the principles of beneficence and nonmaleficence). The concept of deliberately bringing about or contributing to a person's death violates almost every principle of duty ethics that health care providers pledge to uphold. Does this weaken trust between a patient and health practitioners who participate in MAiD?

MAiD and whether it is right or wrong will always depend on an individual's own ethical and moral beliefs and values. The process will continue to pose more questions than answers. In addition, the policies and procedures regarding eligibility still require adjustment. Are there enough safeguards in place to prevent misuse of the process? Will it become "ordinary" so that those assessing eligibility become complacent, creating a slippery slope that could lead to misuse of the process? Should individuals diagnosed with Alzheimer's disease and other forms of dementia be allowed to make arrangements for MAiD while they are still mentally competent? Should those with mental illness be eligible? Should minors be allowed to make such decisions? Is it reasonable to allow someone to have assistance in ending their life to end lifelong suffering, even when death is not imminent?

## Preparation for End-of-Life Decisions

Many individuals, as they get older and who may or may not be suffering from poor quality of life as a result of illness, want some measures in place that will direct their care and end-of-life decisions should they become unable to do so (excluding MAiD, which must be requested by the patient with regard to a current health problem). In the face of deteriorating health, these requests may include specific instructions such as restricting interventions to those that will keep them comfortable, removal from life support (e.g., ventilators), and DNR orders, or they may want all measures aimed at preserving life implemented (although that is not usually the case). There are steps in all provinces and territories that individuals can take to facilitate implementation of their end-of-life decisions, some more complicated than others.

### Do Not Resuscitate Requests

A person entering a health care facility can request a DNR order, usually with the support of their family. The doctor must sign a DNR order, which becomes part of the patient's medical record. In an acute care facility, the attending physicians and staff must be aware of this decision. If a person is transferred from a long-term care facility to an acute care hospital, a DNR order, if applicable, on the chart should be part of the health record transferred with the person. Protocols for making this request may vary with both facilities and jurisdictions. It is important for all those within the person's circle of care to be aware of such requests; if there is not a written, signed order, health professionals are obliged to initiate CPR. If there is a signed order on the patient's chart, health care providers are legally bound to honour such requests, which can be difficult for those who believe that active measures should be taken at all costs. Importantly, a person can reverse their DNR request at any time.

---

### THINKING IT THROUGH

#### *Respecting the Patient's Right to Autonomy*

Currently hospitalized, G.G. suffers a cardiac arrest. Their nurse is in the room at the time and knows that G.G. has a written and signed DNR order because G.G. was constantly reminding the staff of it. However, because of personal and religious beliefs, the nurse feels that saving a person's life takes precedence over everything else. Not resuscitating G.G. is a difficult choice for the nurse to make, even knowing that doing so would violate the patient's request and thus their right to autonomy. Trust also comes into play here. G.G. trusts that the professional staff will honour his wishes.

1. What should the nurse do?
2. What course of action would you take if there was no written or signed DNR order because the family objected, but you knew that was what G.G. wanted?
3. In your jurisdiction, would you be exempt from litigation if you acted on compassionate grounds?

---

### Advance Directives

An advance directive, also called a *living will* or *treatment directive*, specifies the nature and level of treatment a person would want to receive in the event that they become unable to make those decisions at a later time. People prepare advance directives so as to ensure their wishes are known and honoured by family and loved ones and carried out by medical caregivers. Advance directives that appoint a power of attorney for personal care are most likely to result in the person's instructions being followed (see Chapter 8).

## Values History Form

A values history form is a comprehensive document that guides people in thinking about treatment options they would or would not want in the event that they were to become unable to make decisions about their own health care. People can detail their feelings, thoughts, and values as they relate to medical interventions. The form may also assist loved ones who might have to make decisions on the person's behalf, and also clarify the person's choices if disagreements among loved ones occur (Case Example 9.5).

## Levels of Care

*Levels of care* reflects a choice of end-of-life interventions usually assigned to nursing in long-term care facilities. They are discussed with the individual and their family members or proxy decision maker upon admission to a long-term care facility. Once established, the information is entered onto the person's chart. The person (usually called a *resident* in long-term care) or their family members may change their minds at any time. Levels of care most frequently change when a person's state of health begins to deteriorate. Should this occur, the physician or other health care provider along with the nurses almost always consult with the family, updating them on the resident's condition and evaluating options. Although specifics will vary, most facilities offer four options. Note that levels 1 and 2 are congruent with allowing the person to die naturally where they are living at the time.

*Level 1.* The resident wishes to stay in their home (e.g., long-term care or nursing facility), receiving comfort and supportive measures only. This includes pain control, but not usually intravenous therapy for hydration.

*Level 2.* The resident wants to stay in the facility and receive all treatments, medications, and interventions that are possible *at that facility*. This would include pain control and antibiotics if the patient developed an infection, pneumonia, or a urinary tract infection. Other medications may include those to treat cardiovascular problems. Intravenous hydration may or may not be considered. Some long-term care facilities transfer a resident to hospital if they require IV therapy.

*Level 3.* A resident choosing this level of care would be transferred to an acute care facility from their long-term care facility. They would receive recommended imaging and diagnostic tests, an IV if required, antibiotics, and other medications as needed. Level 3 does not include CPR protocol or transfer to the Critical or Intensive Care Unit.

*Level 4.* This level requires the person be transferred to an acute care facility for all active measures required to sustain life.

---

### CASE EXAMPLE 9.5 S.C. and a Values History Form

S.C., a 67-year-old who recently suffered a severe stroke, created an advance directive expressing their wish to receive no active intervention if they have another stroke. However, concerned that another stroke may leave S.C. unable to communicate and on a ventilator, S.C. begins to have doubts about their decision, fearful that if they have a change of heart, they would be unable to communicate it. Many people who have decided against intervention change their minds when actually facing death. Some family members know of S.C.'s recent second thoughts about their advance directive. S.C. decides to complete a values history form to clarify their feelings and thoughts about medical intervention. This form *might* help S.C.'s family if they ever have to make treatment decisions for S.C.

**DID YOU KNOW?**

*Refusing Medications*

Some individuals refuse their daily medications (e.g., antihypertensive medication, diuretics) in an attempt to accelerate their demise. Such refusal is perfectly legal but may pose moral questions for those involved in the individual's care.

## Palliative Care: An Ethical Perspective

Individuals who are facing death, and their families face two challenges: one is the fear of prolonging a person's life unnecessarily, the other is ending a person's life prematurely. From an ethical and moral perspective, the option of palliative care is for many people comforting and in keeping with religious, moral, and ethical values.

Palliative care addresses the physical and emotional needs of those who are dying. Individuals opposed to any kind of interference with the natural course of death believe that palliative care can facilitate a peaceful and painless natural death. Whether delivered in a hospital, in a hospice, or at home, palliative care can aid any person who is in the latter stages of a terminal illness or cannot otherwise cope with their disease without specialized support. Teams of experts work with patients and their families to manage physical discomfort and psychological distress and to meet spiritual needs.

### Palliative Sedation

Sometimes called *conscious sedation*, palliative sedation is typically used when an individual is dying and in severe pain despite all pain management measures. Applied in monitored settings, sedation is administered to induce a state of decreased awareness or to a point where the patient is unconscious. The goal is to relive the patient of the burden of pain. The patient's consent is required (or the consent of an authorized individual, e.g., the person with the power of attorney for personal care). Palliative sedation is typically morally and ethically acceptable to many who oppose MAiD.

## ALLOCATION OF RESOURCES

The term *allocation of resources* refers to who gets what resources, when, and for what reason. Rising health care costs, expensive technologies, and limited access to many services have made the allocation of resources an increasing concern in the health care industry. And limited resources mean that "Who gets what?" becomes a huge ethical problem. A brief discussion of select limited resources follows, with the intent of promoting thought and discussion.

### Organ Transplantation

Organ transplant has become more commonplace with increasing successful outcomes. However, the availability of viable organs remains a scarce resource and continues to involve several ethical issues. Consider Case Example 9.6.

In Case Example 9.6, A.B. has been unable to overcome the disease of alcoholism. Although A.B. has managed to give up drinking for limited periods of time, their ability to maintain sobriety remains questionable. A return to drinking would sharply decrease A.B.'s chances of maintaining even reasonable health with a transplanted liver. Should A.B. therefore be denied a chance at a new life? Another patient lives a healthy lifestyle and develops liver failure as a

## CASE EXAMPLE 9.6   A.B.'s Liver Transplant

A.B., a self-admitted alcoholic, was admitted to hospital in acute liver failure. A.B. has been on the transplant list for a little over a year. For A.B., terms of being a transplant recipient included agreeing to abstain permanently from the use of alcohol. A.B. was required to submit to periodic tests to ensure they remained alcohol free for a year prior to being added to the transplant list. A.B. was alcohol and drug free for 10 months. A.B. had a setback, going on a drinking binge one evening because of some family problems, in addition to the death of a friend. Because of health problems resulting from this binge, A.B. was admitted to hospital. Upon A.B.'s admission assessment, they were no longer considered eligible for a liver transplant, even in the face of failing health. A.B. (and their family) pleaded publicly for a second chance, claiming that one setback should not remove A.B. from the transplant list.

result of an acquired infection. But what if, as is debated in modern medicine, alcoholism was more commonly considered a disease rather than a moral failing? Would A.B. then be in a more favourable position to compete for the liver? Would A.B. be on equal footing with the patient who has liver failure as a result of an acquired infection?

Other considerations from a medical perspective encourage the following questions: Who would be more likely to see significant improvements in their health with the new liver? What damage has alcoholism done to A.B.'s overall health? Alcoholics tend to have lower success rates with transplantation because their general health is usually poorer. A return to drinking would interfere with adherence to the necessary post-transplant treatment regimen, which requires taking immunosuppressant medications. Nonetheless, do any of these factors provide a solid reason to deny A.B.?

## Finances and Resources

In Canada, the demand for health care resources—including finances, health care providers, and medical services such as diagnostic tests and hospital beds—sometimes exceeds supply. The allocation of resources in health care presents an ethical problem because it raises questions about fairness and justness. Priorities should be based on need, but how does a person, organization, or government assess need?

Health care funding in Canada, for the most part, is distributed in such a way that each region can set its own priorities and make decisions about how best to meet the health care needs of the populations it serves. If funds increase, however, how are they distributed? If funds decrease, which services are maintained, and which are sacrificed? How can someone make a decision, for example, to fund expensive treatment for a small group of individuals with a rare disease for which annual treatment is in the hundreds of thousands of dollars for each person if that same amount of money might be spent on cancer treatment that could save thousands of lives? Sometimes, in an attempt to make funding more equitable, the federal government will step in and provide targeted funding for specific areas. This happened when funding was directed toward disease prevention and health promotion in primary care. The healthier the Canadian population is, the fewer health care dollars ultimately need to be spent. Although many consider immunizations among the most important advances in preventive care, others argue that vaccines pose more risks than do diseases such as polio, measles, mumps, typhoid, and rubella, suggesting that immunizations have caused autism in some Canadian children (no definitive proof of this claim exists). Unvaccinated children pose a risk to others in the presence of a disease outbreak (e.g., measles).

Many groups compete for health care dollars—some for treatments for rare conditions that would empty the health care pot of millions of dollars. Teleological theorists, however, would suggest that funds should go to those services that meet the needs of the most people. Most Canadians take the stand that treatment should be available to all Canadians and that governments should ensure such universal availability without imposing financial hardship on an individual or family. How can that happen if financial resources are limited?

---

### THINKING IT THROUGH

#### *Allocation of Resources*

Thousands of Canadians suffer from relatively rare conditions that are incurable but that can be treated with some success. These treatments, however, are often extremely expensive—sometimes medications are not covered by the public plan, and sometimes treatments do not fall within the definition of "medically necessary."

1. Is it ethical to spend a large amount of money on a few individuals when that money could be used to improve health care services for a much larger group?
2. Does each life not deserve the same consideration?
3. Under the *Canada Health Act,* shouldn't the public system be responsible for all costs related to treating an individual? What principles of the *Charter of Rights and Freedoms* might apply here?

---

New technologies continually introduce treatment modalities that preserve and prolong life, and Canadians feel a sense of entitlement to these technologies, most of which are very costly. However, funds are limited; if every life-saving or treatment measure were offered to every person in need, the health care system would collapse. For example, significant (and costly) advancements have been made in sustaining life for very premature babies; however, very premature infants often have little hope of recovery or of having a satisfactory quality of life if they do recover (Case Example 9.7).

Some medications are very costly, such as biologics (see Chapter 4), with a small percentage of the population using a disproportionate amount of money allocated for medications. Is this reasonable, if the money could be used to pay for the cost of medications for thousands of Canadians who cannot afford their prescriptions? With health care costs rising, Canadians may ultimately be asked to consider how their choices will affect costs.

---

### CASE EXAMPLE 9.7   The Cost of Treatment

R.P. gave birth to a baby at 23 weeks' gestation. The baby was transported to the nearest neonatal intensive care unit. Three days later, the doctors told R.P. that the baby had a 20% chance of survival and that if the baby did survive, they would likely be blind, require multiple heart surgeries, suffer from a seizure disorder, and have cerebral palsy. Doctors asked whether R.P. wanted them to continue treatment to attempt to save the baby's life. The cost to the health care system would be enormous, and the quality of life the baby would have would be poor. Left to make a very difficult decision, R.P. had to consider the small margin of hope that the baby would live, and if the baby did survive, the complications the child would have to endure. The last thing on R.P.'s mind was the expense of the treatments—they were covered by the health care system. What decision do you think you would make?

# OTHER ETHICAL ISSUES IN HEALTH CARE

## Abortion

Abortion has been available in Canada without restrictions since 1984 when the Supreme Court of Canada declared that abortion could not legally be forbidden because doing so would violate Section 7 of the *Charter of Rights and Freedoms*. As you may recall, Section 7 states that "everyone has the right to life, liberty and the security of the person and the right not to be deprived thereof except in accordance with the principles of fundamental justice." Further, the court declared that forcing a person to carry a fetus to term is a violation of their "security of the person" (Canadian Charter of Rights and Freedoms, 1982).

The points at which a surgical abortion can be performed vary across the country, but in general, they are not performed if a person is more than 24 weeks' gestation The majority of therapeutic abortions are performed if a person is 12 to 14 weeks pregnant or less. Second-trimester abortions are usually considered only under certain circumstances—for example, when the pregnant person's life is at risk or if it is determined that the fetus has a condition incompatible with life.

As with MAiD, health care providers are not obligated to perform abortions and can refuse to perform them because of religious or moral beliefs. Individuals do not need a reference from a primary care provider to access an abortion clinic.

The moral and ethical issues around abortion concern two main issues: the right of the fetus to life and the right of people to make decisions that involve their own bodies. These issues also include philosophical, religious, cultural, and political components.

Pro-life groups believe that personhood (i.e., the state of being considered a person) begins at conception—the moment the sperm meets the ovum. From a spiritual perspective, some believe that the soul enters the body at this point. Pro-life supporters consider any deliberate interference that threatens the life of this "person" murder, believing that the fetus shares the same rights as all other humans, including the right to life.

Pro-choice groups argue that the pregnant person has the choice to carry the baby to term or to end the pregnancy, maintaining that abortion is a constitutional right and that safe and timely access to hospitals and clinics must be guaranteed. Views among pro-choice groups vary as to when the fetus becomes a person with rights. People who believe that personhood does not begin until the start of the second trimester or later assert that an abortion occurring prior to 13 weeks is both moral and ethical if it reflects the wishes of the pregnant person.

The debate over whether abortion is right or wrong, ethical or unethical, will continue. The argument comes down to personal, moral, religious, and cultural values and beliefs. The availability of abortion services and the related criteria vary somewhat across Canada. In Prince Edward Island, a pregnant person can have a medical abortion if they are 10 weeks pregnant or less (which is fairly standard across Canada), and a surgical abortion if they are no more than 12 weeks pregnant. The person is referred to out-of-province of they are beyond 12 weeks' gestation (Health PEI, 2021). In New Brunswick, an abortion may be performed on a person if they are no more than 14 weeks pregnant, and in Nova Scotia, no more than 16 weeks pregnant.

In the United States, the case *Roe v. Wade* refers to a lawsuit that led to a decision made by the US Supreme Court in 1973 legalizing abortion in that country. The ruling held that a woman had a constitutional right to legally have an abortion. In June 2022, the *Roe v. Wade* ruling was challenged by the State of Virginia in the Supreme Court. The court handed down a ruling reversing the *Roe v. Wade* decision, removing the constitutional right of a woman to have an abortion and leaving abortion laws to be established by the states. Reaction around the country was swift and fierce, sparking protests and challenges at the state level. The decision has also caused reactions among many Canadians, who wonder if this decision could result in upstream implications for the reproductive health of women in Canada. A number of US states moved quickly to make abortion illegal within state boundaries, while others did not tighten their abortion laws, passed amendments to guarantee the right to abortion, and have become safe havens for persons seeking an abortion. States, therefore, have constructed a matrix of laws that codify, regulate, and enact abortion laws within that state. Those restricting or banning abortion determine whether, when, and under what circumstances a person may obtain an abortion.

## Genetic Testing

An increasing number of Canadians are undergoing genetic testing—the examination of one's deoxyribonucleic acid (DNA)—done through a number of online organizations such as www.23andMe.com and www.Ancestry.com, providing direct-to-consumer results. Through genetic testing people can learn whether they carry any genes that put them at a higher risk for disease, such as certain types of cancer (e.g., breast), Alzheimer's disease, and Huntington's disease. Similarly, carrier testing determines whether the potential exists to pass on a genetic disease (e.g., sickle cell anemia and cystic fibrosis) to offspring. A couple who undergo such tests and have positive results must then weigh the severity of the potential disease and the chances of its occurrence when deciding whether to have children. Prenatal diagnostic screening can determine a fetus's risk for certain genetic disorders, aid in earlier diagnosis of fetal abnormalities, and provide prospective parents with important information for making informed decisions about a pregnancy, which may include terminating the pregnancy.

Genetic testing raises a number of moral and ethical questions, however. For instance, if an insurance company obtained records showing that a prospective client carried a gene that put them at risk for developing cancer, would that person be considered uninsurable? Would an employer with access to similar information decide against hiring that person? Some protection is provided for individuals in possession of genetic testing results revealing health concerns that could affect their purchase of insurance policies. Bill S-201 (Genetic Non-Discrimination Act, 2017), an act to prohibit and prevent genetic discrimination, was passed in Canada in early 2017. Under the Act, insurance companies are barred from asking clients to provide them with the results of genetic testing they may have had done when applying for life insurance under the amount of $250,000 or for health insurance. The Act amends the *Canada Labour Code* to prohibit employers from requiring that employees have genetic testing done, or from revealing test results already in the employee's possession. The Act also amends the *Human Rights Code* to prohibit any type of discrimination of a person based on genetic characteristics (e.g., someone with obvious characteristics of Down syndrome). There are still concerns if damaging genetic information somehow fell into the wrong hands, and it can still be requested by insurance companies for more expensive life or health insurance policies. Do you think the fact that Canada has a universal health care system lessens the potential harm of being required to reveal genetic test results when purchasing private health insurance?

What the individual does with the information obtained raises further issues. For example, a woman who learns she has the breast cancer gene might elect to have her breasts and ovaries removed. The American actor Angelina Jolie had a prophylactic double mastectomy based on a family history and on a positive *BRCA* genetic test. Two years after this surgery, Jolie had her ovaries and fallopian tubes removed prophylactically.

## THINKING IT THROUGH

### BRCA1 *and* BRCA2: *Would You Want to Know?*

The presence of the *BRCA1* or *BRCA2* genes can predispose a person with female genitalia to cancer of the breast and the uterus as well. Not all people elect to have any of these surgeries, even if they have either or both of these genes. Instead, some will opt for close monitoring for disease detection.

1. Would you want to know if you or a loved one carried either of these genes?
2. If you or a loved one tested positive, what course of action do you think you would choose?
3. What ethical principles, if any, might affect your decisions?

Canadians are encouraged to think carefully (i.e., to ask what the benefit is in knowing) before having genetic testing for presumed or established conditions. For example, would it help a person to know that they may develop Huntington's disease, an incurable neurological disorder? Such knowledge might provide relief from uncertainty and give a person an opportunity to get their affairs in order. On the other hand, the anxiety produced from living with the risk of developing an incurable disease can be overwhelming and debilitating in itself.

## THINKING IT THROUGH

### *Dementia: Do You Want to Know?*

Assume that several members of your family have suffered from Alzheimer's disease. A genetic test will tell you whether you carry the inherited gene, which would increase your likelihood of developing the disease.

1. Would you want to know if you carried the gene?
2. What advantages and disadvantages exist in either knowing or not knowing?

Although demand for genetic testing in Canada is growing, resources are limited, and individuals who turn to private laboratories usually surrender the advantage of receiving counsel from their own doctors. Results can be indefinite, stressful, damaging to family relationships, and harmful to careers. Genetic tests covered under public insurance in Canada include those for breast and ovarian cancer, colon cancer, high cholesterol, and Alzheimer's disease.

Provincial and territorial governments have questioned the cost-effectiveness of some types of genetic testing (i.e., allocation of resources) and have agreed that the cost-effectiveness depends on the test and resulting benefits. For example, genetic testing for colon or breast cancer is probably cost-effective since individuals who test positive can undergo more intensive screening as a preventative measure. Those at a higher risk for colon cancer, for example, can have periodic colonoscopies, whereas others (considered low risk) can have less expensive screening tests (e.g., fecal immunochemical test—known as *FIT*). Expert genetic counselling accompanies genetic testing in some Canadian jurisdictions, but not all. The aim of genetic counselling is to provide individuals with an understanding of the implications of a positive test, both for themselves and for their relatives, and to ensure individuals make an informed choice about taking the test.

## CRISPR

CRISPR is an acronym for **C**lustered **R**egularly **I**nterspaced **S**hort **P**alindromic **R**epeats (Broad Institute, n.d.). CRISPR is one of several genome editing technology programming systems. The term *CRISPR* is often used to refer loosely to these other systems, including CRISPR-Cas9 and CPS-1, which are genome editing tools. These systems are able to select specific strings of genetic code and edit DNA at targeted points. Genome editing makes it possible for scientists currently working primarily with animal cells and animal models to accelerate research for diseases such as cancer and to identify and modify mutations in the human genome to treat, and perhaps eliminate genetic causes of, certain diseases.

To facilitate research, this technology has been shared with scientists around the world. There is an understanding among scientists globally that this technology is premature and not to be used on humans until adequate research has been conducted in a transparent manner and clinical trials have been completed, shared with other scientists, and peer reviewed. That said, with the technology so widely available, there is no way to monitor what scientists and researchers do with this technology. How far someone might take the research, perhaps advancing to applying it to humans, is unknown.

In 2018, a Chinese biologist by the name of He Jiankui edited the genes of two human embryos to make them resistant to HIV and implanted them into a woman (the mother) who subsequently gave birth to two baby girls. These babies, in theory, are resistant to developing HIV (e.g., if one parent is HIV positive). When He Jiankui made this experiment public it was swiftly and vehemently condemned by scientists around the world. He Jiankui and two individuals who worked with him on the project were charged and subsequently sent to prison.

Numerous ethical concerns arise with the use (or misuse) of CRISPR technology, especially when related to human germline modification. In the case of the twin girls, how safe was the procedure without proper clinical trials? Did the parents understand the risks to the babies? How informed was informed consent? Did the scientist have the moral or ethical right to proceed with this procedure? Even with good intentions, what is there to stop scientists from embarking on other experiments without the proper clinical trials? What is to stop other scientists from using gene editing for other purposes, such as producing "designer" babies? How can the scientific community around the world develop and enforce strict regulatory guidelines for human gene editing? What moral principles and ethical values are involved here?

## SUMMARY

9.1  Ethics is the study of what is right and wrong in how we behave. It encompasses a number of principles including fairness, loyalty, and honesty. The study of ethics examines people's morals, values, and sense of duty. *Ethics* also refers to a code of conduct expected of a person in their professional role. In health care, it is important for health care providers to respect the decisions of others, even when those choices may not be congruent with their personal ethical code.

9.2  Understanding your own moral and ethical beliefs, your values, and your method of making ethical decisions will help you to understand your responses to ethical problems encountered in your professional role. Four ethical theories (teleological theory, deontological theory, virtue ethics, and divine command) define how most people make ethical decisions, providing some explanation for decisions that individuals make about their own health or the health of those they love.

9.3 Six principles (beneficence and nonmaleficence, respect, autonomy, truthfulness, fidelity, and justice) provide the foundation for ethics in health care. Beneficence—doing what is right and good for the patient—dates back as far as the practice of medicine itself as illustrated in the Hippocratic Oath, which has been modernized to be in keeping with changing trends. Although physician oriented, the oath reflects fundamental values expected of most health professionals. Establishing a trusting relationship with patients and being respectful, honest, and truthful allow patients to make their own decisions. This approach also supports the principle of autonomy, or the patient's right to self-determination. In most circumstances, paternalism is no longer acceptable in health care. Patients retain the right to have active treatment withdrawn, to refuse treatment, and to die with dignity.

9.4 A person's right to health care is sometimes ambiguous. Rights generally considered viable include the following: access to one's own health information; the right to confidentiality; the right to informed consent; the right to timely health care deemed medically necessary; and the right to have health care needs addressed in a timely manner.

9.5 Health care providers must establish and maintain therapeutic and respectful relationships with their patients. This includes respecting the patient's right to fair, unbiased care without discrimination. The balance of power that exists between a health care provider and a patient puts the patient in a vulnerable position in which feelings can be misinterpreted. Health care providers faced with a relationship issue must respect the codes of ethics of their profession, their employer, or both.

9.6 The decisions a person makes with respect to end-of-life issues can be both complex and controversial. A person's decisions are usually based on their personal code of ethics and may be influenced by the nature of their illness. A person may decide to refuse treatment or seek active methods to end their life, such as medical assistance in dying (MAiD). Changes made to the legislation governing MAiD expand eligibility criteria and include more safeguards with respect to the procedure. Levels of care offer individuals a choice of what type of interventions they want when their health is deteriorating—a concept that is part of the policies in most long-term care facilities. The first two levels are congruent with allowing a person a "natural" death. Decisions made by the patient, their family, or both can be changed at any time. Do not resuscitate directives must be in the form of an order signed by the physician and present on the patient's medical record. It is important for health care providers to respect the decisions a person makes, even if the decision is incongruent with one they would make for themselves in similar circumstances. This is not always easy, and in some circumstances health professionals can remove themselves from a situation that requires them to act in opposition to their own beliefs and values. This is called *conscientious objection* and can be applied, for example, in cases involving abortion or MAiD.

9.7 With health care costs continuing to rise, provinces and territories have become more conscious about where, when, and how to distribute resources, particularly when related to cost. Should the allocation of resources be based on need, cost-effectiveness, or the principle of equal distribution? Portions of recent funding from the federal government have, in part, been assigned to home care and mental health to improve services in those areas. This is called *targeted funding* and provides some level of assurance that deficits in these areas will be addressed.

9.8 Many areas of health care (e.g., abortion, genetic testing, and MAiD) involve controversy in the application of morals, values, and ethics. For the most part, no right or wrong answers exist—only what beliefs and values dictate. It is essential for health care providers to maintain an open mind, respect the rights of others to make their own decisions, and recognize that such respect can be achieved without compromising one's own beliefs and values. CRISPR is one of several genome editing technology programming systems.

These systems are able to select and modify a person's genetic code with implications to correct defects in human embryos and accelerate research for numerous diseases. The fear is that scientists will use these technologies on humans prematurely and perhaps for less than ethical purposes.

## REVIEW QUESTIONS

1. Explain why ethics and the application of ethical principles are especially important in health care.
2. Giving examples, differentiate among ethics, values, and morals.
3. How do deontological and teleological ethical theories differ?
4. How are paternalism and the principle of autonomy in opposition to each other?
5. Is role fidelity the same thing as functioning within one's scope of practice? Explain.
6. What is meant by the "balance of power" between a health care provider and a patient?
7. Explain the difference between a values history form and an advance directive.
8. Review the stories and videos about Brian Sinclair and Joyce Echaquan. Identify three ethical principles that you think most profoundly affected the way each of these individuals were treated and the tragic outcomes. Give examples to support your choices.
9. Explain the principles involved in medical assistance in dying.
10. Would S.J., who is in the early stages of dementia and has no physical health problems, be eligible for medical assistance in in dying? Why or why not? Discuss implications of this. Would this change if S.J. had a serious medical condition interfering with their quality of life?
11. What is meant by palliative sedation?
12. What is meant by the "allocation of health resources," and why does it present an ethical problem?
13. What are the benefits and drawbacks of having genetic testing done?
14. How would you define personhood?
15. Would it be ethical or moral to make vaccinating children for common childhood diseases mandatory? Support your answer drawing on your own thoughts, beliefs, and values about vaccinations.
16. Following an assault on a nurse by a mentally ill patient, a hospital stipulates that all mentally ill inpatients considered potentially "violent" or with violent tendencies must wear coloured armbands identifying them as such. Is this ethical? Does it violate the patient's rights? If so, which ones and on what grounds? What about the rights of the nurses to a safe environment? Is this policy discriminatory?

## REFERENCES

Broad Institute. (n.d.). *Questions and answers about CRISPR.* https://www.broadinstitute.org/what-broad/areas-focus/project-spotlight/questions-and-answers-about-crispr#:∼:text=A%3A%20%E2%80%9CCRISPR%E2%80%9D%20(pronounced,CRISPR%2DCas9%20genome%20editing%20technology.

Canadian Association of Social Workers. (n.d.). *Code of ethics: Core social work values and principles.* https://www.casw-acts.ca/files/attachements/code_of_ethics_-_printable_poster.pdf.

Canadian Charter of Rights and Freedoms. (1982). *S. 2, Part I of the constitution act, 1982, being Schedule B to the Canada act 1982 (UK) c* (p. 11).

Charlebois, B. (2022). *Canadian governments OK settlement with purdue pharma over opioid addictions.* The Canadian Press. CTV News. https://bc.ctvnews.ca/canadian-governments-ok-settlement-with-purdue-pharma-over-opioid-addictions-1.5968109#:∼:text=B.C.%20settles%20opioid%20lawsuit%

20for%20%24150M&text=A%20proposed%20%24150%2Dmillion%20settlement,of%20opioid%
2Dbased%20pain%20medication.

College of Nurses of Ontario. (2019). *Code of conduct.* https://www.cno.org/globalassets/docs/prac/49040_
code-of-conduct.pdf.

Genetic Non-Discrimination Act (S.C. 2017, c.3). https://laws-lois.justice.gc.ca/eng/acts/G-2.5/FullText.
html.

Government of Canada. (2022). *Suicide in canada.* https://www.canada.ca/en/public-health/services/
suicide-prevention/suicide-canada.html.

Health PEI. (2021). *Abortion services.* https://www.princeedwardisland.ca/en/information/health-pei/
abortion-services.

# 10

# Current Issues and Emerging Trends in Canadian Health Care

## LEARNING OUTCOMES

10.1 Discuss current issues concerning mental health and addiction in Canada.
10.2 Understand the challenges related to homelessness in Canada.
10.3 Describe the status of long-term, home, and community care in Canada.
10.4 Summarize two current health-related concerns of Indigenous people in Canada.
10.5 Explain the significance and management of information technology in health care.
10.6 Outline the most significant changes facing the Canadian health care system.

As noted throughout the book, despite numerous positive features about health care in Canada, there are significant inadequacies as well. These range from the state of mental health and addictions, long-term, and community care across the country to the impact of the COVID-19 pandemic on health and health care services. Currently, the very sustainability of the health care system is challenged, as evidenced by long waits for services and an acute shortage of health human resources.

Although most of these concerns have been addressed on some level throughout this book, this chapter briefly takes a closer look at some of these issues.

## MENTAL HEALTH AND ADDICTION

Every week, at least 500,000 Canadians miss work due to mental illness. Mental illness and issues related to addiction (or both) directly or indirectly affect every Canadian, by association with a family member, a friend, a loved one, or a colleague (Centre for Addiction and Mental Health [CAMH], 2020). Mental illness can affect anyone, regardless of age, sex or gender, educational level or income, culture, or domestic situation.

In any calendar year, one in five Canadians experience some form of mental illness. For those over the age of 40 that figure rises to a surprising one in two (CAMH, n.d.). According to the Centre for Addiction and Mental Health (CAMH), less than half of these individuals will seek support.

Timely access to appropriate mental health care remains a concern. There is an acute shortage of specialized human resources, a lack of strategic planning for collaborative community-based mental health services, and shortfalls in services to support individuals with substance use disorders. Responding to the need for more support for mental health and addiction services, the federal government announced in May 2022 an investment of $3,775,000, with $1,775,000 going toward 13 distress centres across the country and $2 million going to CAMH. The Centre will also help develop resources to support distress centres (Public Health Agency of Canada [PHAC], 2022).

The number of people seeking mental health services has increased since March 2020, with complaints of stress, anxiety, depression, burnout, and post-traumatic stress disorder (PTSD) reported as a result of the COVID-19 pandemic. As the pandemic continued to evolve between early 2020 and 2022, self-rated mental health continued to decrease (Statistics Canada, 2022a).

## THINKING IT THROUGH

### The Mental Health Continuum

Various definitions of mental health are usually wrapped up with those of health and wellness, emphasizing the integration of the different components of health. *Mental health* is the state of well-being in which a person is able to cope effectively with the stresses and challenges of daily living and is able to contribute to society, remain productive, and maintain a sense of self-worth and purpose. A person usually has the flexibility to move along the mental health continuum without illness. For example, the symptoms of sadness, anxiety, stress, and burnout in themselves do not mean a person has a mental illness, but could be warning signs that they need to seek help or support so that their symptoms do not progress to something more serious.

1. How do you cope when you are feeling overly anxious or stressed?
2. At what point would you consider seeking professional help?
3. When would you consider stress, anxiety, or depression or sadness to be a mental illness?

Source: Based on Plouffe, R. A., Liu, A., Richardson, J. D., et al. (2022, May 18). *Validation of the mental health continuum: Short form among Canadian Armed Forces personnel.* Statistics Canada. https://www150.statcan.gc.ca/n1/pub/82-003-x/2022005/article/00001-eng.htm

Burnout can cause significant stress and disruption in people's lives. The term is used loosely by some and more seriously by others. *Burnout* is a form of exhaustion, characterized by a wide range of symptoms including feeling extreme fatigue, discouragement, hopelessness, and futility and the realization of no longer being able to cope with a given situation that may be related to one's personal life or the workplace.

## THINKING IT THROUGH

### Burnout as a Clinical Diagnosis

In 2019, the World Health Organization recognized burnout as a syndrome resulting from chronic stress that has not been successfully managed by other interventions, and included it in the eleventh revision of the International Classification of Disease (ICD-11).

Burnout that many Canadians experience can be related to school, home, the workplace, volunteer or paid work, or a combination of these. A significant number of health care providers—from nurses, doctors, respiratory technologists, and paramedics to those who manage and interpret diagnostic tests—are reporting burnout as a result of the increased pressures added to their professional roles during the COVID-19 pandemic, combined with a sense of lack of respect for the work they do.

1. Have you ever felt overwhelmed or burnout from the pressures at school or work? What were your symptoms? How did you manage them? What resources did you have?
2. Do you feel that this should be a recognized diagnosis? Why or why not?

Sources: World Health Organization. (2019, May 28). *Burn-out an "occupational phenomenon": International Classification of Diseases.* https://www.who.int/news/item/28-05-2019-burn-out-an-occupational-phenomenon-international-classification-of-diseases; Berg, S. (2019, July 23). *WHO adds burnout to ICD-11. What it means for physicians.* https://www.ama-assn.org/practice-management/physician-health/who-adds-burnout-icd-11-what-it-means-physicians#:~:text=Burnout%20is%20now%20categorized%20as,the%20official%20compendium%20of%20diseases

## Structure and Implementation of Services

In Canada, mental health falls primarily under the jurisdiction of the provincial and territorial governments. These governments work with Health Canada, the Public Health Agency of Canada (PHAC), the Canadian Mental Health Association (CMHA), and their jurisdictional counterparts to plan strategies and interventions aimed at caring for people with mental illness and addictions. Provinces and territories share some responsibilities with the federal government for people who require mental health and addiction services when they become involved with the criminal justice system (Correctional Service Canada, 2020). The federal government (as with other aspects of health care) has a direct responsibility for the delivery of mental health services and addiction treatment to populations such as Status Indians and Inuit; the military; veterans; civil aviation personnel; under some circumstances the Royal Canadian Mounted Police (RCMP); inmates in federal penitentiaries; arriving immigrants; and federal public servants. Mental health facilities and the levels of government responsible for different population groups are discussed, in part, in Chapters 2, 3, and 7.

## Community-Based Services

In every province and territory, health organizations provide care and public education. Many jurisdictions offer a centralized point of contact to help people navigate the mental health care system and to provide them with direction about their legal rights (e.g., Alberta's Access Mental Health).

The CMHA and its nationwide branches deliver services and support to those with mental health and addiction challenges. This organization depends heavily on a dedicated team of volunteers to deliver and maintain its community programs. Other organizations such as United Way fund some uninsured services for those unable to pay, although many services remain accessible only to people who can afford them.

Larger hospitals have inpatient psychiatric units for people requiring more intensive care and support, treatment, and services. Patients are usually admitted under the services of a psychiatrist and remain in hospital until their physician considers them able to cope in the community with the appropriate supportive services (which are often inadequate). There are also numerous private facilities across the country that provide services, including specialized ones, such as for substance use or eating disorders. Across the country, as the demand for mental health services grows, availability of even private services is limited. For example, a growing number of referrals for children with eating disorders have been observed since the onset of the pandemic. For these specialized services, in some provinces, wait times for community-based and outpatient programs can be anywhere from 6 to 18 months or longer (Dubois, 2022).

Registered psychiatric nurses (see Chapter 5) continue to provide a wide range of invaluable services to individuals with mental health disorders, in four provinces (Manitoba, Saskatchewan, Alberta, and British Columbia). Services address both mental and developmental health and illness and addiction while also attending to physical, social, and spiritual needs of patients from a holistic perspective (Canadian Institute for Health Information [CIHI], 2022).

Distress centres help individuals connect to a variety of mental health services, including those that offer crisis support, emotional support, crisis intervention, and suicide prevention (PHAC, 2022). These centres are managed by volunteers and operate around the clock, all year round.

## Virtual Mental Health Support Services

The delivery of mental health services has been enhanced through the use of the Internet and related technologies (referred to as *e-mental health*, *virtual*, or *digital mental health services*).

E-health services are rapidly expanding, offering numerous advantages such as connectivity to mental health professionals for treatment and support without having to go to a clinic. Wait times are shorter, and access to services may be obtained in the language one prefers. Numerous apps on mobile devices improve access to web-based support and self-help therapies, which have proven effective in managing disorders such as burnout, depression, anxiety, and PTSD. Mobile device apps can provide mood-tracking options and social media support forums, giving people an improved sense of control over their mental health and treatment. E-mental health options are also valuable in helping to maintain balance and prevent many mental health issues from progressing into something more serious. There are numerous online solutions, including mindfulness exercises to reduce anxiety, that can be done anytime.

### Support Groups

Support groups are available through social media, usually initiated by providers or health organizations, and can be an important part of a person's overall treatment plan. Support groups typically target issues such as grief, mental health, and addiction (see Chapter 7) as well as chronic diseases and cancer. They may be facilitated by a person within the group or be led by a health professional. Support groups help participants cope with their health problems, provide practical advice, and impart a sense of belonging and companionship, or anonymity, as required.

For instance, Alberta Health Services has partnered with Togetherall to establish an entirely anonymous (virtual) peer-to-peer service that is available anytime online. Participants can communicate with larger groups or form smaller ones and have access to a variety of clinically approved resources, including self-guided resources and assessments.

### Wellness Together Canada: Mental Health Support

Wellness Together Canada was created with funding from the federal government in response to an unprecedented rise in mental health and substance use concerns during the COVID-19 pandemic. Wellness Together Canada is designed to be used on demand: the person can choose what services they need as well as the timing (Wellness Together Canada, n.d.). Services range from basic wellness information, to one-on-one sessions with a counsellor, to participating in group sessions. Organizations supporting Wellness Together Canada include Bell Let's Talk and the Canadian Psychological Association.

### MindBeacon

MindBeacon is an online therapist-guided program for Ontario residents over the age of 16 years that helps participants address and deal with such issues as stress, anxiety, and depression. To register, a person must complete an online form detailing information about themselves and their issues and expectations. Through secure, direct messaging, a therapist works with the applicant to address their concerns during a 12-week individualized program that is based on cognitive behavioural therapy (MindBeacon, n.d.). Funding for MindBeacon was reduced by approximately 85% in August 2022 (King, 2022). As a result, the program changed from being a self-referral, free program to one wherein a person must have a specialized referral for it to remain free of charge. Others wanting to enroll in the program are required to pay a fee of $525.

### Substance Use Disorders

Approximately one-fifth of Canadians experience a substance use disorder at some time in their lives (CMHA, n.d.). The most commonly used substances are alcohol, cannabis, cocaine, methamphetamines, and opioids. Opioids include oxycodone, hydrocodone (Vicodin), morphine, methadone, and fentanyl.

The COVID-19 pandemic has contributed to the existing and ongoing national public health overdose crisis in the use of opioids and other stimulants. Increased use of drugs during the pandemic has been attributed to more people experiencing elevated levels of stress, anxiety, feelings of isolation, and a corresponding lack of mental health services. The result has been increased mortality rates and other harms across Canada. During the first year of the pandemic, there was a 96% increase in apparent opioid toxicity deaths (April 2020 to March 2021) compared to the year before (Government of Canada, 2022a). The majority of opioid toxicity deaths were from nonpharmaceutical fentanyl. Most deaths occurred in British Columbia, Alberta, Manitoba, and Ontario, largely due to toxic drug supplies and limited access to mental health and other services, including harm reduction sites (many of which were closed during the pandemic because of public health restrictions).

### Harm Reduction Sites

Harm reduction sites are also referred to as *safe injection sites* or *supervised consumption sites or clinics*. They are guided by strategies, practices, and procedures that reduce the harm to individuals caused by substance use and addiction.

Harm reduction sites offer a variety of services that vary among provinces and territories. These services include testing drugs for impurities or containments (additives), providing clean needles, responding to overdoses, and, in some jurisdictions, distributing prescription-grade heroin. Many sites also offer counselling services and access to rehabilitation facilities. Harm reduction sites can be found in almost every community across the country. Some are temporary, others more permanent. Establishing a clinic requires permission from either municipal or provincial or territorial governments. Clinic locations are carefully selected in collaboration with the relevant community. More recently, the focus has been on alleviating harm related to the misuse of opioids such as methadone, oxycodone, hydromorphone, fentanyl (one of the most toxic opioids), and heroin.

Because of an increasing supply of contaminated street drugs, an innovative strategy using machines that dispense prescription-grade hydromorphone tablets (initially introduced in British Columbia in 2016) has recently been expanded on a trial basis in Ontario and Nova Scotia (see Box 10.1).

---

### DID YOU KNOW?

#### *Street Drugs*

Many street drugs are illegally produced with the addition of various combinations of drugs that add to the potency and response unpredictability. For example, carfentanyl (sometimes used by veterinarians as a sedative in large animals such as elephants) is often compounded into pills, making it very difficult, if not impossible, to differentiate it from a prescription opioid. Because of its high toxicity, a very small amount of carfentanyl can cause a severe overdose and often death. The antidote (which reverses the effect of the opioid) is Narcan or naloxone, which is now widely available across the country, from pharmacies to libraries. Narcan comes as an injection or in the form of a nasal spray. It takes between 30 seconds and 2 minutes to work.

---

***Prescription opioids.*** Since October 2018, Health Canada has made it mandatory that pharmacists alloy bright yellow stickers to all medication containers containing dispensed opioids, stating that "opioids can cause dependence, addiction and overdose." In addition, a pamphlet outlining the risks of the drug is given to the patient by the pharmacist. Pharmaceutical companies must also implement risk management plans for the opioids they produce that indicate the dangers related to their use (addictive properties) and signs of addiction (Health Canada, 2018).

BOX 10.1 **MySave Dispensing Terminals**

Between 2016 and 2020, approximately 80% of overdose deaths in British Columbia were attributed to a contaminated drug supply. One effort to combat this trend is a dispensing machine that resembles an ATM that is stocked with hydromorphone tablets. The machine, called MySafe, which was installed in Vancouver's East Side in 2020, identifies designated users by scanning the vein pattern in their hands. Once the person's identity is verified, the machine dispenses their prescription on a predetermined schedule. People who use opioids and have a history of overdosing undergo prescreening and medical assessment before acceptance into the program; they also commit to regular follow-up with a medical professional.

In 2021, federal funding allowed for expansion of the MySafe project to another site in Vancouver and one each in Victoria (British Columbia), Dartmouth (Nova Scotia), and London (Ontario).

Source: Based on Watson, B. (2020, January 17). *Vancouver's drug-dispensing machine: Why it exists and how it works*. CBC News. https://www.cbc.ca/news/canada/british-columbia/vancouver-drug-dispensing-machine-opioids-overdoses-1.5429704

***New legal agreement for British Columbia.*** In May 2022, British Columbia became the first jurisdiction in Canada to negotiate an agreement with the federal government to allow people to possess up to 2.5 grams of designated illegal drugs, for personal use, without fear of being criminally charged (Health Canada, 2022a). These drugs include heroin, morphine, fentanyl, cocaine, methamphetamine, and MDMA (Ecstasy). Individuals must be over 18 years old and found to have no intent to traffic the drugs in their possession. Instead, those found in possession of one of these substances are given information on health-related resources and help accessing these services.

This trial, which began in January 2023, was initiated by the province to address the high mortality rate and related harms from the use of illegal drugs. The exemption was granted under Section 56 of the *Controlled Drugs and Substances Act*. Other jurisdictions have voiced interest in establishing a similar agreement with the federal government, but the arrangement is only with British Columbia until the trial is complete, in January 2026.

## MENTAL HEALTH AND HOMELESSNESS IN CANADA

The causes of homelessness are multiple and complex. Almost without exception, predisposing factors include socioeconomic inequities. Simply being homeless can have such detrimental effects on a person that it can precipitate a mental illness or intensify the seriousness of an existing or pre-existing condition exclusive of other socioeconomic factors including poverty, social isolation, and personal issues. Homeless people experience a higher prevalence of mental illness than the general population (up to 50%) in addition to disproportionately high rates of substance use and altered physical health (Homeless Hub, n.d.). That said, it must be noted that not all people experiencing homelessness have or will ever develop a mental health condition.

Community services play an important role in helping homeless people access services and stay connected with mental health support workers. This support is critical as individuals who have no permanent address are further disadvantaged because they often have no sustainable means of communication and establishing or maintaining treatment plans for mental health support.

The emergency department (ED) is a frequent point of care for people with homelessness, who are usually disconnected from their primary care practitioner (if they ever had one) and who may not be close to their original community.

## Reducing Homelessness

Strategies to reduce homelessness vary with the province or territory and community. They are determined on the basis of available resources, demographics, and varying needs in each community. Resources available may or may not include government funding, fundraising events, planners and policymakers, service providers, medical and mental health authorities, community groups, and volunteers.

### Housing First

Housing First is a framework widely used across Canada for developing housing programs for people who are experiencing homelessness. Housing First provides accommodation, clinical services (access to community services), and additional support—for example, helping people find employment and educational opportunities and integrate into the community. One of the key elements of the Housing First framework is providing permanent housing without setting preconditions or eligibility criteria; for example, applicants do not have to be sober or attend treatment sessions before being considered for permanent housing.

Providing people with housing through programs like Housing First dramatically reduces visits to the ED and improves residents' general health. Seven cities in Alberta reported that, as a result of the program, overall lengths of hospital stays were reduced by 64% and numbers of visits to the ED by 60% (7 Cities, 2018). In Medicine Hat, Alberta, the Housing First initiative, in conjunction with other community agencies, has all but eliminated homelessness in that city. The initiative aims to have every person who is homeless or at risk of homelessness connected with a support worker, on average within 3 days, and move into permanent housing within 10 days (Lawrynuik, 2017). By doing so, the city of Medicine Hat became the first in Canada to functionally eliminate chronic homelessness in the community in 2021 (Ranney, 2021). Many of these strategies are now embedded in strategies used by Canada's national homeless strategy (Infrastructure Canada, 2022). However, in 2022, Medicine Hat faced some renewed challenges finding accommodation for increased numbers of homeless people.

### Reaching Home: Canada's Homeless National Housing Strategy

A national housing strategy called *Reaching Home* was announced for the first time in the fall of 2017. Building on past frameworks, the federal government pledged to invest more than $40 billion over a 10-year time frame into housing programs for vulnerable populations (Infrastructure Canada, 2022). Reaching Home delivers funding to reduce homelessness in urban, Indigenous, and remote communities, addressing the specific needs of each community. The primary goals of the national strategy are ambitious, including to reduce homelessness by half by 2028.

Some of the funding was earmarked to reduce homelessness among Indigenous people. In consultation with Indigenous communities and leaders, culturally safe resources and support are provided to meet the unique needs of vulnerable individuals within that population base.

Members of the committee recommending ways to reduce homelessness were from diverse backgrounds and included individuals with actual lived experience of homelessness to ensure that strategies embraced demographic and cultural needs. It is important to note that these strategies have considered the jurisdictional barriers (both historic and current) identified by the Truth and Reconciliation Commission (2015) and acknowledged that implemented practices must be consistent with the Commission's Calls to Action.

Funding goes directly to municipalities and local service providers. Although there are some guidelines, the federal government does not specifically dictate how funds are to be used in each community. Some funding does target Housing First programs as well as those organizations that provide emergency shelters and services when housing is unavailable. Housing First programs are encouraged to adapt their programs to respond to the unique needs of youth, Indigenous people, women seeking refuge from intimate partner violence, and Armed Services veterans. Under the restructured framework, communities not already receiving support can apply for funding. The strategy will provide ongoing support in terms of information, advice, and the tools needed to structure and deliver system-based plans to reduce homelessness in a coordinated manner, utilizing services and resources within their communities. For example, the national strategy uses the Homeless Individual and Families Information System, a data collection and case management platform that enables numerous service providers within a community to access real-time information for promoting coordination of services and daily operations, in addition to the collection and development of a national picture of homelessness. Available reports generated by this system include an analysis of shelter capacity and use as well as the nationally coordinated Point-in-Time Counts (which provide a national picture of homelessness at any given time).

Despite a national strategy, eliminating homelessness in any community will always be difficult. Some of the reasons include the high cost of housing in many cities; inflation, affecting the cost of labour and building materials; the shortage of housing and rental units; stigma, with people not wanting shelters or assisted housing in their neighbourhoods; existing lack of funding and of coordinated, effective strategies; and an increased incidence of mental illness and addictions, with inadequate mental health services to address these concerns.

Currently, Canada's National Housing Strategy is the largest undertaken by the federal government to date. The federal government will invest over $70 billion to improve access to affordable housing for Canadians across the country. This money is in addition to $13 billion proposed through the 2020 Fall Economic Statement. One of the main goals of this strategy is to cut chronic homelessness by 50% within 10 years and to initially focus on the most vulnerable people in the country (Government of Canada, 2020).

There will always be individuals who require emergency shelters, many of whom won't find a bed because of shortages in hostels and shelters, forcing individuals to stay outside. During the winters, street-involved people are particularly vulnerable. Cities across Canada scramble to provide accommodation, sometimes opening facilities as temporary sanctuaries. In 2023, advocates in some communities pushed to have warming centres opened around the clock during the cold weather months (not just overnight). Alternatively, outreach workers canvas known locations to provide food, warm drinks, blankets, and sleeping bags (Advisory Committee on Homelessness, 2018).

Numerous organizations across Canada provide temporary or emergency shelter, for example, the Salvation Army (operating in over 4000 communities across Canada); Out of the Cold Foundation (a network of churches and other religious organizations rotating available facilities); the Scott Mission (providing family accommodation in Toronto, Ontario); Young Parents No Fixed Address (focusing on pregnant youth and those with children in Toronto); Inn from the Cold (which opened Calgary's first emergency shelter); Hope Mission (also operating a 24-7 rescue van supplying blankets, lunches, and necessary supplies to people who are homeless in Edmonton); Bissell Centre (which provides shelter and warm meals in Edmonton); and the Lighthouse (operating emergency shelters and affordable housing plus other services in Saskatoon).

In 2021, the Government of Québec invested $280 million through an initiative called *S'allier devant l'itinerance* to provide short- and long-term support for homeless people in the province (Québec Ministry of Health and Social Services, 2021). The intent is to afford a stable source of funding for organizations addressing homelessness. Some of the money is allocated for those at immediate risk of homelessness, Indigenous people, and homeless women.

## Effects of COVID-19 on Homelessness

Individuals experiencing homelessness have been disproportionately affected by the COVID-19 pandemic because of their medical comorbidities and the lack of access to preventive care and health services (Baral et al., 2021). A 2021 6-month study of 30,000 individuals in Ontario found that people experiencing homelessness were approximately 20 times more likely to be hospitalized with COVID-19, 10 times more likely to require intensive care treatment, and more than 5 times likely to die within 21 days of testing positive for COVID-19 (Booth et al., 2021).

During the pandemic, shelters already stretched beyond capacity, struggled to adhere to infection prevention and control measures necessary to reduce transmission of the virus. In an attempt to meet public health guidelines, communities did their best to increase shelter capacity by any means possible, such as renting rooms in hotels and motels. Crowded conditions in shelters and outright lack of any accommodation motivated many homeless individuals to join homeless encampments, which were already abundant in both rural and urban settings across the country.

## THINKING IT THROUGH

### Homeless Encampments

Encampments (also referred to as *tent cities*) vary in size, sometimes accommodating well over 100 people. Encampments may be under overpasses, on green spaces near exit ramps to highways, or in parks. Encampments are not limited to larger cities, existing in small communities and rural areas. Factors that contribute to homelessness and hence the number of people living in encampments include low wages and pensions, lack of affordable housing, and discrimination due to mental illness or addictions, which affect peoples' ability to hold down a job and thus afford a place to live. According to one human rights report, "Ultimately, encampments are a reflection of Canadian governments' failure to successfully implement the right to adequate housing" and are a public health crisis (Farha & Schwan, 2020).

Even though encampment life is hard, with year-round exposure to the elements and a lack of sanitation that is challenging, even deadly, some residents feel safer there than in shelters, where there is some social support.

The number of encampments increased dramatically during the pandemic as people fled overcrowded shelters. Encampments are, for the most part, illegal and unwanted by cities and most communities because of health concerns (e.g., lack of basic services such as toilets and showers) and lack of safety for those in the encampment as well as the surrounding community. Although most people agree that encampments are neither safe nor sustainable, viable solutions remain elusive. When encampments are forcibly disbanded, often by the police, alternatives for where residents can go are not offered. What's more, people's trust in service providers is negatively affected, making it harder to convince people to move into shelters.

1. How would you feel about a homeless encampment in your community? Explain your answer.
2. What alternatives or suggestions would you make to address solutions for these encampments?

The Royal Society of Canada has proposed ways to reduce or even prevent negative outcomes from COVID-19 and future respiratory outbreaks in the homeless population (Adams & Tremblay, 2020). Short-term goals include reacting promptly in coordinating a response; ensuring adequate supplies of personal protective equipment and tests; coordinating access to available vaccines; having in place contact management strategies; ensuring adequate structural resources to implement isolation protocols; and reducing congestion in shelters. Long-term goals include the provision of adequate subsidized and supportive housing through such initiatives as Housing First.

## HOME, COMMUNITY, AND LONG-TERM CARE

Well before the pandemic, there was general agreement that Canada needed a national strategy to develop Canada-wide standards of care that address the needs of an aging population in order to provide equality and consistency of care (Canadian Home Care Association, 2018). Establishing national standards of care for an aging population necessitates adopting a best practices approach for both home and community care and long-term care across the country. This process includes developing programs for healthy aging, devising strategies to combat ageism, improving coordination of health and social services, and establishing more clearly defined and transparent methods for older Canadians to navigate the health care system. There also needs to be in place a national mechanism to evaluate system performance so that strategies are research-based, logical, and effective. Existing services and programs need to be improved to address the requirements of Canada's culturally diverse population as well.

### Long-Term and Residential Care

COVID-19 has affected industry, businesses, organizations, and the health care system, as well as the lives of every Canadian in one way or another. But it presented perhaps some of the greatest challenges to residential and long-term care (LTC) facilities. Residents in LTC have been disproportionately affected by the pandemic in terms of both morbidity and mortality rates. An analysis, which includes data from both the CIHI and the National Institute on Ageing, shows that during the first three waves of the pandemic, individuals living in LTC facilities accounted for 3% of all COVID-19 infections and 43% of COVID-19 deaths. Between May 2020 and March 2021 alone there were more than 15,000 COVID infections among LTC residents and approximately 22,000 infections among staff members, resulting in over 14,000 deaths (among staff and residents) (CIHI, 2021). It is interesting to note that in early 2021, approximately 95% of individuals in LTC facilities across Canada received their first vaccination compared with about 3% of the general population. As a result, both COVID-related infections and deaths in these facilities dropped by over 90%. Table 10.1 illustrates COVID-19 deaths in LTC facilities by province occurring during the first three waves of the pandemic.

Capacity, staffing shortfalls, quality of care, and built-environment issues related to LTC have persisted over many years in all jurisdictions. During the pandemic these issues were exacerbated. These factors, plus the gaps in infection prevention and control (IPAC) measures, contributed to the disproportionate morbidity and mortality rates among residents in LTC facilities across the country. Frontline health care workers were also adversely affected; most did their best to care for residents under very difficult conditions while navigating the risk of acquiring the infection themselves and balancing their own safety and that of their families. Other caregivers simply left, abandoning their patients and responsibilities for many of the same reasons.

The alarming number of infections and the unprecedented mortality rates among LTC residents during the first wave of the pandemic resulted in the Chief Science Advisor assembling a task force to advise on strategies to limit the spread of COVID-19 among staff and residents in facilities and improve residents' health outcomes (Office of the Chief Science Advisor of Canada, 2020). The task force comprised experts in related fields from across the country. The first part of the report, released in April 2020, outlined short-term goals and recommended actions that addressed these priority concerns. Priority areas requiring immediate action identified by the task force included the following:

- Providing adequate staffing levels to meet the care needs of all residents
- Ensuring that staff have the mix and level of skills that correspond with residents' needs

**TABLE 10.1   COVID-19 Deaths in Long-Term Care per 100,000 Population**

| Province | Wave 1: March 1 to August 31, 2020 (6 months) | Wave 2: September 1, 2020 to February 28, 2021 (6 months) | Wave 3: March 1 to August 15, 2021 (5.5 months) |
|---|---|---|---|
| Nova Scotia | 5.9 | 0.0 | 0.0 |
| New Brunswick | 0.3 | 1.1 | 0.9 |
| Québec | 43.2 | 17.3 | 1.6 |
| Ontario | 13.5 | 13.9 | 0.4 |
| Manitoba | 0.2 | 32.7 | 0.9 |
| Saskatchewan | 0.2 | 6.6 | 0.7 |
| Alberta | 3.2 | 15.7 | 0.4 |
| British Columbia | 2.6 | 12.8 | 0.7 |

Notes: In Alberta, long-term care is defined as any site with long-term care spaces, including sites with co-located supportive living spaces.
There were no long-term care cases in Prince Edward Island, Yukon, the Northwest Territories, or Nunavut.
**Source:** Canadian Institute for Health Information. (2021, December 9). *COVID-19's impact on long-term care*. https://www.cihi.ca/en/covid-19-resources/impact-of-covid-19-on-canadas-health-care-systems/long-term-care

- Making sure that hospitals provide adequate coordination and support for LTC facilities (In some jurisdictions, hospitals were asked to assist LTC facilities with IPAC protocols and testing at times and respond to other needs such as staffing, care of residents, organization, and administrative requirements.)
- Evaluating and improving IPAC measures so that they are current and effective (The same year, the task force endorsed the Public Health Agency of Canada's *Infection Prevention and Control for COVID-19: Interim guidance for long-term care homes*, which was updated in June 2021.) (Government of Canada, 2022b)

The second part of the report addressed existing issues exacerbated by the pandemic, which included the following:

- Long-standing inattention and inaction in assessing and improving LTC facilities and how they deliver care
- Lack of consistency in facilities in terms of structural and operational functions
- Inadequate resources, especially during times of crisis
- A built environment that contravenes IPAC procedures and policies (e.g., close contact of residents, often with two or three residents living in one room, and staff), increasing the infectivity rate

The task force noted that LTC facilities in different regions operate in different contexts, but suggested the same recommendations be applied to any setting where older persons live (e.g., retirement, residential, and group homes). The recommendations provided by the task force became part of the wider national strategy for reforming the LTC system.

## National Standards for Long-Term Care

In 2021, the Standards Council of Canada (SCC), Health Standards Organization (HSO; associated with Accreditation Canada), Canadian Standards Association (CSA) Group, and over 18,000 Canadians collaborated to develop two new national standards for LTC in Canada. The standards address both new and existing problems (identified in other reports) brought to light during the COVID-19 pandemic (Health Standards Organization, 2022). They include the delivery of high-quality care that is safe, predictable, and reliable in addition to operational components of LTC facilities and IPAC policies and procedures.

Enactment of these recommended changes requires ongoing collaboration and cooperation at all levels of government working with the LTC sector across jurisdictions. Implementation of the standards also requires sustained and predictable funding in addition to recruiting and training health human resources (Canadian Association for Long-Term Care, 2022). A draft of the recommendations was released for public comments and feedback by the CSA Group and HSO in February 2022. The final report was released in late 2022. The report, *National Standard of Canada for Operation and Infection Prevention and Control of Long-Term Care Homes,* focuses on safe operational practices and the development of IPAC measures. The categories of topics under this umbrella include organizational commitments, operations, IPAC design, LTC home systems, information and technology, and training (Health Standards Organization, 2022).

Guidance for improving standards of care and facilitating a strong, reliable, and competent workforce as well as upholding governance standards and practices were developed by HSO's Long-Term Care Services Standard Technical Committee. A link to the standards is available on the EVOLVE site for this book.

## Home and Community Care

Most people want to maintain their independence for as long as possible. Living at home with the proper support is often a better option than living in long-term or continuing care, and a more economical one. Although home care is more cost-effective, many obstacles to this exist: insufficient numbers of trained home care workers; limited provincial and territorial insurance coverage for these services; inconsistent, poorly coordinated, and poor-quality care; and scheduling or communication issues among caregivers (Canadian Home Care Association, 2017). Most families provide a certain amount of care for family members (in addition to care provided by homecare agencies). Known as *informal caregivers*, they play an important role in keeping family members and loved ones at home, but they can only do so much.

### Informal Caregivers

The number of Canadians who cannot manage independent living is expected to double within the next 30 years (Arrigada, 2020). Because of lack of capacity in the health care system, more and more families may have to assume responsibilities for their loved ones. Conditions that older Canadians are coping with include aging, cancer, Alzheimer's disease or dementia, cardiovascular disease, and mental illness, in order of prevalence. Each condition has its unique set of challenges, which are compounded by comorbidities.

In 2018, about one-quarter of Canadians over 15 years old were providing some level of care for family members or friends in their homes. What's more, 25% of caregivers were over 65 years old, often themselves coping with altered health.

## THINKING IT THROUGH

### *Informal Caregivers*

The COVID-19 pandemic intensified the responsibilities assumed by informal caregivers and highlighted the importance of their contributions in providing care in the home *as well as* in long-term care facilities. During the pandemic, many informal caregivers found they had to increase the hours of care they provided to the people they were caring for because of the decreased capacity of the public system and other organizations to provide the level of care they did before the pandemic.

1. How do you think the public system could best support informal caregivers other than providing some monetary support and job protection if they must take time off from work?
2. What other suggestions can you make that would help older persons stay out of long-term care facilities?

### What Is Next for Home Care?

All jurisdictions have a mandate to improve home care services with the targeted funding received from the federal government in 2017 as well as any other funds they receive (federally or from within the jurisdiction). This includes developing policies, procedures, and strategies to address problems (see Chapters 3 and 5). It is important to remember that the demographics of an older population vary with jurisdiction, resulting in variation in funding formulas as well as in the specific needs and concerns in each community. For example, more older Canadians live in Québec, New Brunswick, Saskatchewan and British Columbia (Statistics Canada, 2022b).

Although Canada lacks a national legislative platform for home care standards, a pan-Canadian framework of standards has been proposed through the Canadian Home Care Association after consultation with home care policy planners, health care providers, patients, and caregivers. These standards are based in part on the Harmonized Principles for Home Care, which is a statement of home care values that are shared across Canada. The Harmonized Home Care Principles underpin quality standards acknowledged by national accreditation bodies, specifically Accreditation Canada's Qmentum program. Ministries of Health in Alberta, British Columbia, Manitoba, New Brunswick, Nova Scotia, and Yukon have expressed support for principle-based home care standards. These standards include care that is evidence-informed, accessible, sustainable, integrated, person- and family-oriented, and accountable.

Even with national standards of care as a guideline, establishing an efficient, cost-effective, and comprehensive home care system in each province and territory will take time. Effective use of home care services and a collaborative framework will optimize current resources, organizing services and managing inventory to avoid duplication and taking steps to reduce supply wastage. Improving communication and organization of scheduling can ensure that the same care provider stays with the same care recipient as long as possible, improving the efficiency, quality, and continuity of care a person receives.

### Provincial and Territorial Actions

Jurisdictions are doing what they can to address the challenges of home and community care and long-term and continuing services in general, as well as in the aftermath of the pandemic. In April 2022, the federal government gave Ontario $375 million through the Safe Long-Term Care fund (Health Canada, 2022b). The money will be used for such measures as improving IPAC management, ensuring adequate supplies of personal protective equipment and testing, and to strengthen staff recruitment and retention. In May 2022, Ontario repealed the *Home Care and Community Services Act* replacing it with the *Connecting People to Home and Community Act* with the purpose of modernizing the framework for delivering home and community care.

In its 2022 budget, Alberta allotted $204 million to update existing continuing care facilities in the province over 3 years and added additional spaces for Indigenous people and other communities based on need (Government of Alberta, 2022). In addition, funds from the 2022 operating budget were to be directed toward home care, continuing care, and continuing or long-term care improvements.

All jurisdictions are balancing protocols to keep older persons safe, whether it is in the community or in long-term or continuing care facilities. Protocols will continue to be fluid, adjusting as required to threats imposed by the pandemic and other challenges.

## CURRENT ISSUES FOR INDIGENOUS PEOPLE

Issues facing Indigenous people in Canada (such as those discussed throughout this book) have remained relatively constant for decades, with modest improvements in some areas and very few in others. The lack of clean water on many reservations and the continued trauma caused by the discovery of unmarked graves on the grounds of some residential schools are addressed here.

### Clean Water

Canada has the third-largest renewable freshwater supply in the world, yet there are many Indigenous communities (particularly reserves) in Canada who do not have access to clean water and remain under "boil water" advisories (some communities for up to 25 years) (Lillo et al., 2021). Can you imagine growing up under these conditions? Not being able to turn on the tap and know the water is safe to bath or cook with, let alone to drink? And yet, access to clean water is considered a basic human right.

Progress has been made with respect to improving access to clean water on reserves, with a majority of communities having some form of water treatment system. However, these treatment systems often do not work properly or do not serve an entire community because of lack of infrastructure. As a result, residents must rely on water from private wells and stand pipes that are vulnerable to contamination from *E. coli* and other microorganisms. In many First Nations communities, water has elevated levels of heavy metals, including iron and manganese, which cannot be removed by boiling.

In 2015, the federal government promised that all long-term boil water advisories in First Nations reserves would be ended by 2021. Although progress has been made, this goal has not been met for several reasons. One is the fact that Indigenous Services Canada's financial support is chronically inadequate because of an outdated funding policy for the operation and maintenance of water systems. A salary gap makes it difficult to retain trained and certified water system operators (Office of the Auditor General Canada, 2021). Until such time as deficiencies in the management and maintenance of water treatment systems are adequately addressed, many communities will continue to experience boil water advisories as well as need drinking water brought into the community.

As of January 2023, 32 short-term drinking water advisories were in place in Canada (not including British Columbia and the territories), and 34 long-term advisories were in place in 32 communities, not including the territories. (Government of Canada 2023a; Government of Canada 2023b). Note that these figures fluctuate as advisories are lifted or reimposed with alarming frequency.

In December 2022, the federal government settled an $8 billion lawsuit launched in 2019 by Indigenous communities concerning prolonged drinking-water advisories on First Nations reserves across the country. The settlement includes compensation for individuals as well as First Nations who endured drinking water advisories lasting at least one year between November 1995 and June 2021. Of this, $1.5 billion went to individuals deprived of clean drinking water during that time frame (First Nations Drinking Water, n.d.)

For a comprehensive understanding of the challenges Indigenous people face with respect to a precarious supply of clean water and the effects it has on them as individuals and as a community, consider watching *Broken Promises*, an investigation into water quality issues in First Nations communities. This video was produced by students at the School of Journalism at the University of Regina, with research contributions from students at First Nations University of Canada. A link to this video and others is found on the Evolve site for this book.

### Unmarked Graves on the Grounds of Residential Schools

In May 2021, the Tk'emlúps te Secwépemc First Nation discovered 215 unmarked graves on the grounds of a former residential school outside of Kamloops, British Columbia. The revelation sent shock waves across the country, validating what many former students had described experiencing and witnessing in these institutions (Hopper, 2021). The next month, the Cowessess First Nation found 751 unmarked graves on the grounds of a former residential school east of Regina, Saskatchewan. Similar unmarked graves continue to be discovered across the country (Eneas, 2021).

Approximately 150,000 children are thought to have attended residential schools (see Chapter 1). Of these, the Truth and Reconciliation Commission estimated that at least 3200 died at these schools, but it may have been as many as 6000. Causes of death include accidents, infectious diseases such as pneumonia and tuberculosis, and malnutrition as well as suicide. Records of the children who died were poorly maintained, if at all, and were often incomplete. School officials may have recorded the death of a child but little or no information about them—not even their gender. Some families never heard from nor saw their children again—a source of unimaginable grief and trauma.

Many former residential school students continue to re-experience the trauma they endured. Their descendants may live with intergenerational trauma, having learned adaptive "survival" behaviour, passed on through generations, that limits their ability to thrive because they lack a sense of safety and security. People experiencing intergenerational trauma often have extreme reactivity to stress and hypervigilance; a heightened sense of vulnerability and helplessness; increased anxiety and guilt; low self-esteem; depression, suicidal thoughts, and substance use disorders; as well as difficulty with relationships and in regulating aggression (Journey Counselling, 2021; Limmena, 2021).

---

### DID YOU KNOW?

#### *Telephone Helpline*

In the four days following the finding of unmarked graves in Kamloops, crisis lines saw a 265% increase in calls. Crisis support lines across the country are staffed with people trained to provide mental health support. The Hope for Wellness Helpline (https://www. hopeforwellness.ca/), for example, provides direct support for Indigenous people who require immediate, culturally competent counselling, crisis intervention, or both for recently triggered painful memories or for current or past incidents. Another resource is the Indian Residential Schools Resolution Health Support Program, which provides mental health, emotional, and cultural support services for survivors of the residential school system and their families (Indigenous Services Canada, 2022).

During the coming years, technical teams will work to find more answers regarding these unmarked graves, identify remains where possible, and repatriate these to their rightful resting places. Please view the related video on the Evolve site, as it explains much about the discovery of these unmarked graves (stressing that they are not mass graves), who else might be resting in these grave sites, and the reasons why at least some of these graves are unmarked.

## The Way Forward

The discovery of these unmarked graves has served as a wake-up call to many non-Indigenous people in Canada, providing proof of the horrors that Indigenous people have described witnessing and enduring at residential schools. In an interview with CBC television in June 2022, singer/song writer Buffy Sainte-Marie said of the discovery of unmarked graves, "the good news about the bad news is more people know about it" (Hobbs, 2022). Perhaps the shock will also promote a better understanding of the inequities that Indigenous people cope with on a daily basis in terms of systemic racism within health care and in many Canadian institutions.

Improving the health and wellness of Indigenous populations goes well beyond treating individuals; it is necessary to recognize the devastating effects of the residential school system, the Sixties Scoop, and other effects of colonization on the health and well-being of Indigenous people (see Chapter 6). While no short-term solutions exist, we cannot afford to delay any further action, with all levels of government, agencies, and organizations working across disciplines.

The broader challenges are complex. At the forefront is a multilayered and multifaceted health care system managed by multiple partners and levels of government; a lack of trust, understanding, and vision among stakeholders; cultural complexities; resource limitations (financial and physical); and the length of time it takes to implement change. Progress requires a sound commitment from all stakeholders and a willingness to build trust, maintain open minds, and employ innovative thinking to meet the challenges. Most importantly, Indigenous people themselves must be involved at all levels of health care—from identifying health problems to participating in solutions for appropriate services and care that is culturally safe.

The *Truth and Reconciliation Commission of Canada: Calls to Action* report (2015) identifies key health care areas that must be addressed in Calls to Action 18 through 24. Six years after the release of the Truth and Reconciliation Commission's report, fewer than one-fifth of the 94 Calls to Action have been completed, with the actual number varying between 11 and 17 according to the source—Indigenous organizations or the federal government (Jewell & Mosby, 2020). In health care, there has been limited progress. For example, one of the Canadian Institutes of Health Research (CIHR), the Institute of Indigenous Peoples' Health (IIPH), oversees national health research (in collaboration with Indigenous leaders and communities) to garner information on identifying and analyzing core problems that continue to affect the health and well-being of Indigenous peoples (CIHI, 2018). In 2017, the IIPH founded the Indigenous Health Research Support Office to support other projects, including Pathways to Health Equity for Aboriginal Peoples. Their mandate includes research on mental wellness, tuberculosis, diabetes and related obesity, as well as oral health.

In addition, each jurisdiction has implemented programs specific to their own needs, policies, and procedures, many in collaboration with the federal government. Universities such as the University of British Columbia, the University of Saskatchewan, the University of Alberta, and the University of Manitoba have expanded their educational programming to include culturally based curricula recommended in the Calls to Action.

# INFORMATION TECHNOLOGY AND ELECTRONIC HEALTH RECORDS

Information technology (IT) has changed the face of health care, with advances occurring sometimes daily with the promise of efficiencies that improve patient care and connectivity across the health care spectrum. Until recently, however, the Canadian health care system has lagged behind in terms of technological advances, despite the high volume of health information created, accessed, and exchanged every day in medical offices, hospitals, and other facilities across the country. For example, many facilities are still using fax machines, which, some claim, are cumbersome and time-consuming to use and outdated when it comes to transferring information; others feel the fax machine offers advantages that digital technology does not (Davis, 2019).

IT connectivity in health care benefits hospitals, clinics, health care providers and primary care groups, and patients (sometimes in a life-saving capacity). Digitalization provides endless options, allowing health care providers to rapidly access and share X-rays, scans, and laboratory and other diagnostic test results of hospitalized and clinic patients from their offices and share documents. This speeds up the process of information exchange, limiting the risk of misplacing documents, reducing the quantity of paper used, and vastly increasing the efficiency or productivity of medical practice. Digitalization also enables remote monitoring of health conditions and maintaining electronic health records (EHR) and electronic medical records (EMR), enhancing continuity of care. E-prescriptions reduce errors due to illegible handwriting and enable storing of a pharmacological history; the pharmacist at any point of service (where connectivity exists) can monitor a person's medications, thus avoiding harmful medication interactions and reducing prescription abuse.

**THINKING IT THROUGH**

*M.T. and Electronic Health Records*

M.T. a 32-year-old New Brunswick resident, was brought into the emergency department at the Foot Hills Medical Centre in Calgary. M.T. had been hit by a car and sustained a serious and painful leg injury. In the emergency department, M.T. was semiconscious and incoherent—a condition not congruent with the injury. The nurses located M.T.'s provincial health card and accessed their medical health records and found a history of diabetes and allergic reactions to a number of medications.
1. What information was most important for the physician to have?
2. What possible problems might have occurred if health care providers had not been able to access M.T.'s electronic health records?

## The Use of Electronic Information Systems in Hospitals

Almost every phase of the hospital experience, from admission to discharge, is supported electronically. Patient charts in most facilities are completely computerized, including the writing of doctors orders referred to as Computerized Provider Order Entry (CPOE). Using CPOE, the practitioner records all patient orders into the facility's integrated software system, which then sends each order to the appropriate destination (e.g., medication orders to the pharmacy, blood work to the laboratory department, diet orders to nutritional services). Hospital electronic health information systems also function as safeguards to care, identifying and tracking infections, and notifying individuals of medication errors and other adverse events. CPOE alerts physician prescribers to the potential for drug interactions, if the patient is allergic to a prescribed medication or its ingredients, when tests have been duplicated, or if there is a critical lab value for a patient.

Computerized charts are accessible at the bedside, enabling care providers to view orders, laboratory results, and medications and enter notes at point of care. Most hospital pharmacies prepare medications using robot technology. Once prepared, the patient's medications are transferred to a secure electronic medication cabinet where nurses can retrieve the patient's medications when they are due to be given. Three of the most commonly used hospital information systems are Cerner, Epic, and Meditec.

Hospitals are continually working to find interfaces that will allow computer systems among a variety of care partners to "talk" to each other, using interfaces such as H7 (Health Level Seven International). This communication protocol facilitates the transfer of information from point of entry to an intended destination. Consider Z.O., who is a complex-care patient with several organizations caring for him at home. Z.O. comes into the emergency department (ED), and Z.O.'s demographic information is entered into the hospital system. The hospital system will automatically contact surrounding organizations to see if Z.O. is in their system. If he is, the computer through the H:7 interface will send Z.O.'s community care plan to the ED. With that information, the physician may be able to send this patient back home, knowing that he has the proper supports in place. This type of coordination of services is sometimes referred to as *transitions of care*. Unfortunately, hospitals often use operating systems that are incompatible with those used by care partners, which impedes this hoped-for connectivity.

## Cybersecurity

Cybersecurity of health information is a top priority for hospitals and is an area where costs are increasing, along with the risks of security breaches. Many facilities outsource their cybersecurity, especially smaller hospitals or clinics. For smaller health facilities, it is difficult (and expensive) to both hire and retain individuals with the IT talent and experience to efficiently manage hospital IT security, in addition to having the tools they need to accomplish this.

Hospital IT security scans identify hacking agents almost daily. Hospital information systems contain information of all the people who interface with a hospital. Each registered patient provides significant personal data upon registration—their health card number, address, date of birth, and insurance information. Every detail about their health history, the reason for each admission, all medications, interventions, treatment, and diagnostic and lab test results are contained in their electronic hospital chart. To cyberhackers, this information is a goldmine.

At the same time, hospitals are part of an interoperable system that exchanges health information with providers, pharmacies, diagnostic facilities, other hospitals, and long-term care facilities (with whom they share a network), to name a few. One weak link in the security chain can make all connecting sources of information vulnerable. In addition, many hospitals have portals allowing a patient to access their online medical records; this alone has the potential to put a hospital in a vulnerable position with respect to IT security.

### Security Protocols

Hospitals have security protocols, procedures, and policies that all employees, physicians, and care providers are expected to be familiar with and adhere to. An employee, not the security system, is more likely to be responsible for a security breach. The potential harm that can result from one mistake is far-reaching and is likely not limited to one computer but can affect an entire system. It is important for employees to not only follow the rules but to always be alert for anything suspicious that might lead to a virus infection or entry for a hacker.

Hospital IT departments sometimes test employees' awareness and how well they scrutinize Internet sites, emails, and messages. For example, some facilities conduct what is called a "phishing expedition" to see how employees respond to a bogus email with an inviting link (e.g., sale of equipment in the hospital with a link to details of the sale). One hospital had over 60% of their employees click on the link, which could have contained a virus. The link brought them to the IT department. There were hidden clues within the link and email that the IT department thought employees would have taken the time to check out, such as subtle differences in the hospital logo and language that was not quite right. Employees who clicked on the link were invited to a refresher seminar on security protocols.

For the most part, hospitals have several separate networks: an external one for the public (such as Wi-Fi that patients and visitors can log onto); an internal one for use when carrying out work-related responsibilities; and another internal one that is more secure, providing access to highly confidential information, including medical charts. Hospital employees who want to use their own electronic devices in the hospital must give the IT department permission to scan their devices for viruses and allow the IT department access to their devices at any time should they think there is a threat. This protocol is called *mobile device management*.

Hospital IT security also has software that continually scans for security breaches within the facility and can identify individuals attempting to access charts and other information for which they do not have clearance. Only a health care practitioner within a person's circle of care is allowed to access their health information. IT can also flag the charts of patients in the public domain (sometimes identified as "VIPs," short for "very important persons") to ensure that only those people sanctioned to access that person's health information can do so. For example, if a celebrity was admitted, some staff might not be able to resist having a quick look at the reason for admission. Any staff member breaching this protocol is usually suspended or terminated on the spot for unethical behaviour.

If a facility is hacked, the hospital must respond quickly, assess the damage, and report any breaches to the proper authorities. Sharing information related to hacking attempts or actual hacks with other facilities can limit the harm done. If a hospital system is hacked or infected with ransomware, the entire facility may need to be shut down temporarily, with the cancellation of appointments, tests, and surgeries, as happened in Newfoundland and Labrador in fall 2021. Everyone who is believed to have been compromised must be notified of the incident and of potential risks. A facility can never assume its IT systems are safe. A popular quote in the information security industry, credited to former FBI Director Robert Mueller, is that there are two types of organizations, "those that know they have been compromised, and those that don't" (TaoSecurity Blog, 2018).

### Physicians' Sites

A growing number of Canadian physicians have a practice website that offers patients access to their health information through secure portals. A person can review their medication profile, lab and diagnostic test results, and immunization history, among other things. Some portals allow the patient to exchange secure email with the health care team, change contact information, request prescription refills (although many prescribers ask patients to call their pharmacy for prescription repeats or refills), and access educational materials and more detailed information about their health conditions, treatment options, and potential treatment plans. A bonus is that individuals can come to appointments more informed about their health problem or condition, without necessarily having resorted to searching for information from potentially dubious sources.

***Physician reviews.*** People can look up information about their physicians and other providers on rating websites and submit comments. Information on these websites may not be accurate. Some people will post opinions and relate experiences that are more subjective in nature than fact-based.

***Scheduling appointments.*** Although most physicians work in an electronic environment, with only some offices still using a mix of paper and electronic charts, virtually all are using computers for scheduling appointments. Self-scheduling programs are also available. An example is Click4Time, an award-winning self-scheduling appointment and resource booking system that is growing in popularity.

The major laboratories have websites through which people can also book appointments for tests, making the process easier and more convenient for individuals and their health care providers. Shortly after the results are processed, most laboratories send them electronically to the ordering provider and allow patients to see the results online. Shoppers Drug Mart Corporation is one pharmacy that has set up a portal through which physicians and nurse practitioners can access drug reimbursement information and other clinical tools (e.g., health information, handouts about selected conditions). Individuals can also log in to their accounts and request prescription refills online.

### A National Electronic Health Record System: Is it Achievable?

An effective interoperable system for managing EHRs within communities, provinces, and territories has not yet been realized, let alone one that is pan-Canadian. The goal of a nationwide EHR system is ambitious at best, and the challenges are multiple, differing in each jurisdiction. A significant barrier is the lack of systemwide architecture to support breaking down the siloed health information systems (i.e., different systems that operate in isolation without the ability to "talk" to other systems) that exist in most jurisdictions.

At present, although the situation is improving, there is no effective technological framework that can facilitate the connectivity of health records among multiple users (e.g., primary care, acute care, hospitals, home and community care, diagnostic facilities, public health). This is in part because there are limited ways in which to build an applied programming interface (API) for existing primary care physician medical record systems, hospital record systems, and those used in home and community care. Today, with the implementation of team-based approaches to health care, it is more important than ever that practitioners, caregivers, and agencies have the ability to access, share, update, amend, and coordinate patient health information to provide the right care at the right time and in the right place.

Improving and implementing a national EHR system requires the following:

1. Continued commitment of all stakeholders to share in the vision and embrace the technology
2. Collaborative efforts by all levels of government and health care organizations
3. Continual responsible financing for provincial and territorial initiatives, including funds to encourage all stakeholders to adopt and promote interoperable electronic medical solutions
4. A public that trusts that their health information will be managed respectfully and securely
5. Foolproof tracking and security systems that can identify who accesses what information in case of security breaches, and laws that specifically address privacy violations
6. Computer software programs that message each other without connectivity problems
7. Support systems at the federal, provincial/territorial, and municipal levels that work to ensure seamless information exchange

8. A uniform vocabulary of technical language to increase the effectiveness of system use
9. Clearly defined laws governing the use and exchange of health information across provincial and territorial boundaries, including specific guidelines to clarify who bears responsibility for the information and what fees are charged for services provided

Connectivity to various points of care is one of the major obstacles to successfully implementing a pan-Canadian EHR system. Electronic systems must be capable of networking with local and provincial or territorial systems. Few jurisdictions have standardized options, so compatibility with other systems is also a concern. Canada-wide digital solutions, such as those established or still being implemented by the Canada Health Infoway, would minimize these problems, but care partners are under no obligation to sign on to these networks.

Computerization and EHRs also extend to home and community care organizations. However, determining a definitive timeline to reach the goal of a fully integrated electronic health care system is next to impossible. Connectivity even within communities is imperfect. In fact, it may never be completely achieved. Hybrid systems (a mix of electronic and paper) will probably always coexist with completely electronic environments.

## THE HEALTH CARE CRISIS IN CANADA

Problems plaguing the health care system in Canada are on the minds of most Canadians, many of whom believe it is on the brink of collapse. The acute shortage of human health resources across the health care spectrum has recently dominated the news and affected every aspect of health care. Health care workers are stressed, exhausted, and experiencing burnout mitigated by working throughout the pandemic, most under unimaginably horrific conditions. Many are also feeling demoralized as they cannot give the quality of care they want to give, experiencing moral distress, and as time has passed, many health care workers have been berated, harassed, and threatened with violence as groups of people protested vaccination mandates and other public health measures both online and outside clinics and hospitals. Large numbers of health workers are continuing to leave their careers (particularly frontline providers), simply unable or unwilling to cope with the stress any longer. This leaves an overworked, discouraged, and depleted workforce to provide what care they can to those who need it and to cope with the demands of system backlogs.

The recent, albeit limited, closure of some EDs, clinics, and Intensive Care Units because of a shortage of physicians and nurses is unprecedented. The same can be said for the fact that the availability of ambulances to respond to emergency calls in some communities has been severely limited and at times nonexistent. Paramedics, along with their ambulances, are held up in emergency bays because they cannot off-load their patients as there is no room for them in the ED. In most jurisdictions, paramedics must keep their patients in the ambulance until such time as they are seen in the ED. That said, in Nova Scotia, as of June 2022, a direct-to-triage initiative allows paramedics to transfer care of their low-risk patients to the waiting area where they are assessed; this frees up the ambulance to attend to other calls.

On October 6, 2021, representatives from the Canadian Medical Association (CMA) and the Canadian Nurses Association (CNA) hosted an emergency COVID-19 summit to discuss the pandemic and its devastating effects on the health care system and workforce (Canadian Medical Association, 2021). The goals of the meeting were to form immediate and long-term action plans to deal with workforce burnout and staffing shortages. This meeting was followed up with another on March 9, 2022 where the CMA and the CNA were joined by approximately 40 health organizations. Priorities for action included the creation of a data source of health human resources, a national strategy for health human resources across related disciplines, and a concrete commitment to restructure the health care system.

Despite, or perhaps in addition to, these suggestions, some people have proposed that what is needed is increased funding from the federal government. Others feel that money is not the answer but instead restructuring how health care is delivered, as well as offering more support and improved working conditions for health care providers. Some provinces such as Ontario have plans of their own. Ontario plans to move selected outpatient surgeries to private clinics (addressing the backlog of surgeries resulting from the pandemic), something that has been done by other jurisdictions. These procedures would be covered by the public health plan. Amidst fierce opposition, Ontario also passed a controversial plan allowing hospitals to discharge patients occupying acute care beds and transfer them to alternative accommodation, up to 150 km away from their community depending on where they live. This can be done without the person's consent if needed. If the person refuses to go, they will be formally discharged from the hospital and have to pay a daily fee for accommodation to remain. The person would be transferred back to a facility of their choice when a bed becomes available. In January 2023, Ontario introduced legislation allowing healthcare providers who are registered/licensed in their province of origin to practice in Ontario upon arrival—a first in the country.

Early in 2023, the goverment of Nova Scotia announced a plan to provide extra resources and other changes to relieve the strain on emergency departments following the untimely deaths of two women who had waited hours for care.

As part of a five-point plan, the Northwest Territory Health Department is offering contracts to paramedics to work in health centres along with nurses to provide acute care to remote communities (Hudson, 2022). New Brunswick is placing emphasis on recruitment and measures to retain health care workers.

In August 2022, the 13 provincial and territorial premiers met in British Columbia for a health care conference. Part of the agenda was dedicated to sharing concerns and potential solutions regarding the apparent health care crisis from both a regional and national perspective. On the Evolve site, you will find a link to a video of the post-meeting press-conference. Here, the premiers answer numerous questions about their concerns and make suggestions for future strategies.

Also in August 2022, the federal government announced a reinstatement of a Chief Nursing Officer as well as the Office of Nursing Policy under the umbrella of Health Canada's Strategic Policy Branch, which had been eliminated in 2012 (see Chapter 2) (Health Canada, 2022c; personal correspondence with Marie-France Proulx, Office of the Honourable Jean-Yves Duclos, Minister of Health). According to the federal government, this reinstatement is to "recognize their (nurses in Canada) expertise and increase their input in decisions affecting our health care system" (Health Canada, 2022c).

The appointee (Dr. Leigh Chapman) will provide strategic advice from a nursing perspective to Health Canada and participate in the development of broad health policies and programs regarding workforce planning; mental health; long-term, home, and palliative care; as well as nursing scope of practice and competencies. The person in this position will also represent the federal government at public forums at home and abroad (Tasker, 2022). Bearing in mind that health care is not under federal jurisdiction, the person in this role will act in a collaborative, advisory capacity to provinces and territories. How the reinstatement of this position will benefit the health care system remains to be seen.

## TRENDING FORWARD

Revisit the questions asked at the beginning of Chapter 1 and then review the principles of comprehensiveness, universality, and accessibility of the *Canada Health Act* discussed in the same chapter. Have your answers changed? Are these principles being met in your community? Health care in Canada *should* be high quality, accessible, comprehensive, and universal, no matter who is delivering it, where it is delivered, or who is receiving it. Most Canadians would tell you that our health care system falls far short of meeting these standards.

Disruptions in health care services have affected all of us in one way or another and will continue to do so for the foreseeable future. Finding solutions is complicated and will take time, and there is no universal "fix." Communication, collaboration, and flexibility are necessary components to promoting a unified approach to finding solutions while addressing the uniqueness of provincial and territorial needs.

## SUMMARY

10.1 In any calendar year, one in five Canadians experience some form of mental illness or a substance use disorder. There has been a dramatic rise in the number of people with mental health issues since the onset of the COVID-19 pandemic, particularly for such complaints as stress, anxiety, depression, and burnout. Burnout was recognized as a clinical diagnosis in 2019 by the World Health Organization and was added to the eleventh revision of the International Classification of Disease (ICD-11). Since the beginning of the pandemic there has also been an increase in substance use and increased mortality rates from drug-related deaths. Responsibilities for mental health and addiction services are managed jointly by federal, provincial, and territorial governments. Strategies to address substance use in Canada include implementation of harm reduction sites, which are also referred to as safe injection sites or supervised consumption sites/clinics. They are guided by strategies, practices, and procedures that reduce the harm to individuals caused by substance use and addiction. Contaminated drugs are in part responsible for an alarming number of drug-related deaths across the country. Narcan kits used to reverse the effects of overdoses are widely available in all jurisdictions.

10.2 Homelessness, the causes of which are both multiple and complex, is experienced by people from all walks of life and in both urban and rural settings across the country. Somewhere between 23 and 67% of individuals who are homeless may have a mental illness, a substance dependency, or both, many relying on community social support services. Almost without exception, predisposing factors include socioeconomic inequities. Strategies to reduce homelessness vary with the province or territory and community. They are determined on the basis of available resources, demographics, and varying needs in each community. Resources available may or may not include government funding, fundraising events, planners and policy makers, service providers, medical and mental health authorities, community groups, and volunteers.

10.3 For decades there has been a need for a national strategy for home and community care, as well as for long-term care. The pandemic shined a light on many of the weaknesses in both systems, but perhaps more so on long-term care. The number of residents who died from COVID-19 in long-term care facilities is staggering and was due to understaffing, lack of personal protective equipment and IPAC protocol, and a built environment that contravenes almost every IPAC recommendation. A national strategy recently developed to manage long-term care is meant to provide a platform for effective reform. Home care is recognized as a critical component of primary health care, keeping people functioning more independently for a longer period of time and out of long-term care facilities. As with long-term care, there is an acute shortage of health human resources available to work in the home care system. A significant number of individuals requiring home care rely on family, friends, and volunteers, many of whom are aging themselves and with health problems of their own.

10.4 Indigenous people in Canada face inequities at a level often not experienced by non-Indigenous people, largely due to the social and economic determinants of health. Almost all of these are related in some manner to the impact of residential schools on survivors and on subsequent generations who experience intergenerational trauma. A significant inequity is the number of Indigenous communities (particularly reserves) who have little or no access to clean water for drinking, bathing, or cooking. Some communities have been under boil water advisories for over 25 years. Although significant progress has been made to construct water treatment plants in many communities, they are plagued with problems such as maintenance that requires the community to revert back to boil water advisories and use bottled water brought in by road or air to drink. In addition, the discovery of unmarked graves on the grounds of residential schools has caused significant emotional trauma for many Indigenous people as they mourn the loss of so many children who were sent to these schools. The outcomes of these discoveries are far from being realized, as unmarked graves continue to be discovered and investigations continue. So many questions remain unanswered.

10.5  All facilities have security measures in place to protect health information. Some hospitals outsource information technology (IT) security to companies specializing in that field, while others (especially larger hospitals) have an entire department devoted to identifying threats from within and outside the facility. Hospitals and other facilities are a virtual goldmine of information for hackers, storing almost every demographic detail and health status of patients (including their health care number). Hospitals also have internal security systems in place to address security breaches by, for example, employees who access patient information without authorization. In addition, employees do not always adhere to policies and protocols, and those who are not alert to cyber intrusions pose a significant risk to the system's security. Something as seemingly benign as clicking on an unrecognized link in an email can expose the entire hospital to a cyberattack.

10.6  Canada's health care system is in crisis mode. Many of the problems are not new but have been exacerbated by the pandemic. The lack of human health resources is front and centre. There has been an exodus of health professionals leaving a number of the health professions as a result of the stresses and exhaustion they experienced during the pandemic. A shortage of human health resources affects every aspect of health care and health care delivery. Provincial and territorial leaders met in Victoria, British Columbia in August 2022 to discuss strategies to address current issues. All agree that increased funding from the federal government is a starting point, but others feel that more money will not fix the health care system.

## REVIEW QUESTIONS

1. Explain the concept of burnout.
2. The federal government is responsible for mental health and illness for what population groups?
3. Briefly explain the role of the Canadian Mental Health Association (CMHA) and United Way with respect to mental health and addiction services.
   a. Describe three services for mental health and addiction that are available in your community.
   b. In your opinion, why does the stigma of mental illness prevent individuals from seeking help?
4. State three advantages of online or virtual mental health support.
   a. Identify two online or virtual supports available for mental health and addiction in your jurisdiction or community.
5. What are three contributing factors to the increased use of drugs during the pandemic? Which jurisdictions saw the highest mortality rates?
6. In what ways do harm reduction sites benefit individuals using drugs?

7. What legal agreement did the province of British Columbia make with the federal government regarding possession of opioids? Why was this agreement made?

8. Briefly describe the purpose of Canada's National Homeless Strategy, considering its goals, target populations, and funding.

9. What are three factors contributing to the high morbidity and mortality rates in long-term care facilities during the pandemic?

10. Explain two reasons why sone Indigenous communities in Canada are still under boil water advisories (some transitory).

11. How has the discovery of unmarked graves affected Indigenous people in Canada?

12. What are three benefits of electronic health records?

13. Why do some smaller hospitals and facilities hire outside organizations to provide IT security?

14. How can hospital employees reduce the risks of an IT security breach?

15. What are three contributing factors to the shortage of human health resources in Canada? Explain the context behind each factor.

16. Why is there a shortage of ambulance services in some communities?

17. What are three responsibilities of the federally appointed Chief Nursing Officer?

18. In small groups, discuss three major issues facing health care in your jurisdiction (or a community within your jurisdiction).
    a. How have these issues impacted the delivery of health care?
    b. What steps have been taken to address these concerns?
    c. What issues or concerns do you see regarding health care and health care delivery over the next year?

19. Investigate and summarize what negotiations or agreements are *currently* in place between the federal government and all jurisdictions regarding increased financing for healthcare.

## REFERENCES

7 Cities. (2018). *Ending homelessness*. https://www.7cities.ca/ending_homelessness.

Adams, T. L., & Tremblay, P. F. (2020, August 5). *Harsh realities and new opportunities: Royal society of canada members on the impact of COVID-19 on Canadian society*. RCS COVID-19 Series. Publication #34. https://rsc-src.ca/en/voices/harsh-realities-and-new-opportunities-royal-society-canada-members-impact-covid-19-canadian

Advisory Committee on Homelessness. (2018). *Final report of the Advisory Committee on Homelessness on the homelessness partnering strategy*. Employment and Social Development Canada. www.canada.ca/en/employment-social-development/programs/communities/homelessness/publications-bulletins/advisory-committee-report.html.

Arrigada, P. (2020, November 24). *The experiences and needs of older caregivers in Canada*. https://www150.statcan.gc.ca/n1/pub/75-006-x/2020001/article/00007-eng.htm.

Baral, S., Bond, A., Boozary, A., et al. (2021, June 10). Seeking shelter: Homelessness and COVID-19. *FACETS, 6*, 925–958. https://doi.org/10.1139/facets-2021-0004.

Booth, R. L., Rayner, J., Clemens, K. K., et al. (2021). Testing, infection and complication rates of COVID-19 among people with a recent history of homelessness in Ontario, Canada: A retrospective cohort study. *CMAJ Open, 9*(1), E1–E9. https://doi.org/10.9778/cmajo.20200287.

Canadian Association for Long-Term Care. (2022, January 27). *New national standards an opportunity, but shared approach needed for transformational change*. https://caltc.ca/2022/01/new-national-standards-an-opportunity-but-shared-approach-needed-for-transformational-change/.

Canadian Home Care Association. (2017, June). *Harmonized principles for home care*. https://cdnhomecare.ca/wp-content/uploads/2021/08/CHCA_Harmonized-Principles-2017-web-b.pdf.

Canadian Home Care Association. (2018, March). *A framework for national pri*nciple-based home care standards. content/uploads/2021/08/CHCA-IIome-Care-Standards-Framcwork-B.pdf.

Canadian Institute for Health Research (CIHI). (2018). *Action plan: Building a healthier future for First Nations, Inuit, and Métis peoples.* Canadian Institutes of Health Research. https://www.cihr-irsc.gc.ca/e/50372.html.

Canadian Institute for Health Information (CIHI). (2021, December 9). *COVID-19's impact on long-term care.* https://www.cihi.ca/en/covid-19-resources/impact-of-covid-19-on-canadas-health-care-systems/long-term-care.

Canadian Institute for Health Information (CIHI). (2022). *November 17).* Registered psychiatric nurses. https://www.cihi.ca/en/registered-psychiatric-nurses.

Canadian Medical Association (CMA). (2021, October 5). *Emergency COVID-19 summit tonight: Canada's doctors and nurses meet to discuss devastating impact on health system.* https://www.cma.ca/news-releases-and-statements/emergency-covid-19-summit-tonight-canadas-doctors-and-nurses-meet.

Canadian Mental Health Association. (n.d.). Substance use and addiction. https://ontario.cmha.ca/addiction-and-substance-use-and-addiction/.

Centre for Addiction and Mental Health CMAH). (n.d.) Mental illness and addiction: Facts and statistics. www.camh.ca/en/driving-change/the-crisis-is-real/mental-health-statistics#:~:text=Prevalence,Canadians%20experiences%20a%20mental%20illness.&text=By%20the%20time%20Canadians%20reach,have%20had%20%E2%80%93%20a%20mental%20illness.

Centre for Addiction and Mental Health (CAMH). (2020, January 6). *Workplace mental health: A review and recommendations.* https://www.camh.ca/-/media/files/workplace-mental-health/workplacemental health-a-review-and-recommendations-pdf.

Correctional Service Canada. (2020). *Health services.* https://www.csc-scc.gc.ca/health/092/MH-strategy-eng.pdf.

Crown-Indigenous Relations and Northern Affairs Canada. (2022, June 22). *Government introduces legislation to establish National Council for Reconciliation.* https://www.canada.ca/en/crown-indigenous-relations-northern-affairs/news/2022/06/government-introduces-legislation-to-establish-national-council-for-reconciliation.html.

Davis, J. (2019, November 14). *90% of healthcare providers still rely on fax machines, posing privacy risk.* Health IT Security. https://healthitsecurity.com/news/90-healthcare-providers-still-rely-on-fax-machines-posing-privacy-risk.

Dubois, S. (2022, August 1). *Wait times for eating disorder treatment in Canada grow during the pandemic.* CBC News. https://www.cbc.ca/news/health/wait-times-for-eating-disorder-treatment-in-canada-grow-during-the-pandemic-1.6533635.

Eneas, B. (2021, June 24). *Sask. First Nation announces discovery of 751 unmarked graves near former residential school.* CBC News. https://www.cbc.ca/news/canada/saskatchewan/cowessess-marieval-indian-residential-school-news-1.6078375.

Farha, L., & Schwan, K. (2020, April 30). *A national protocol for homeless encampments in Canada.* UN Special Rapporteur on the Right to Housing. https://www.make-the-shift.org/wp-content/uploads/2020/04/A-National-Protocol-for-Homeless-Encampments-in-Canada.pdf.

First Nations Drinking Water. (n.d.). FAQs. https://firstnationsdrinkingwater.ca/index.php/help-support/faqs/#:~:text=The%20%248%20billion%20settlement%20includes,1995%20and%20June%202020%2C%202021.

Government of Alberta. (2022). *Continuing Care Capital Program.* https://www.alberta.ca/continuing-care-capital-program.aspx#:~:text=in%20the%20future.-,Funding,this%20one%2Dtime%20grant%20funding.

Government of Canada. (2020). *What is the national housing strategy?* www.placetocallhome.ca/what-is-the-strategy#:~:text=The%20National%20Housing%20Strategy%20is,access%20a%20safe%2C%20affordable%20home.

Government of Canada. (2022a). *Opioid- and stimulant-related harms in Canada.* https://health-infobase.canada.ca/substance-related-harms/opioids-stimulants.

Government of Canada. (2022b). *Infection prevention and control for COVID-19: Interim guidance for long-term care homes.* https://www.canada.ca/en/public-health/services/diseases/2019-novel-coronavirus-infection/prevent-control-covid-19-long-term-care-homes.html.

Government of Canada. (2023a). *Short-term drinking water advisories.* https://www.sac-isc.gc.ca/eng/1562856509704/1562856530304.

Government of Canada. (2023b). *Remaining long-term drinking water advisories.* https://www.sac-isc.gc.ca/eng/1614387410146/1614387435325.

Health Canada. (2018). *New regulations to provide better information for patients on the safe. use of opioid medication.* [News release]. https://www.canada.ca/en/health-canada/news/2018/05/new-regulations-to-provide-better-information-for-patients-on-the-safe-use-of-opioid-medications.html

Health Canada. (2022a). *Exception from controlled drugs and substances act: Personal possession of small amounts of certain illegal drugs in british columbia. January 31, 2023 to January 31, 2026)* https://www.canada.ca/en/health-canada/services/health-concerns/controlled-substances-precursor-chemicals/policy-regulations/policy-documents/exemption-personal-possession-small-amounts-certain-illegal-drugs-british-columbia.html.

Health Canada. (2022b). *Government of Canada invests more than $379 million to support Canadians living in long-term care in Ontario.* https://www.canada.ca/en/health-canada/news/2022/04/government-of-canada-invests-more-than-379-million-to-support-canadians-living-in-long-term-care-in-ontario.html.

Health Canada. (2022c). *Government of Canada announces chief nursing officer for Canada.* https://www.canada.ca/en/health-canada/news/2022/08/government-of-canada-announces-chief-nursing-officer-for-canada.html.

Health Standards Organization. (2022, February 11). *CSA group and HSO release new national long-term care standards for public review.* https://healthstandards.org/general-updates/csa-group-hso-release-new-national-long-term-care-standards-public-review/#:~:text=The%20National%20Long%2DTerm%20Care,centred%2C%20high%2Dquality%20care.

Hobbs, G. (2022, June 21). *Buffy Sainte-Marie wants more than just and apology from the Pope.* CBC News. https://www.cbc.ca/news/canada/buffy-sainte-marie-residential-schools-1.6489384.

Homeless Hub. (n.d.). Substance use and addiction. https://www.homelesshub.ca/about-homelessness/topics/substance-use-addiction.

Hopper, T. (2021, May 29). *Why so many children died at Indian residential schools.* National Post https://nationalpost.com/news/canada/newly-discovered-b-c-graves-a-grim-reminder-of-the-heartbreaking-death-toll-of-residential-schools.

Hudson, A. (2022, August 18). *Paramedics to help out at NWT health centres as territory contends with staff shortages.* CBC News. https://www.cbc.ca/news/canada/north/nwt-health-staff-recruitment-retention-initiatives-paramedics-1.6555426.

Indigenous Services Canada. (2022). *Indian residential schools resolution health support program.* https://www.sac-isc.gc.ca/eng/1581971225188/1581971250953.

Infrastructure Canada. (2022). *About reaching home: Canada's homelessness strategy.* https://www.infrastructure.gc.ca/homelessness-sans-abri/index-eng.html.

Jewell, E., & Mosby, I. (2020, December). *Calls to Action accountability: A 2020 status update on reconciliation. Yellowhead Institute.* https://yellowheadinstitute.org/wp-content/uploads/2020/12/yi-trc-calls-to-action-update-full-report-2020.pdf.

Journey Counselling. (2021). *Intergenerational trauma of indigenous communities.* [Blog post]. https://journeycounselling.ca/blog/intergenerational-trauma-of-indigenous-communities/

King, A. (2022, August 12). *Ontario cuts funding by 85% for online therapy program introduced during the pandemic.* CBC News. https://www.cbc.ca/news/canada/toronto/ontario-icbt-program-cuts-covid19-1.6548962.

Lawrynuik, S. (2017). *Medicine Hat maintaining homeless-free status 2 years on.* CBC News. https://www.cbc.ca/news/canada/calgary/medicine-hat-homeless-free-update-1.3949030.

Lillo, A., Champagne, E., Touchant, L., et al. (2021, April 29). *Canada has 20 percent of the world's freshwater reserves — this is how to protect it. The Conversation.* https://theconversation.com/canada-has-20-per-cent-of-the-worlds-freshwater-reserves-this-is-how-to-protect-it-159677.

Limmena, M. R. (2021). *How intergenerational trauma affects Indigenous communities.* https://blog.scienceborealis.ca/how-intergenerational-trauma-affects-indigenous-communities/.

MindBeacon. (n.d.). It's time for you. Mental Health support that fits your life. https://www.mindbeacon.com/?utm_campaign=Ontario&utm_source=google&utm_medium=sem&utm_content=performance&gclid=CjwKCAjw7vuUBhBUEiwAEdu2pHuJghTyogSiU44GXglEOHFxujTZmcT9cirLZnUJ-9t8k21jvQAZNxoC6A8QAvD_BwE.

Office of the Auditor General. (2021, February 25). *Report 3—access to safe drinking water in First Nations communities—Indigenous Services Canada.* https://www.oag-bvg.gc.ca/internet/English/att__e_43754.html.

Office of the Chief Science Advisor of Canada. (2020). *Long-term care and COVID-19: Report of a special task force prepared for the Chief Science Advisor of Canada.* https://www.ic.gc.ca/eic/site/063.nsf/vwapj/Long-Term-Care-and-Covid19_2020.pdf/$file/Long-Term-Care-and-Covid19_2020.pdf.

Public Health Agency of Canada (PHAC). (2022, April 25). *Government of Canada invests in mental health and distress centres.* https://www.canada.ca/en/public-health/news/2022/04/government-of-canada-invests-in-mental-health-and-distress-centres0.html.

Québec Ministry of Health and Social Services. (2021, October 18). *Joining forces on homelessness—nearly $280 million for the implementation of the 2021–2026 interdepartmental homelessness action plan.* https://www.msss.gouv.qc.ca/ministere/salle-de-presse/communique-3214/.

Ranney, K. (2021, July 12). *Medicine Hat becomes first city in Canada to end chronic homelessness.* Community Solutions https://community.solutions/case-studies/medicine-hat-becomes-first-city-in-canada-to-end-chronic-homelessness/.

Statistics Canada. (2022a). *Self-rated mental health decreases after another year of the COVID-19 pandemic.* https://www150.statcan.gc.ca/n1/daily-quotidien/220607/dq220607e-eng.htm.

Statistics Canada. (2022b). *A portrait of Canada's growing population aged 85 and older from the 2021 Census.* https://www12.statcan.gc.ca/census-recensement/2021/as-sa/98-200-X/2021004/98-200-X2021004-eng.cfm.

TaoSecurity Blog. (2018, December 18). *The origin of the quote "There are two types of companies".* https://taosecurity.blogspot.com/2018/12/the-origin-of-quote-there-are-two-types.html.

Tasker, J. P. (2022, August 23). *Chief nursing officer appointed to help deal with health care 'crisis': Minister.* CBC News. https://www.cbc.ca/news/politics/chief-nursing-office-appointed-1.6559588.

Truth and Reconciliation Commission of Canada. (2015). *Calls to Action.* www.trc.ca/websites/trcinstitution/File/2015/Findings/Calls_to_Action_English2.pdf.

Wellness Together Canada. (n.d.). About Wellness Together Canada. https://www.wellnesstogether.ca/en-CA/about.

# GLOSSARY

## A

**Aboriginal:** Refers to the original inhabitants of a country or a land. Used in Canada initially to refer to Indigenous people. Although the term is no longer acceptable (in favour of *Indigenous*), it still appears in some legal documents.

**Accredited program:** A program that meets standards requisite for its graduates; usually, the standards are set by the profession's governing body, which may be national or provincial or territorial.

**Act:** A comprehensive body of laws passed by Parliament or a provincial or territorial legislature.

**Active euthanasia:** The taking of deliberate steps to end a dying person's life.

**Active ingredients:** Those ingredients in a drug that have therapeutic value meant to cure, palliate, or otherwise treat a health problem.

**Advance directive:** A legal document that specifies the nature and level of treatment a person would want to receive in the event of later being unable to make those decisions. Also called a *living will* or *treatment directive*.

**Affiliating body:** An association that provides, among other things, direction, support, continuing education, and networking opportunities for its professional members (who may be regulated or nonregulated).

**Allied health professional:** A health care provider other than a doctor, nurse, or, according to some sources, a pharmacist or dentist who provides supportive health care, including direct patient care, technical care, therapeutic care, and support services.

**Alternate levels of care (ALC):** Inpatient care in a facility or part of a facility in which the level of care provided meets the physical, mental, and emotional needs of the patient.

**Aseptic technique:** A procedure performed under sterile conditions to reduce the risk of infection.

**Autonomy:** The right to self-determination.

## B

**Band:** A term imposed on First Nation's people under the Indian Act defining a 'governing unit' of Indians under the Act.

**Beneficence:** The act of doing good or being kind.

**Block transfer:** One payment from the federal to the provincial and territorial governments to cover all services.

**Branch:** A division of a main office offering extended or supportive functions.

**Bureau:** Government department responsible for a specific entity or duty.

## C

**Canada Health Act:** Legislation passed in 1984 that governs and guides the delivery of equal, prepaid, and accessible health care to Canadians.

**Capitation-based funding:** A funding formula to pay physicians who participate in some type of primary health care reform group. The doctor receives a set amount (determined by the age and health status of each patient) for each rostered patient per year.

**Cardiovascular disease:** Disease that affects the heart and vascular system (i.e., blood vessels).

**Catastrophic drug costs:** Prescription drug costs that cause undue burden on individuals with serious health conditions or illnesses.

**Cerebrovascular disease:** A number of conditions that affect the flow of blood to the brain, the most serious of which is a stroke.

**Civil law:** A legal system in which laws governing civil rights and relationships within society, between people and property, and within families are written rather than being determined by judges.

**Code of ethics:** A set of values and responsibilities serving to guide the behaviour of the members of an organization or a profession.

**Common law:** Laws established over time by judges on the basis of decisions made on similar cases; sometimes referred to as *case law*.

**Community-based care:** Care provided for the client in the home (e.g., incorporating visits from nurses or physiotherapists) or on an outpatient basis rather than in the hospital or another health care facility.

**Compassionate interference:** The act of imposing treatment against a patient's will when deemed in the best interests of the patient.

**Compensation:** That part of the health—illness continuum in which a person is neither in good nor poor health, is able to accommodate a malady, and is continuing on with daily life.

**Confidential:** Kept private or shared only with authorized individuals (e.g., in health care, shared only with those authorized to have health information about a patient).

**Conflict of interest:** The possible clash of two or more concerns. For example, a personal financial interest in a business may influence one's professional decisions.

**Constitutional law:** The area of law dealing with legislation derived from or related to Canada's Constitution.

**Continuity of care:** Health care based on treating practitioners having all required information to optimize the care the patient receives. Having access to the individual's health records and maintaining excellent communication among all parties involved in the patient's care are ways to ensure continuity of care.

**Contract law:** The branch of law dealing with agreements between parties, including the interpretation or enforcement of agreements when there is a dispute.

**Controlled act:** An act that, as specified in the *Regulated Health Professions Act*, may be performed only by authorized regulated health care providers.

***Controlled Drugs and Substances Act:*** Federal legislation addressing Canada's drug laws, including a classification system for drugs.

**Copayment:** A predetermined dollar amount or percentage of the cost of a health care service or medication that an individual must pay.

**Criminal law:** The field of law dealing with crimes against the state or against society. Criminal law defines offences and controls the regulations concerning the apprehension,

charging, and trying of those believed to have committed a criminal offence.

**Culture:** Common elements of a social group, including its beliefs, practices, behaviours, values, and attitudes. Culture can relate to a society or to subgroups within a society.

## D

**Deductible:** The amount of money that an individual or family is required to pay toward health care costs before an insurance plan will take over.

**Delegated act:** A controlled act that a physician authorizes another health care provider, either regulated or unregulated, to do in their stead and under supervision.

**Delisted:** The removal of an item from a list or a registry. In Canada, the term is frequently used when a medical service is no longer considered medically necessary and is removed from the government's list of insured services.

**Deontological theory:** An ethical theory that calls for a moral and honest action to be taken, regardless of the outcome.

**Disability:** A physical or mental incapacity that differs from what is perceived as normal function. A disability can result from an illness or accident or be genetic in nature.

**Disease:** A disorder or medical condition affecting a system or organ. The condition can be mental, physical, or genetic in origin. *Disease* also refers to a deviation from how the body normally functions.

**Disease burden:** The impact of a health problem, measured by financial cost, mortality, morbidity, or other indicators.

**Disease prevention:** Used in conjunction with health promotion. Information initiatives

aimed at encouraging individuals, especially those in high-risk population groups (e.g., with a family history of diabetes or heart disease), to adopt strategies to prevent diseases.

**Dispensing fee:** A service fee charged by a pharmacy for dispensing a prescription medication (i.e., reading the prescription and preparing the medication for the patient).

**Divine command ethics:** An ethical theory believing that ethical philosophies and rules are set out by a higher power.

**Double effect:** Acting in a manner that brings about the most good or the least harm.

**Drug identification number (DIN):** A unique number assigned to each medication approved by Health Canada for use in Canada.

**Duties:** Obligations a person has in response to another's claims on them. A duty may result from a professional or personal obligation or may relate to one's own morals or values.

**Duty of care:** The obligation to act in a competent manner according to the standards of practice.

## E

**Electronic health record (EHR):** Health information collected by more than one facility and shared electronically among health care service providers (e.g., a doctor's office, emergency department, and pharmacy).

**Electronic medical record (EMR):** Health information obtained and stored at one facility, perhaps a dentist's, chiropractor's, or doctor's office.

**Eligible:** Qualified for inclusion because of meeting certain criteria or requirements.

**Enhanced services:** Optional health services, such as choice in hospital rooms, enhanced medical goods and services, and services not covered by the public health insurance system, offered to the patient at a cost.

**Ethical principle:** An acceptable, usually highly valued and moral standard of human behaviour—for example, honesty, truthfulness, and fairness.

**Ethical theory:** A framework of ideas that provides a template for making decisions to justify a set of actions.

**Ethics:** The knowledge of and rules about behaving according to set values, duties, and moral principles.

**Ethnicity:** A social group that shares certain common elements, such as traditions, history, religion, culture, and language.

**Etiology:** The study of causes. In medicine, *etiology* refers to the origin or cause of a disease.

**Evidence-informed:** Proven, through high-quality scientific studies, to be effective.

**Exacerbation:** A period of time when a disease (usually chronic) is active and the person has symptoms. *Exacerbation* may also refer to an increase in the severity of a disease.

**Extra billing:** An additional fee, considered a contravention of the *Canada Health Act*, charged to the user by a health care provider for a service covered under the terms of a provincial or territorial health insurance plan.

### F

**Fidelity:** The quality of being faithful.

**Fiduciary duty:** A duty that binds professionals to act with honesty and integrity and in the best interests of their patients with regard to their professional practice.

**Fiduciary relationship:** A relationship based on trust.

**First ministers:** The premiers of the provinces and territories.

**First Nations:** Refers to one of three Indigenous population groups in Canada (the other two groups are Metis and Inuit). It also refers to the ethnicity of First Nations people in Canada. First Nation used in the singular format refers to a band, a reserve-based community, or a large tribal grouping including status Indians who are part of these groups. First Nation can also refer to various/geo-cultural groups (e.g. Cree or Ojibwe).

**Food insecurity:** Poor or no physical or economic access to nutritious foods required to maintain a healthy state.

**Forensic psychiatric hospitals:** Hospitals that assess and treat individuals referred by the Canadian courts, and those requiring a secure inpatient facility due to a risk for harm to self or others.

**Formulary list:** A list of prescription medications (often generic brands) selected for coverage by a public or private health insurance plan.

### G

**Geriatrics:** The branch of medicine dealing with the physiological characteristics of aging and the diagnosis and treatment of diseases affecting older persons.

**Good Samaritan law:** A law protecting individuals who attempt to offer help to a person in distress.

### H

**Health accord:** A legal agreement between the federal and provincial and territorial governments on health care funding.

**Health behaviour:** The activities a person engages in to acquire and maintain good physical and psychological health.

**Health beliefs:** Things people believe to be true about their personal health and susceptibility to illness and about illness, prevention, and treatment in general.

**Health care provider:** A person who has graduated from a health-related college or university program and is accredited by a professional or regulating body. Often the person must be licensed by a provincial or territorial government.

**Health indicators:** Measurements that help to gauge the state of health and wellness of a population.

**Health model:** A concept of an approach to care, including the development of a treatment plan and involvement and communication with a patient.

**Health promotion:** Initiatives that inform people about things they can do to remain healthy and to prevent disease and illness.

**Holistic:** Refers to being whole. In health care, a holistic approach treats the whole person, not an individual part of the person. For example, a holistic approach to treating a person with a heart condition would consider the patient's emotional state, diet, and fitness level, not just their heart problem.

**Hospice:** A facility that provides supportive and compassionate care to individuals who are usually in the final stages of a terminal illness. Care providers address the physical needs of patients, including pain management as well as the spiritual, social, and psychological needs of patients and their loved ones.

**Hypoglycemia:** A response to a drop in blood sugar levels. The symptoms may include mild weakness or dizziness; headache; cold, clammy, or sweaty skin; problems concentrating; shakiness; uncoordinated movements or staggering; blurred vision; irritability; hunger; fainting; and loss of consciousness.

## I

**Immigrant:** A person who comes to another country to live, usually to join family members or for economic reasons. Immigrants are not forced to leave their country of origin under the same conditions as refugees are.

**Implied consent:** Consent assumed by the patient's actions, such as their seeking out the care of a health care provider or their failure to resist or protest treatment.

**Incident report:** A legal document outlining all relevant information concerning any negative occurrence in the workplace.

*Indian Act*: The most significant Act affecting First Nations, signed in 1976. Although it has been amended several times, it remains largely the same as the original Act. The *Indian Act* is a Canadian federal law that governs matters relating to Indian status and reserves. It is managed by Crown-Indigenous Relations and Northern Affairs Canada (CIRNAC).

**Indigenous people:** Refers to the original inhabitants of a land and their descendants. In Canada, *Indigenous* refers to First Nations, Inuit, and Métis people living within Canadian borders.

**Inequities in health:** Unfair and unequal distribution of health resources in relation to resources available and the population involved.

**Infant mortality:** The death of an infant (i.e., within the first year of life).

**Informed consent:** A formal agreement signed by a patient consenting to a treatment, procedure, or test administered by a health care provider after the patient has been fully informed of all related risks and benefits.

**Interprofessional collaboration:** Multiple health care workers from a variety of professions working together to deliver evidence-informed, patient-centred health care.

**Intersectoral cooperation:** Joint action among the public, the government, and non-governmental or community-based organizations.

**Intubate:** The passing of a tube into a person's trachea to facilitate breathing.

**Inuit:** Indigenous people in northern Canada, generally living above the tree line in the Northwest Territories, Northern Québec, and Labrador.

**Inuk:** A member of any Inuit people, singular for *Inuit*.

**Involuntary euthanasia:** A person's bringing about the death of another person without their express consent and possibly against their wishes (e.g., when a patient is unconscious and their wishes are not known or are unclear).

## L

**Laparoscopic surgery:** A type of surgical procedure in which a small incision is made in the body, through which a viewing tube (laparoscope) is inserted. A small camera in the laparoscope allows the doctor to examine internal organs.

Other small incisions may be made to insert instruments to perform surgery.

**Life expectancy:** The number of years a population or parts of a population are expected to live as determined by statistics.

**Longitudinal care:** A holistic approach to individualized health care in which a plan of care is developed that includes health promotion, disease prevention, and both short- and long-term treatment goals.

## M

**Malpractice:** Illegal, negligent, or substandard treatment (failing to meet the treatment standards of one's profession) by a medical practitioner. Malpractice may be intentional or unintentional wrongdoing that may or may not result in injury to a patient.

**Medical assistance in dying (MAiD):** The taking of one's own life with means provided by a doctor.

**Medically necessary:** A clinical judgement made by a physician regarding the necessity of a service provided under a provincial or territorial health plan to maintain, restore, or palliate (i.e., ease symptoms, such as pain, without curing the underlying disease).

**Medicare:** The informal name for Canada's national health insurance plan. Note that the term's use in Canada differs from that in the United States, where *Medicare* refers to a federally sponsored program for individuals over the age of 65.

**Morality:** A code of conduct defined by a group of people, culture, society, or religion. Individuals may have a moral code that governs the way they live, behave, and interact with others.

**Morals:** A person's beliefs about right and wrong regarding how to treat others and how to behave in an organized society.

**Morbidity:** The occurrence of disease or impairment resulting from accidents or environmental causes—for example, the number of people injured in a multiple-vehicle accident or the number of people who have a particular disease, such as cancer (but who have not died).

**Mortality:** The occurrence of deaths resulting from disease, accidents, or environmental causes—for example, the number of people killed in a multiple-vehicle accident or the number of people who died from a particular disease, such as cancer.

### N

**Negligence:** The failure of a health care provider, whether intentional or unintentional, to meet the standards of care required of their profession; also sometimes referred to as *malpractice*, especially when resulting in harm or injury to the patient.

**Nonmaleficence:** Doing no harm.

**Nonprofit organizations (NPOs):** Organizations that return surplus revenue (profits) back to the facility for purposes of maintaining or improving the facility and its operations; usually managed by a board as opposed to private owners.

**Non-Status Indians:** First Nations people registered in Canada's official record (the *Indian Act of Canada*), sometimes referred to as *Treaty Indians*.

### O

**Oral consent:** Verbal agreement from a patient to undergo a treatment, procedure, or test performed by a health care provider.

**Orphan patient:** A person without a family doctor.

### P

**Palliative care:** Care for the dying. Palliative care services, offered in the home or another facility (e.g., palliative care unit in a hospital or a hospice), may include nursing care, counselling, and pain management and may involve those individuals close to the patient.

**Pandemic:** A sustained, worldwide human-to-human transmission of disease.

**Passive euthanasia:** The process of allowing a person to die by removing life support or other life-sustaining treatment.

**Patented drugs:** Drugs that are legally protected from generic production for a period of 20 years from the date of filing.

**Paternalism:** The attempt to control or influence another's decision regarding medical care. Paternalism does not honour the patient's right to autonomy.

***Personal Information Protection and Electronic Documents Act (PIPEDA):*** A federal act ensuring the protection of personal information in the private sector.

**Population health:** A framework for gathering and analyzing information about conditions that affect the health of a population. The aim is to both maintain and improve the health of the entire population and to reduce inequities in health status among population groups.

**Positron emission tomography (PET) scanner:** A scanning device that uses nuclear imaging techniques to obtain 3-D images of parts of the body.

**Power of attorney:** A legal document naming a specific person or persons to act on behalf of another in matters concerning personal care, personal estate, or both.

**Practice setting:** The context and environment in which health care is delivered.

**Precarious worker:** People who are underemployed, or unemployed and who work in low-satisfaction or high-stress jobs tend to have poorer health

**Precontact era:** That period of time before people Indigenous to what is now called Canada had contact with individuals from other parts of the world.

**Prepaid health care:** Access to medically necessary hospital and physician services on a prepaid basis, and on uniform terms and conditions.

**Primary care:** Frontline care, direction, and advice provided by interprofessional health care teams. Primary care also involves initiatives that seek to improve access to, quality of, and continuity of care; patient and health care provider satisfaction; and cost-effectiveness of health care services.

**Primary care organizations:** Groups of health care professionals from a variety of disciplines who work together as an interprofessional team to provide patients with comprehensive high-quality health care. Each team member brings their unique skills to the organization, offering the patient a wide range of primary care services.

**Primary care setting:** The organizational and physical environment in which a person receives point-of-entry care (e.g., a doctor's office, walk-in clinic).

**Primary health care:** Health care with an emphasis on individuals and their communities. It includes essential medical and curative care received at the primary, secondary, or tertiary levels and involves health care providers as well as community members delivering, within the community, care that is cost-effective, comprehensive, and collaborative (i.e., uses a team approach).

**Primary health care reform:** Changes to the delivery of primary health care with the goal of providing all Canadians access to an appropriate health care provider 24 hours a day, 7 days a week, no matter where they live.

**Privacy:** The patient's right to control access to their body and personal information.

**Professional misconduct:** Behaviour or some act or omission that falls short of what would be proper in professional circumstances. Examples include deviating from a profession's standards of practice or violating the boundaries of a professional–patient relationship.

**Protein-specific antigen (PSA):** A protein marker that can be identified in a blood test which, if elevated, indicates that there may be a malignancy of the prostate gland.

**Public health:** The use of health information from a variety of resources (e.g., Statistics Canada; the World Health Organization; provincial, territorial, and regional sources) to improve the health of communities. Public health programs often carry out recommendations made by population health studies.

**Publicly funded health care:** Health care services whose finances are managed by the government or a government agency for the good of the entire population.

## Q

**Qualitative research:** A method of research that examines the way a population group thinks and behaves. The analysis is largely subjective in nature.

**Quantitative research:** A method of research that deals with the measurement of data, such as the number of deaths from cancer.

**Quarantine:** The enforced isolation of people having or suspected of having a contagious disease.

*Quarantine Act*: Updated in 2005, this legislation gives the federal government powers to assess individuals and detain those who may pose a health risk to Canadians.

## R

**Racism:** Occurs when an individual or group of people judge another because of their physical appearance, such as skin colour, texture of their hair, or physical features different from their own.

**Rationalization:** A strategy wherein a health system centralizes or co-locates similar services within a given geographic location.

**Rationalization of services:** Any changes that increase the effectiveness and efficiency of health care services—clinical, administrative, or financial.

**Refraction:** Testing of the eyes to evaluate their ability to see. An ophthalmologist or optometrist does a refraction to determine the type of lens a patient needs in their glasses to maximize vision.

**Refugee:** A person who seeks refuge in a country other than their country of origin because of political turmoil, economic distress, or regional or ethical issues. Refugees fear for their safety if they remain in or return to their own country.

**Refugee claimants:** People who, feeling unsafe in their home country, seek protection in another country.

**Regionalization:** The organization and integration of a health care system so that a regional group or body assumes responsibility for providing and administering health care services within a given geographic area.

**Regulation:** A form of law made by persons or organizations (e.g., an administrative agency) awarded such authority within an act (whether federal, provincial, or territorial) that has the binding legal power of an act.

**Regulatory law:** Laws made not by Parliament or by a legislature but by authorized persons or organizations to govern a particular group; these laws are ultimately subject to the provincial, territorial, or federal act that governs the administrative body, organization, or tribunal.

**Remission:** A period of time during which a chronic disease is neither active nor acute and the person has no obvious symptoms.

**Renal dialysis:** A process that filters waste and fluid from the blood in a way similar to kidneys. Individuals whose kidneys are not functioning must undergo this procedure several times a week to stay alive while waiting for a kidney transplant.

**Reserve:** Land set aside by the Crown and designated for the use and occupancy of Indigenous people.

**Residential care:** Refers to living accommodations that offer a variety of support needs, usually for older persons. These accommodations include lodges (public or private), assisted living, or supportive services in the community and long-term care facilities.

**Rights in health care:** Entitlements, or things that can and should be expected of health care providers and the health care system. Rights may be tangible (e.g., the right to receive a vaccination covered under the provincial or territorial plan) or intangible (e.g., the right to be treated with respect).

**Risk assessment:** The assessment or examination of a condition or a situation to determine the potential harm or hazards (risk) related to it (e.g., the risk of having an accident if you drive a car in a snowstorm).

**Role fidelity:** In health care, meeting the reasonable expectations of members of the health care team, patients, their families, and employers by being loyal, truthful, and faithful; showing respect; and earning and maintaining trust.

**Rostering:** The registering of a patient in a primary health care reform group. Patients sign a nonbinding form stating that they will seek care only from a specific doctor or primary care group. Also called *patient attachment* or *formal registration*.

**Royal assent:** The final stage a bill passes through before becoming law. Largely symbolic in nature, this approval is given by the Governor General as a representative of the Crown.

### S

**Scope of practice:** A range of skills, learned in school or through on-the-job training, that a practitioner can perform competently and safely. From a professional perspective, legal parameters usually, but not always, dictate what a practitioner may or may not do, based on the profession's education, training, and licensure.

**Self-determination:** The freedom to make one's own decisions.

**Self-imposed risk behaviours:** Actions such as smoking tobacco that a person willfully engages in despite knowing these actions pose a danger to their health.

**Severe acute respiratory syndrome (SARS):** A severe form of pneumonia that first swept across parts of Asia and the Far East before spreading worldwide in 2003.

**Sick role behaviour:** A person's response to disease or illness. Removed from normal societal expectations and responsibilities, the sick person may respond to situations differently from when they are well. Sick role behaviour is usually temporary in nature.

**Signs:** Those things related to an illness that a person or examiner can see (e.g., a rash).

**Social movements:** Advancements by advocacy or interest groups to promote a common interest by acting together to influence public policy.

**Specialist:** A physician trained in a specific field, usually concerning body systems or organs—for example, cardiology, internal medicine, orthopedic surgery—although some specialties (e.g., geriatrics) have a socioeconomic focus.

**Status Indians:** Individuals recognized by the federal government as being registered under the *Indian Act*.

**Statutory law:** Written law, formally created or established by the legislature.

**Symptoms:** Those conditions that a person feels that may relate to an illness (e.g., fatigue, a headache). Symptoms are sometimes referred to as *clinical signs*.

**Syndrome:** A name given to a group of symptoms (clinical manifestations) that are usually connected and for which there is no clear diagnosis.

### T

**Telehealth:** A telephone help system, usually available 24/7 and funded by the provincial or territorial government, used to provide professional health care advice to Canadians who cannot readily access a doctor or other primary care provider.

**Teleological theory:** An ethical theory that defines an action as right or wrong depending on the results it produces; also called *consequence-based theory*.

**Title protection:** Legal restrictions around and guidelines for the use of a professional title.

**Tort:** A civil wrong committed against a person or their property.

### U

**Upstream investments:** Actions that can be taken to improve the health of a population or to prevent illness when the potential for a health problem is first recognized.

**Urodynamic:** Referring to tests and assessments done to measure the function of the bladder and urinary tract.

**User charges:** A fee imposed for an insured health service that the provincial or territorial health care insurance plan does not cover.

### V

**Values:** Something a person holds dear, such as a quality or a standard by which to act or behave (e.g., loyalty, honesty).

**Values history form:** A document that helps people think about the health care choices they would want made for them.

**Virtue ethics:** An ethical theory that operates under the belief that a person of moral character will act wisely, fairly, and honestly and will uphold ethical principles.

**Voluntary euthanasia:** A person's bringing about the death of a dying person with the dying person's consent.

## W

**Wellness:** Good health and a sense of well-being on many levels (i.e., emotional as well as physical) as described or experienced by an individual.

**Wellness—illness continuum:** A method of measuring one's state of health at any given point in time. A person's health state may range from optimum health at one end to death at the other end.

**Whistleblower:** An individual who assumes responsibility for publicly divulging information about a wrongdoing or misconduct by another individual or an organization.

**Workplace Hazardous Materials Information Systems (WHMIS) legislation:** A group of laws, rules, or statutes enacted by a government (federal, provincial, territorial, or municipal) to ensure safety in the workplace.

# INDEX

Note: Page numbers followed by *f* indicate figures, *t* indicate tables, and *b* indicate boxes.